AF180720

Gynaecological cancers: biology and therapeutics

RCOG PRESS

Since 1973 the Royal College of Obstetricians and Gynaecologists has regularly convened Study Groups to address important growth areas within obstetrics and gynaecology. An international group of eminent clinicians and scientists from various disciplines is invited to present the results of recent research and to take part in in-depth discussions. The resulting volume, containing enhanced versions of the papers presented, is published within a few months of the meeting and provides a summary of the subject that is both authoritative and up to date.

SOME PREVIOUS STUDY GROUP PUBLICATIONS AVAILABLE

Disorders of the Menstrual Cycle
Edited by PMS O'Brien, IT Cameron and AB MacLean

Infection and Pregnancy
Edited by AB MacLean, L Regan and D Carrington

Pain in Obstetrics and Gynaecology
Edited by A MacLean, R Stones and S Thornton

Incontinence in Women
Edited by AB MacLean and L Cardozo

Maternal Morbidity and Mortality
Edited by AB MacLean and J Neilson

Lower Genital Tract Neoplasia
Edited by Allan B MacLean, Albert Singer and Hilary Critchley

Pre-eclampsia
Edited by Hilary Critchley, Allan MacLean, Lucilla Poston and James Walker

Preterm Birth
Edited by Hilary Critchley, Phillip Bennett and Steven Thornton

Implantation and Early Development
Edited by Hilary Critchley, Iain Cameron and Stephen Smith

Contraception and Contraceptive Use
Edited by Anna Glasier, Kaye Wellings and Hilary Critchley

Multiple Pregnancy
Edited by Mark Kilby, Phil Baker, Hilary Critchley and David Field

Heart Disease and Pregnancy
Edited by Philip J Steer, Michael A Gatzoulis and Philip Baker

Teenage Pregnancy and Reproductive Health
Edited by Philip Baker, Kate Guthrie, Cindy Hutchinson, Roslyn Kane and Kaye Wellings

Obesity and Reproductive Health
Edited by Philip Baker, Adam Balen, Lucilla Poston and Naveed Sattar

Renal Disease in Pregnancy
Edited by John M Davison, Catherine Nelson-Piercy, Sean Kehoe and Philip Baker

Cancer and Reproductive Health
Edited by Sean Kehoe, Eric Jauniaux, Pierre Martin-Hirsch and Philip Savage

Reproductive Ageing
Edited by Susan Bewley, William Ledger and Dimitrios Nikolaou

Reproductive Genetics
Edited by Sean Kehoe, Lyn Chitty and Tessa Homfray

Maternal and Infant Deaths: Chasing Millennium Development Goals 4 and 5
Edited by Sean Kehoe, James P Neilson and Jane E Norman

Current Management of Polycystic Ovary Syndrome
Edited by Adam Balen, Stephen Franks, Roy Homburg and Sean Kehoe

Gynaecological cancers: biology and therapeutics

Edited by

Sean Kehoe, Richard J Edmondson, Martin Gore
and Iain A McNeish

RCOG
PRESS

Sean Kehoe MD FRCOG
Convenor of Study Groups, Lead Consultant in Gynaecological Oncology, Oxford Gynaecological Cancer Centre, Churchill Hospital, Oxford OX3 7LJ and Fellow of St Peter's College, University of Oxford

Richard J Edmondson MD
Consultant and Senior Lecturer in Gynaecological Oncology, Northern Gynaecological Oncology Centre, Queen Elizabeth Hospital, Gateshead NE9 6SX and Northern Institute for Cancer Research, Newcastle University, Newcastle NE2 4HH

Martin Gore PhD FRCP
Professor of Cancer Medicine, The Royal Marsden Hospital, 203 Fulham Road, London SW3 6JJ and Institute of Cancer Research, London

Iain A McNeish PhD FRCP
MRC Senior Clinical Fellow and Professor of Gynaecological Oncology, Barts Cancer Institute, Queen Mary University of London, John Vane Science Centre, Charterhouse Square, London EC1M 6BQ

CAMBRIDGE
UNIVERSITY PRESS

University Printing House, Cambridge CB2 8BS, United Kingdom

Published in the United States of America by Cambridge University Press, New York

Cambridge University Press is part of the University of Cambridge.

It furthers the University's mission by disseminating knowledge in the pursuit of education, learning and research at the highest international levels of excellence.

www.cambridge.org
Information on this title: www.cambridge.org/9781906985448

First published 2011
Second Edition 2012
Reprinted 2013

A catalogue record for this publication is available from the British Library

ISBN 978-1-906-98544-8 Paperback

A machine-readable catalogue record for this publication can be obtained from the British Library [www.bl.uk/catalogue/listings.html]

Front cover image courtesy of Andrea Rockall: PET/CT image of a nodal metastasis along the left pelvic side wall in a woman with recurrent cervical cancer

Contents

Participants

Ahmed Ashour Ahmed
Clinical Reader in Gynaecological Oncology, Nuffield Department of Obstetrics and Gynaecology and Department of Oncology, University of Oxford, Old Road Campus Research Building, Headington, Oxford OX3 7DQ, UK.

Susana Banerjee
Specialist Registrar in Medical Oncology, The Royal Marsden NHS Foundation Trust, Downs Road, Sutton SM2 5PT, UK.

James D Brenton
Group Leader and Honorary Consultant in Medical Oncology, Functional Genomics of Ovarian Cancer Laboratory, Cancer Research UK Cambridge Research Institute, Li Ka Shing Centre, Robinson Way, Cambridge CB2 0RE, UK.

Robert Brown
Professor of Translational Oncology, Epigenetics Unit, Ovarian Cancer Action Research Centre, Department of Surgery and Cancer, IRDB 4th Floor, Hammersmith Hospital, Du Cane Road, London W12 0NN, UK.

Dennis S Chi
Associate Professor, Gynecology Service, Department of Surgery, Memorial Sloan-Kettering Cancer Center, 1275 York Avenue, New York, NY 10065, USA.

Andrew Clamp
Senior Lecturer and Honorary Consultant in Medical Oncology, The Christie NHS Foundation Trust and University of Manchester School of Cancer and Enabling Sciences, Wilmslow Road, Manchester M20 4BX, UK.

Nandita M deSouza
Co-Director, Cancer Research UK and EPSRC Cancer Imaging Centre, Institute of Cancer Research and Royal Marsden NHS Foundation Trust, Downs Road, Sutton SM2 5PT, UK.

Yvette Drew
Cancer Research UK Clinical Fellow and Specialist Registrar – Medical Oncology, Northern Institute for Cancer Research, Paul O'Gorman Building, Framlington Place, Newcastle University, Newcastle upon Tyne NE2 4HH, UK.

Richard J Edmondson
Consultant and Senior Lecturer in Gynaecological Oncology, Northern Gynaecological Oncology Centre, Queen Elizabeth Hospital, Gateshead NE9 6SX and Northern Institute for Cancer Research, Newcastle University, Newcastle NE2 4HH, UK.

Hani Gabra
Professor of Medical Oncology and Director, Ovarian Cancer Action Research Centre, Department of Surgery and Cancer, Imperial College London, Hammersmith Campus, Du Cane Road, London W12 0NN, UK.

Martin Gore
Professor of Cancer Medicine, The Royal Marsden Hospital, 203 Fulham Road, London SW3 6JJ and Institute of Cancer Research, London, UK.

Sean Kehoe
Convenor of Study Groups, Lead Consultant in Gynaecological Oncology, Oxford Gynaecological Cancer Centre, Churchill Hospital, Oxford OX3 7LJ and Fellow of St Peter's College, University of Oxford, UK.

Tito Lopes
Consultant Gynaecological Oncologist, Royal Cornwall Hospital, Truro TR1 3LJ, UK.

Tim Mould
Consultant Gynaecological Oncologist, UCLH Gynaecological Cancer Centre, 2N, 250 Euston Road, London NW1 2PG, UK.

W Glenn McCluggage
Consultant Gynaecological Pathologist, Department of Pathology, Royal Group of Hospitals, Grosvenor Road, Belfast BT12 6BA, UK.

Iain A McNeish
MRC Senior Clinical Fellow and Professor of Gynaecological Oncology, Barts Cancer Institute, Queen Mary University of London, John Vane Science Centre, Charterhouse Square, London EC1M 6BQ, UK.

Melanie Powell
Consultant Clinical Oncologist, Department of Radiotherapy, Barts and The London NHS Trust, London EC1A 7BE, UK.

Andrea Rockall
Consultant Radiologist, Imaging, Barts Cancer Centre, King George V Wing, St Bartholomew's Hospital, London EC1A 7BE, UK.

Gordon Rustin
Director of Medical Oncology, Mount Vernon Cancer Centre, Rickmansworth Road, Northwood HA6 2RN, UK.

Timothy A Yap
Cancer Research UK Clinical Research Fellow and Specialist Registrar in Medical Oncology, Cancer Research UK Cancer Therapeutics Unit, Royal Marsden NHS Foundation Trust and The Institute of Cancer Research, Downs Road, Sutton SM2 5PT, UK.

Additional contributors

Robert C Bast Jr
Professor, Department of Experimental Therapeutics, The University of Texas MD Anderson Cancer Center, Houston TX 77030, USA.

Aiste Cerbinskaite
Cancer Research UK Clinical Research Fellow in Gynaecological Oncology, Northern Institute for Cancer Research, Newcastle University, Newcastle NE2 4HH, UK.

Nicola J Curtin
Professor of Experimental Cancer Therapeutics, Northern Institute for Cancer Research, Newcastle University, Newcastle NE2 4HH, UK.

Christina Fotopoulou
Associate Professor, European Competence Center for Ovarian Cancer, Department of Gynecology, Charité, Campus-Virchow-Clinic/University Hospital, Augustenburger Platz 1, 13353 Berlin, Germany.

Janet Graham
Specialist Registrar in Medical Oncology, Beatson West of Scotland Cancer Centre, Great Western Road, Glasgow G11 0YN, UK.

Stan B Kaye
Cancer Research UK Professor of Medical Oncology, Section of Medicine, Institute of Cancer Research, Royal Marsden Hospital, Downs Road, Sutton SM2 5PT, UK.

Stefan Knapp
Professor of Structural Biology, Nuffield Department of Clinical Medicine, SGC, Oxford OX3 7DQ, UK.

Stavroula Kyriazi
Clinical Research Fellow, Cancer Research UK and EPSRC Cancer Imaging Centre, Institute of Cancer Research and Royal Marsden NHS Foundation Trust, Downs Road, Sutton SM2 5PT, UK.

Angus McIndoe
Consultant Gynaecological Oncologist, West London Gynaecological Cancer Centre, Queen Charlotte's and Hammersmith Hospital, Imperial College Healthcare NHS Trust, Du Cane Road, London W12 0NN, UK.

Leena Mukherjee
Specialist Registrar, Mount Vernon Cancer Centre, Rickmansworth Road, Northwood HA6 2RN, UK.

Asima Mukhopadhyay
Clinical Research Fellow in Gynaecological Oncology, Northern Gynaecological Oncology Centre, Queen Elizabeth Hospital, Gateshead NE9 6SX and Northern Institute for Cancer Research, Newcastle University, Newcastle NE2 4HH, UK.

Christine A Parkinson
NIHR Clinical Lecturer in Medical Oncology, Functional Genomics of Ovarian Cancer Laboratory, Cancer Research UK Cambridge Research Institute, Li Ka Shing Centre, Robinson Way, Cambridge CB2 0RE, UK.

Evis Sala
Lecturer and Honorary Consultant Radiologist, University Department of Radiology, Box 218, Level 5 Addenbrooke's Hospital, Hills Road, Cambridge CB2 0QQ, UK.

Jalid Sehouli
Professor and Head of Department, European Competence Center for Ovarian Cancer, Department of Gynecology, Charité, Campus-Virchow-Clinic/University Hospital, Augustenburger Platz 1, 13353 Berlin, Germany.

Susan Shanley
Consultant in Clinical Cancer Genetics, The Royal Marsden NHS Foundation Trust, Downs Road, Sutton SM2 5PT, UK.

Anil K Sood
Professor, Department of Gynecologic Oncology, The University of Texas MD Anderson Cancer Center, 1155 Herman Pressler, Houston, TX 77030, USA.

Karen Tipples
Specialist Registrar in Clinical Oncology, Department of Radiotherapy, Barts and The London NHS Trust, London EC1A 7BE, UK.

Oliver Zivanovic
Gynecology Service, Department of Surgery, Memorial Sloan-Kettering Cancer Center, 1275 York Avenue, New York, NY 10065, USA.

DECLARATIONS OF PERSONAL INTEREST

All contributors to the Study Group were invited to make a specific Declaration of Interest in relation to the subject of the Study Group. This was undertaken and all contributors complied with this request. Robert Bast is a member of the Scientific Advisory Boards for Fujirubio Diagnostic, Inc., Vermillion, Illumina, Ovary Cancer Action and Ovarian Cancer National Alliance. He receives royalties for CA125 from Fujirebio Diagnostics, Inc. James Brenton was previously the vice-chair of the Cancer Research UK Biomarkers and Imaging Discovery and Development (BIDD) Committee, and a member of the Target Ovarian Cancer Pathfinder Study Advisory Panel. Robert Brown's department receives financial support from AstraZeneca. Andrew Clamp is a member of the Advisory Board for PharmaMar on trabectedin and a member of the NCRI Gynaecological Cancers Clinical Studies Group. Nandita deSouza is a consultant to the NCRI Gynaecological Clinical Studies Group. Martin Gore is a member of the Advisory Boards for AstraZeneca and GlaxoSmithKline, and is a prinicipal investigator for Ovarian Cancer Action. Sean Kehoe is a senior medical adviser to Ovacome and is president of the British Gynaecological Cancer Society. Glenn McCluggage is a member of the Ovacome Medical Advisory Board. Gordon Rustin is a member of the Advisory Boards for Oxygene and Roche. Evis Sala is a member of the NCRI Gynaecological Oncology Clinical Studies Group.

Preface

The 60th RCOG Study Group focused on gynaecological cancers, a spectrum of cancers affecting over 16 000 women each year in the UK alone. There is a lack of real understanding of these conditions compared with other malignancies, possibly owing to their relative rarity when viewed as individual diseases, which can influence the desire to invest in research.

The objective of the Study Group was to try to examine as many biological aspects of these cancers as possible, including therapies, both surgical and non-surgical. A wide remit, without doubt, and inevitably not all aspects could be covered in the desired detail.

While a great deal of research is still needed, it is also clear that progress in therapy is occurring, with new agents such as PARP inhibitors targeting specific defects found only in the cancer cell. This is an approach that is opening a new route to therapy besides the normal direct approach to cell destruction. The knowledge that some pathologies previously considered as a primary ovarian disease are in fact of primary fallopian tube origin may not immediately have an effect on patient care but does have implications for research and clinical trials that will ultimately result in better directed therapies.

Advances in multimodal therapies, imaging and targeted and individualised treatments, as well as the role of surgical approaches, are all also covered in this book.

Experts from the UK and abroad have dedicated their time to discuss the varied aspects of these malignancies and I am grateful to all involved.

Sean Kehoe
Convenor of Study Groups

Section 1

Biology of gynaecological cancers: our current understanding

Chapter 1

Morphological sub-types of ovarian carcinoma: new developments and pathogenesis

W Glenn McCluggage

Introduction

In most developed countries, ovarian carcinoma is the second most common malignancy of the female genital tract, following endometrial carcinoma. Most cases present at an advanced stage and the overall prognosis is poor. Although clinically often considered as one disease, there is an increasing realisation that the various morphological sub-types of ovarian carcinoma are associated with distinct molecular alterations and have different natural history and prognosis.[1–3] Most studies lump the various morphological sub-types of ovarian carcinoma together, with the result that it is difficult to tease out the behaviour of the various tumour sub-types; with our current state of knowledge, this is not appropriate. Given these factors, and the realisation that some tumour sub-types, for example clear cell, mucinous and low-grade serous, do not respond well to traditional ovarian chemotherapeutic agents and that continuing trials are investigating the efficacy of various agents in some of these tumour sub-types, it is clear that accurate pathological typing of ovarian carcinomas will be critical in the future in directing therapy. To this end, it is recommended that central pathology review becomes mandatory in ovarian carcinoma (and other gynaecological tumours) trials when treatment is dependent on the morphological sub-type or some other pathological parameter. In the UK, this should be organised by the British Association of Gynaecological Pathologists (BAGP) representative on the National Cancer Research Institute (NCRI) Gynaecological Cancer Clinical Studies Group.

In this review, I cover the major morphological sub-types of ovarian carcinoma, including their pathogenesis, and discuss problematic areas in typing. Although sub-typing of most cases is possible on morphology alone, immunohistochemistry may assist in problematic cases. Before discussing the major sub-types of ovarian carcinoma, I cover some general issues regarding the relative frequencies of the various tumour types and tumour grading.

Major morphological sub-types of ovarian carcinoma and relative frequencies

The major morphological sub-types of ovarian carcinoma are serous, endometrioid, clear cell and mucinous.[4] Two relatively recent population-based studies[5,6] that included central pathology review have provided updated information regarding the relative frequencies of the major sub-types (Box 1.1). It can be seen that serous is the most common, followed by clear cell, endometrioid and mucinous in that order. This represents a change from many older studies where mucinous carcinoma was the second most common sub-type and accounted for approximately 12% of primary ovarian carcinomas,[7] a much higher frequency than in the two more recent studies; reasons for this apparent reduction are discussed later. These recent studies also indicate an increase and a decrease in the frequency of serous and of endometrioid carcinoma, respectively; this is probably a reflection of the fact that the distinction between a high-grade serous and an endometrioid carcinoma was previously poorly reproducible[8–12] and there is now a realisation that many neoplasms that were previously diagnosed as advanced stage, high-grade endometrioid carcinoma were, in fact, of serous type (discussed later). When divided into early stage (stage I–II) and late stage (stage III–IV), it can be seen that serous, clear-cell and endometrioid carcinomas are approximately equally represented in early stage whereas almost all advanced stage neoplasms are serous in type (Table 1.1). To put it another way, a high percentage of clear-cell, endometrioid and mucinous carcinomas are early stage and in fact these tumour types (especially endometrioid and mucinous) are usually confined to the ovary at diagnosis (stage I).

The traditional management of advanced stage ovarian carcinoma has for many years been surgical debulking followed by adjuvant chemotherapy. However, in some cases, upfront chemotherapy is administered, especially in women with miliary disease or widespread metastasis where optimal debulking is not considered feasible;

Box 1.1 Relative frequencies of sub-types of ovarian carcinoma based on two recent population-based studies[5,6]

- 68–71% serous
- 12–13% clear cell
- 9–11% endometrioid
- 3% mucinous
- 1% transitional
- 6% mixed

Table 1.1 Early-stage (I/II) versus late-stage (III/IV) distribution of sub-types of ovarian carcinoma based on two recent population-based studies[5,6]

Sub-type	Stage I/II	Stage III/IV
Serous	36%	88%
Clear cell	26%	5%
Endometrioid	27%	3%
Mucinous	8%	1%

this should then followed by surgery after three cycles, with a further three cycles of postoperative chemotherapy. The morphological features of ovarian carcinomas treated by chemotherapy often differ markedly from native tumours. Post-chemotherapy, many ovarian carcinomas have abundant clear or eosinophilic cytoplasm and the nuclear features are often bizarre.[13,14] There may be no residual tumour or it may be difficult to identify tumour cells owing to a pronounced chemotherapy effect with marked fibrosis, necrosis, inflammation, cholesterol cleft formation, haemosiderin deposition and dystrophic calcification. Unless there is no or minimal response, it can be very difficult to type an ovarian carcinoma following chemotherapy and there is a tendency to misdiagnose some as clear-cell carcinoma owing to the abundant clear cytoplasm.[13,14] If upfront chemotherapy is being administered, a pre-chemotherapy tissue biopsy (usually a percutaneous radiologically guided biopsy) should be considered the standard of care for definitive typing, rather than relying on cytology of the ascitic fluid in combination with serum CA125 levels and imaging. This is also the recommendation in the National Institute for Health and Clinical Excellence (NICE) guideline on ovarian cancer.[15] The procurement of a tissue biopsy also means that material is available for additional studies in the future; for example, targeted therapies are likely to be developed against specific proteins and if tissue is available this will be useful in assessing whether the target protein is present in the tumour cells. Tissue obtained at various stages in treatment may also be useful in assessing tumour progression and response to therapy.

Grading of ovarian carcinomas

Several grading systems for ovarian carcinoma are in use but pathological grading is often poorly performed.[16] Most of the grading systems are universal in that they can be applied to all the major morphological sub-types of ovarian carcinoma.[17,18] However, there is an increasing tendency to use different grading systems for different morphological sub-types of ovarian carcinoma and this practice has been recommended in the Royal College of Pathologists Cancer Datasets in the UK.[19] Grading of the various sub-types of ovarian carcinoma is discussed with each specific tumour type.

Serous carcinoma

The perceived relationship between benign, borderline and malignant ovarian serous neoplasms was controversial and a source of confusion for many years. It has always been tempting to speculate that a continuum of ovarian serous neoplasia exists, from benign to borderline to malignant. However, pathological evidence for this is lacking and, until recently, it was generally assumed that there was no firm relationship between borderline and malignant serous neoplasms, although occasionally the two were found to coexist. Recent studies have shed significant light on this and have convincingly demonstrated that there are two distinct types of ovarian serous carcinoma, low grade and high grade.[20–25] Although termed low-grade and high-grade serous carcinoma, it is important to emphasise that these are not two grades of the same neoplasm but rather two distinct tumour types with different underlying pathogenesis, molecular events, behaviour and prognosis. High-grade serous carcinoma is much more common than low grade. Low-grade serous carcinoma is thought to arise in many cases in a stepwise fashion from a benign serous cystadenoma through a serous borderline tumour to an invasive low-grade serous carcinoma. Thus, there is a well-defined adenoma–carcinoma sequence. However, it is relatively uncommon to see areas of invasive low-grade serous carcinoma within a serous borderline tumour and, conversely, in many low-grade serous carcinomas a borderline component is not seen. It is thus not proven that all low-grade serous carcinomas arise from a pre-existing borderline tumour and it is possible that some or many do not. In contrast, high-grade serous carcinoma is not related to serous borderline tumour and was thought until recently to arise directly from the ovarian surface epithelium or the epithelium of cortical inclusion cysts with no well-defined precursor lesion. There is now emerging and quite compelling evidence (discussed in the next section) that many high-grade ovarian serous carcinomas actually originate from the epithelium of the distal fimbrial portion of the fallopian tube.[26–31] Instead of grading ovarian serous carcinoma using a three-tiered system (well, moderate, poor; grade 1, 2 or 3), there is now a growing tendency to classify these as either high grade or low grade; this is the recommendation in the Royal College of Pathologists Dataset on ovarian neoplasms[19] and the classification of a serous carcinoma as low grade or high grade has been shown to be highly reproducible among pathologists.[32] Almost all serous carcinomas that would have previously been classified as moderately or poorly differentiated represent high-grade neoplasms, while those that would have been classified as well differentiated may be either low grade or high grade using the current classification. Although two distinct tumour types, on rare occasions a low-grade serous carcinoma may transform into a high-grade carcinoma or a high-grade serous carcinoma may arise directly from a serous borderline tumour.[33] However, most low-grade serous carcinomas, when they recur, do so as low-grade neoplasms. Some use the term invasive micropapillary serous carcinoma as an alternative to low-grade serous carcinoma; I would not recommend this terminology since some low-grade serous carcinomas do not have a micropapillary architecture while, conversely, many high-grade serous carcinomas do have a micropapillary growth pattern. Figure 1.1 illustrates the postulated pathways of development of low-grade and high-grade serous carcinoma.

The underlying molecular events differ between low-grade and high-grade serous carcinoma. Low-grade serous carcinoma is associated with *KRAS* or *BRAF* mutation in approximately two-thirds of cases.[26–31] These mutations occur early in the evolution of low-grade serous carcinoma since they are also found in borderline and benign areas within the same neoplasm. *KRAS* and *BRAF* mutations appear to be mutually exclusive; in other words one, but not both, may be present in a

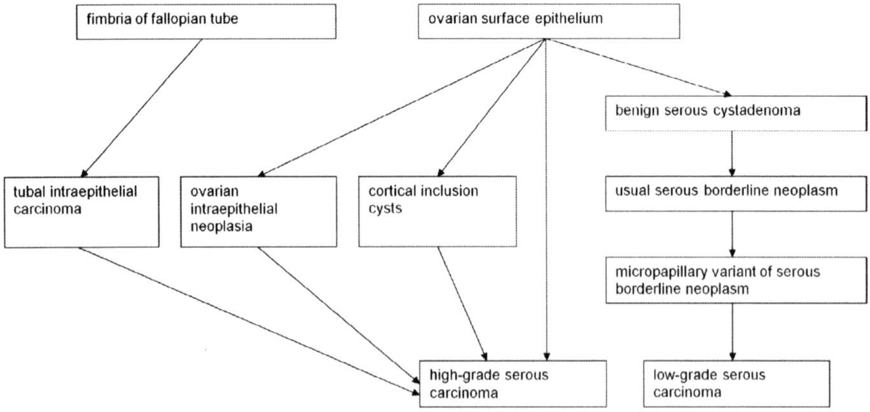

Figure 1.1 Postulated development of low-grade and high-grade ovarian serous carcinoma

particular neoplasm. Low-grade serous carcinoma is not associated with abnormalities of p53.[26–31] In contrast, high-grade serous carcinomas almost universally harbour p53 (*TP53*) mutations and this appears to occur early in neoplastic development;[26–31] these tumours are only rarely associated with *KRAS* or *BRAF* mutation. A study published in 2010 that used stringent techniques identified p53 dysfunction, nearly always representing mutation, in 97% of ovarian high-grade serous carcinomas.[34]

Evidence for the origin of high-grade pelvic serous carcinoma from the fallopian tube

There is convincing and accumulating evidence that many serous carcinomas of the ovary, fallopian tube and peritoneum currently classified as high grade (collectively referred to as high-grade pelvic serous carcinomas) are derived from the fimbria of the fallopian tube.[26–31,35] The initial evidence for this came from prophylactic salpingo-oophorectomy specimens from women with germline *BRCA1* or *BRCA2* mutation, who have a high risk of developing ovarian high-grade serous carcinoma. In initial studies, small high-grade ovarian serous carcinomas were occasionally identified. However, when pathologists began examining the fallopian tube in its entirety, it was found that there was more likely to be a small *in situ* or invasive high-grade serous carcinoma involving the fimbria of the fallopian tube; the *in situ* lesions are referred to as serous tubal intraepithelial carcinoma (STIC). This is relatively uncommon but is occasionally seen in prophylactic salpingo-oophorectomy specimens from women with *BRCA1* or *BRCA2* mutation. Further studies carefully examined the fallopian tubes in women with sporadic high-grade ovarian serous carcinoma and found similar lesions, usually STIC, involving the fimbria in a significant percentage of cases.[26,29] Furthermore, identical p53 mutations were demonstrated within the ovarian and tubal lesions. While this does not unequivocally prove that the origin is within the fallopian tube (this could represent a tumour within the ovary spreading along the fallopian tube), there is accumulating evidence that many high-grade pelvic serous carcinomas arise from the tubal fimbria. A p53 signature has also been identified in the fallopian tube.[26–31] This takes the form of small foci of intense p53 staining involving the secretory cells, most commonly of the fimbria, in the absence of morphological changes. p53 mutations have been demonstrated in some of these p53 signatures and these may represent the earliest stage of development of high-grade pelvic serous carcinoma. However, p53 signatures are extremely common in the fallopian tube even in women with benign disease and no hereditary predisposition to developing ovarian cancer and it is clear that only a small proportion will ever develop into a STIC.

It is probable that not all high-grade pelvic serous carcinomas are derived from the fallopian tube. A study published in 2010 that systematically examined the fallopian tubes in a consecutive series of ovarian carcinomas identified STIC in nearly 60% of high-grade ovarian serous carcinomas but not in other morphological sub-types of ovarian carcinoma.[29] It is possible that some high-grade serous carcinomas do arise from the ovarian surface epithelium or the epithelium of cortical inclusion cysts, the latter being lined by ciliated epithelium identical to that lining the fallopian tube. Another possibility in those cases in which no pre-malignant or malignant lesion is found in the fallopian tube is that tubal epithelium may exfoliate and become incorporated into the ovary and subsequently give rise to a high-grade serous carcinoma.

In summary, there is accumulating evidence that most high-grade pelvic serous carcinomas (high-grade serous carcinomas that are currently classified as ovarian, tubal or peritoneal in origin) arise from the fimbria of the fallopian tube. In most cases, the malignant cells exfoliate from the fimbria into the pelvis and abdomen and result in the formation of an ovarian mass or masses with or without disease elsewhere in the pelvis and abdomen; this is conventionally referred to as ovarian high-grade serous carcinoma. In other cases, the malignancy remains localised to the fallopian tube, resulting in a fallopian tube high-grade serous carcinoma, or gives rise to extensive peritoneal disease in the absence of significant ovarian or tubal involvement; this is conventionally referred to as primary peritoneal high-grade serous carcinoma. It is likely that what are currently referred to as high-grade serous carcinomas of the ovary, fallopian tube and peritoneum are all different manifestations of the same disease and the designation high-grade pelvic serous carcinoma may be more appropriate. A consequence of these observations is that screening programmes for ovarian carcinoma may be relatively ineffective in downstaging high-grade serous carcinomas since these are most probably disseminated from the outset. However, it is possible that screening could be of value in picking up serous carcinomas when the burden of disease is lower. Future studies investigating the underlying molecular events in the development of high-grade pelvic serous carcinoma should concentrate on the distal fallopian tube.

Mucinous carcinoma

As mentioned above, primary ovarian mucinous carcinomas are relatively uncommon, with the two studies referred to earlier[5,6] suggesting that these account for only about 3% of primary ovarian carcinomas, a significantly lower percentage than in older studies. The reasons behind the apparent marked decline in primary ovarian mucinous carcinomas are well known. In older studies, it is likely that many presumed primary ovarian mucinous carcinomas, especially of advanced stage, were metastases from elsewhere. Advances in imaging, serum markers and preoperative workup have resulted in better recognition of metastatic ovarian neoplasms. Moreover, pathologists are now better at recognising the morphological features of metastatic mucinous carcinoma in the ovary,[1,36–42] including the well-known maturation phenomenon resulting in areas resembling benign and borderline mucinous cystadenoma. The use of differential cytokeratin staining and other immunohistochemical markers[43–50] has also improved the situation, although problems still exist. It is now clear that ovarian mucinous neoplasms associated with pseudomyxoma peritonei are almost always of appendiceal origin,[51–53] with the very rare exception of primary ovarian intestinal-type mucinous neoplasms arising in a dermoid cyst.[54] There has also been a redefinition of the criteria for diagnosis of a well-differentiated mucinous carcinoma with so-called expansile or non-destructive invasion and the distinction of this from a mucinous borderline tumour at the upper end of the spectrum with intraepithelial carcinoma;[1,36–38,55,56] this still represents a somewhat poorly reproducible area among pathologists and results in some variation in the reported prevalence of primary ovarian mucinous carcinomas between centres.

Most primary ovarian mucinous carcinomas are stage I and advanced stage neoplasms are extremely uncommon. In this scenario, a secondary neoplasm should always be strongly considered. One point I wish to make is that, although metastatic mucinous carcinomas in the ovary are still sometimes misdiagnosed as a primary ovarian mucinous carcinoma or even a mucinous borderline tumour owing to the pronounced maturation effect seen with some secondary mucinous carcinomas in the ovary, we have to some extent come full circle in that, in my opinion, there is now a tendency to overplay the possibility of a secondary neoplasm even when the pathological features are obviously those of a primary ovarian neoplasm. I feel that, in a large majority of cases, the distinction between a primary and secondary mucinous carcinoma in the ovary can be achieved by careful pathological examination encompassing both the gross and microscopic findings and taking into account the distribution of the disease. It has been stated that, when a mucinous carcinoma is diagnosed in the ovary, further investigations such as colonoscopy and detailed imaging of the upper abdomen should be undertaken to exclude a primary neoplasm elsewhere. I feel this is unnecessary in most cases since, as discussed, basic pathological examination is usually sufficient to distinguish between a primary and secondary ovarian mucinous neoplasm.

Most primary ovarian mucinous carcinomas (and borderline tumours) are of the so-called intestinal (enteric or non-specific) type. A much more uncommon Müllerian type also exists.[57,58] Ovarian mucinous neoplasms of intestinal type comprise a spectrum or continuum from benign through borderline to malignant. In other words, intestinal-type ovarian mucinous carcinomas, like low-grade serous carcinomas, are thought to arise through a well-defined adenoma–carcinoma sequence from a benign cystadenoma through a borderline tumour to a mucinous carcinoma.[1,36–38] Similarly to low-grade serous carcinomas, ovarian mucinous tumours of intestinal type commonly exhibit *KRAS* mutations and identical mutations have been demonstrated in benign, borderline and malignant areas within the same neoplasm, suggesting that *KRAS* mutation is an early event in the evolution of these tumours.[59–61] Unlike the case with low-grade serous carcinomas, *BRAF* mutations are not a feature of ovarian mucinous neoplasms of intestinal type.

Invasion in primary ovarian mucinous carcinomas can be either expansile (non-destructive or confluent glandular) or infiltrative (destructive) in type;[1,36–38,55,56] the former is more common and is associated with a good prognosis. It may be difficult to diagnose a mucinous carcinoma with expansile invasion owing to the orderly growth pattern and absence of a stromal reaction and, as discussed, this is an area where there is significant inter-observer variability among pathologists. My criteria for the distinction between a borderline mucinous tumour with intraepithelial carcinoma and a carcinoma exhibiting expansile invasion are that the latter contains closely packed small- to intermediate-sized glands with a confluent back-to-back arrangement and no or minimal intervening stroma. A labyrinthine or cribriform growth pattern is also common and the epithelium should be cytologically malignant.[1]

Establishing a diagnosis of a mucinous carcinoma with infiltrative stromal invasion is straightforward but a secondary neoplasm should always be considered. It is stressed that primary ovarian mucinous tumours of intestinal type are commonly large and may be extremely heterogeneous within an individual neoplasm. It is not uncommon to see benign, borderline, borderline with intraepithelial carcinoma, and malignant areas side by side within the same neoplasm. Thorough pathological sampling is mandatory in such cases so that a small focus of invasion is not missed. Although there is no evidence base, the Royal College of Pathologists Ovarian Cancer Datasets recommend that primary ovarian mucinous carcinomas be graded in the same way as endometrioid carcinomas (see next section). Most primary ovarian mucinous carcinomas are well differentiated (grade 1), confined to the ovary and have a favourable prognosis. Advanced stage primary ovarian mucinous carcinomas have a very poor prognosis but are extremely uncommon.

As discussed above, most primary ovarian mucinous carcinomas (and borderline tumours) are of so-called intestinal type. The presence of goblet cells is not a prerequisite for an intestinal-type mucinous tumour and many of these exhibit gastric or pancreaticobiliary differentiation.[62] Intestinal-type ovarian mucinous neoplasms, although typically positive with CK7, also commonly express, either focally or diffusely, enteric markers such as CK20, CDX2, CEA and CA19.9 and are negative with hormone receptors, CA125 and WT1.[63,64] CA19.9 especially is often diffusely positive and there may be elevation in the serum level of this marker.[65] Serum CA19.9 levels may be extremely high and are of no value in predicting preoperatively whether an ovarian mucinous neoplasm is benign, borderline or malignant.[65]

Endometrioid adenocarcinoma

Most, but not all, ovarian endometrioid adenocarcinomas are low grade and low stage (usually confined to the ovary). They often, although not always, arise from endometriosis (especially an endometriotic cyst) or a pre-existing borderline adenofibroma.[66,67] The reported prevalence of primary ovarian endometrioid adenocarcinoma is lower in recent than in older studies.[5,6] This is almost certainly due to the recognition that many neoplasms that would previously have been diagnosed as high-grade and high-stage endometrioid carcinomas are, in fact, serous in type. This is an area where previously there was poor reproducibility among pathologists and where WT1 staining may be useful (discussed later). With an endometrioid adenocarcinoma involving the ovary, there is not uncommonly a synchronous endometrioid proliferation, either pre-malignant or malignant, within the uterine corpus.[68]

In the Royal College of Pathologists Ovarian Cancer Dataset,[19] it is recommended that ovarian endometrioid adenocarcinomas be graded using the International Federation of Gynecology and Obstetrics (FIGO) system used to grade uterine endometrioid adenocarcinomas. Although less extensively studied, endometrioid adenocarcinomas of the ovary exhibit similar molecular events to those occurring in uterine endometrioid adenocarcinomas; these events include *PTEN*, β-catenin, *KRAS* and *PIK3CA* mutations and microsatellite instability.[69]

Clear-cell carcinoma

Clear-cell carcinomas have a characteristic morphological appearance typically consisting of an admixture of architectural arrangements including tubulocystic, glandular, solid and papillary. Hobnail cells and eosinophilic stromal hyalinisation are common. It is this admixture of architectural patterns that is more characteristic of clear-cell carcinoma than the presence of clear cells per se, cells with clear cytoplasm sometimes being a feature of both serous and endometrioid carcinomas. Most clear-cell carcinomas are diagnosed at early stage (stage I or II) and the majority arise in endometriosis. Careful pathological sampling, especially concentrating on cystic areas, will often reveal background endometriosis.

It is recommended that clear-cell carcinomas of the ovary be automatically graded as grade 3.[19] Since these neoplasms are often well differentiated architecturally, have a low cytological grade and are mitotically relatively inactive, formal grading may result in these being categorised as grade 1 or 2. The underlying molecular events in ovarian clear-cell carcinoma have not been extensively investigated[70] but a study published in 2010 identified *ARID1A* mutations in a significant percentage of cases.[71] It is generally assumed that clear-cell carcinomas are relatively resistant to the traditional chemotherapeutic agents used in the treatment of ovarian carcinoma and it is possible that this is because these neoplasms exhibit a low proliferation index.

Transitional carcinoma

In my opinion, primary ovarian transitional carcinomas are rare, although they do occur.[72] I feel that most tumours that are diagnosed as transitional carcinoma represent variants of high-grade serous carcinoma and that transitional carcinoma is a poorly reproducible diagnosis. Other cases so diagnosed may represent endometrioid adenocarcinomas with a transitional-like growth pattern. Transitional carcinomas of the ovary express Müllerian and not urothelial markers and are usually positive with WT1,[73] a point in favour of many being variants of high-grade serous carcinoma. Some ovarian transitional carcinomas recur or metastasise as serous carcinoma and this is further evidence that many are variants of the latter.

Undifferentiated carcinoma

The World Health Organization definition of an undifferentiated ovarian carcinoma is a primary ovarian carcinoma with no differentiation or only small foci of differentiation.[4] These are uncommon but not rare. Most probably represent the extreme end of the spectrum of high-grade serous carcinoma since undifferentiated areas are not uncommonly seen in the latter. With a seemingly undifferentiated carcinoma, further pathological sampling may reveal areas more diagnostic of high-grade serous carcinoma. Gene expression studies support the hypothesis that most undifferentiated ovarian carcinomas are related to high-grade serous carcinoma.[3] WT1 staining also supports this since many, although not all, undifferentiated ovarian carcinomas exhibit nuclear staining with this marker that is ubiquitously expressed in ovarian serous carcinoma.[1,3] A smaller number of undifferentiated ovarian carcinomas may represent dedifferentiation within a low-grade endometrioid carcinoma.[74]

Mixed carcinomas

In my experience, true mixed carcinomas of the ovary (unlike in the uterus) are relatively uncommon, although they do occur. A combination of endometrioid and clear-cell carcinoma occurs since both tumour types commonly arise within endometriosis. Cases that are diagnosed as mixed serous and endometrioid or mixed serous and clear-cell carcinoma mostly, in my opinion, represent high-grade serous carcinomas with areas that mimic endometrioid or clear-cell carcinoma; I feel that the combination of serous and endometrioid or serous and clear-cell carcinoma is uncommon. This is discussed in the next section. The combinations of serous and undifferentiated or endometrioid and undifferentiated carcinoma have already been discussed.

Problematic areas in sub-typing of ovarian carcinomas

From personal experience, sub-typing of ovarian carcinomas is reproducible for well-differentiated tumours of the four most common types – serous, endometrioid, clear cell and mucinous. However, there are problems with regard to typing poorly differentiated carcinomas; I feel that this situation has improved over the past few years. Many of the difficulties relate to the categories of high-grade serous, high-grade endometrioid and undifferentiated carcinoma in which there is morphological overlap. Another source of disagreement is the categorisation of clear-cell areas within ovarian carcinomas, specifically whether these represent a clear-cell carcinoma or component of clear-cell carcinoma or clear cells within a serous, endometrioid or undifferentiated carcinoma.

Some pathologists tend to diagnose poorly differentiated ovarian carcinomas as serous in type while others classify them as endometrioid or mixed serous and endometrioid. My opinion is that the vast majority of these are serous carcinomas. In making the distinction, WT1 immunohistochemical staining may be of value.[75–78] Most primary ovarian (as well as primary peritoneal and tubal) serous carcinomas exhibit diffuse nuclear positivity with WT1, while most endometrioid adenocarcinomas are negative or focally positive.[75–78] In problematic cases, I would recommend WT1 staining as an adjunct to help distinguish between a high-grade serous and a high-grade endometrioid adenocarcinoma.

Characteristically in ovarian clear-cell carcinoma, an admixture of growth patterns is present, as discussed previously. Most clear-cell carcinomas are diagnosed without difficulty but there is a tendency to overdiagnose clear-cell carcinoma or a clear-cell carcinoma component owing to the presence of clear cells within serous and to a lesser extent endometrioid adenocarcinomas. The presence of more typical areas of serous or endometrioid adenocarcinoma are useful pointers in diagnosis (sometimes a combination of clear-cell and endometrioid adenocarcinoma occurs) and it is stressed that the mere presence of clear cells does not constitute a clear-cell carcinoma. WT1 is usually negative in ovarian clear-cell carcinoma. Estrogen receptor (ER) may also be of value in that most clear-cell carcinomas are negative while many serous and most endometrioid adenocarcinomas are positive.

The concept of type I and type II ovarian carcinoma

Given the significant advances in our knowledge regarding the pathogenesis of the major sub-types of ovarian epithelial malignancy, we can now think of a broad dualistic pathway of ovarian epithelial carcinogenesis; similarly to the uterus, the terms type I and type II ovarian carcinoma have been proposed.[2] This does not imply that the terms type I and type II carcinoma should replace the specific histologic designations or that all type I and type II carcinomas have a similar behaviour and natural history but, like the dualistic pathway relating to the pathogenesis of uterine carcinomas, this terminology is concerned with broad mechanisms of tumour development. Type I tumours are considered to arise via a well-defined adenoma–carcinoma sequence from a benign precursor lesion, such as a borderline tumour or endometriosis, and to evolve in a stepwise fashion. They are associated with a variety of genetic abnormalities, as discussed earlier. Type I tumours are, in general, slow-growing and indolent neoplasms and include low-grade serous, endometrioid, mucinous and clear-cell carcinoma. There are obvious parallels with type I endometrial cancers that are also, in general, indolent and arise from a well-defined precursor, atypical hyperplasia. In contrast, type II ovarian carcinomas are high-grade clinically aggressive neoplasms. Most represent high-grade serous carcinoma. Carcinosarcoma and undifferentiated carcinoma (both essentially variants of high-grade serous carcinoma) are also included in this category. They are often associated with p53 mutations and there is emerging evidence that many arise from the epithelium of the distal fallopian tube. Again, there are obvious parallels with type II endometrial cancers. In rare cases, a type I ovarian carcinoma can transform into a type II carcinoma; for example, I have seen low-grade serous carcinomas recur as high-grade serous or undifferentiated carcinoma, although this is uncommon.

References

1. McCluggage WG. My approach to and thoughts on typing of ovarian carcinomas. *J Clin Pathol* 2008;61:152–63.
2. Shih IeM, Kurman RJ. Ovarian tumorigenesis: a proposed model based on morphological and molecular genetic analysis. *Am J Pathol* 2004;164:1511–18.
3. Gilks CB. Subclassification of ovarian surface epithelial tumors based on correlation of histologic and molecular pathologic data. *Int J Gynecol Pathol* 2004;23:200–5.
4. Tavassoli FA, Devilee P, editors. *World Health Organization Classification of Tumours. Pathology and Genetics: Tumours of the Breast and Female Genital Organs.* Lyon: IARC Press; 2003.
5. Seidman JD, Horkayne-Szakaly I, Haiba M, Boice CR, Kurman RJ, Ronnett BM. The histologic type and stage distribution of ovarian carcinomas of surface epithelial origin. *Int J Gynecol Pathol* 2004; 23:41–4.
6. Köbel M, Kalloger SE, Huntsman DG, Santos JL, Swenerton KD, Seidman JD, *et al.* Differences in tumor type in low-stage versus high-stage ovarian carcinomas. *Int J Gynecol Pathol* 2010;29:203–11.
7. Koonings PP, Campbell K, Mishell DR Jr, Grimes DA. Relative frequency of primary ovarian neoplasms: a ten year review. *Obstet Gynecol* 1989;74:921–6.
8. Bertelsen K, Holund B, Andersen E. Reproducibility and prognostic value of histologic type and grade in early epithelial ovarian cancer. *Int J Gynecol Cancer* 1993;3:72–79.
9. Baak JP, Langley FA, Talerman A, Delemarre JF. Interpathologist and intrapathologist disagreement in ovarian tumor grading and typing. *Anal Quant Cytol Histol* 1986;8:354–7.
10. Cramer SF, Roth LM, Ulbright TM, Mazur MT, Nunez CA, Gersell DJ, *et al.* Evaluation of the reproducibility of the World Health Organization classification of common ovarian cancers: with emphasis on methodology. *Arch Pathol Lab Med* 1987;111:819–29.
11. Lund B, Thomsen HK, Olsen J. Reproducibility of histopathological evaluation in epithelial ovarian carcinoma: clinical implications. *APMIS* 1991;99:353–8.
12. Sakamoto A, Sasaki H, Furusato M, Suzuki M, Hirai Y, Tsugane S, *et al.* Observer disagreement in histological classification of ovarian tumors in Japan. *Gynecol Oncol* 1996;54:54–8.
13. McCluggage WG, Lyness RW, Atkinson RJ, Dobbs SP, Harley I, McClelland HR, *et al.* Morphological effects of chemotherapy on ovarian carcinoma. *J Clin Pathol* 2002;55:27–31.
14. Miller K, Price JH, Dobbs SP. An immunohistochemical and morphological analysis of post-chemotherapy ovarian carcinoma. *J Clin Pathol* 2008;61:652–7.
15. National Institute for Health and Clinical Excellence. *Ovarian Cancer: the Recognition and Initial Management of Ovarian Cancer.* London: NICE; 2011. [http://guidance.nice.org.uk/CG122].
16. Silverberg SG. Histopathologic grading of ovarian carcinoma: a review and proposal. *Int J Gynecol Pathol* 2000;19:7–15.
17. Shimizu Y, Kamoi S, Amada S, Hasumi K, Akiyama F, Silverberg SG. Toward the development of a universal grading system for ovarian epithelial carcinoma. I. Prognostic significance of histopathologic features–problems involved in the architectural grading system. *Gynecol Oncol* 1998;70:2–12.
18. Shimizu Y, Kamoi S, Amada S, Akiyama F, Silverberg SG. Toward the development of a universal grading system for ovarian epithelial carcinoma: testing of a proposed system in a series of 461 patients with uniform treatment and follow-up. *Cancer* 1998;82:893–901.
19. Wilkinson N, McCluggage WG. *Datasets for the Histopathological Reporting of Neoplasms of the Ovaries and Fallopian Tubes and Primary Carcinomas of the Peritoneum.* London: Royal College of Pathologists; 2010 [www.rcpath.org/index.asp?PageID=1605].
20. Russell HE, McCluggage WG. A multistep model for ovarian tumorigenesis: the value of mutation analysis in the *KRAS* and *BRAF* genes. *J Pathol* 2004;203:617–19.
21. Singer G, Kurman RJ, Chang HW, Cho SK, Shih IeM. Diverse tumorigenic pathways in ovarian serous carcinoma. *Am J Pathol* 2002;160:1223–8.
22. Singer G, Shih IeM, Truskinovsky A, Umudum H, Kurman RJ. Mutational analysis of K-ras segregates ovarian serous carcinomas into two types: invasive MPSC (low-grade tumor) and conventional serous carcinoma. *Int J Gynecol Pathol* 2003;22:37–41.
23. Singer G, Stohr R, Cope L, Dehari R, Hartmann A, Cao DF, *et al.* Patterns of p53 mutations separate ovarian serous borderline tumors and low and high grade carcinomas and provide support

for a new model of ovarian carcinogenesis: a mutational analysis with immunohistochemical correlation. *Am J Surg Pathol* 2005;29:218–24.
24. Ho C-L, Kurman RJ, Dehari R, Wang TL, Shih IeM. Mutations of *BRAF* and *KRAS* precede the development of ovarian serous borderline tumors. *Cancer Res* 2004;64:6915–18.
25. Sieben NLG, Macropoulos P, Roemen GMJM, Kolkman-Uljee SM, Jan Fleuren G, Houmadi R, *et al.* In ovarian neoplasms, *BRAF*, but not *KRAS*, mutation are restricted to low-grade serous tumours. *J Pathol* 2004;202:336–40.
26. Kindelberger DW, Lee Y, Miron A, Hirsch MS, Feltmate C, Medeiros F, *et al.* Intraepithelial carcinoma of the fimbria and pelvic serous carcinoma: evidence for a causal relationship. *Am J Surg Pathol* 2007;31:161–9.
27. Lee Y, Medeiros F, Mindelberger D, Callahan MJ, Muto MG, Crum CP. Advances in the recognition of tubal intraepithelial carcinoma: applications to cancer screening and the pathogenesis of ovarian cancer. *Adv Anat Pathol* 2006;13:1–7.
28. Medeiros F, Muto MG, Lee Y, Elvin JA, Callahan MJ, Feltmate C, *et al.* The tubal fimbria is a preferred site for early adenocarcinoma in women with familial ovarian cancer syndrome. *Am J Surg Pathol* 2007;30:230–6.
29. Przybycin CG, Kurman RJ, Ronnett BM, Shih IeM, Vang R. Are all pelvic (nonuterine) serous carcinomas of tubal origin? *Am J Surg Pathol* 2010;34:1407–16.
30. Lee Y, Miron A, Drapkin R, Nucci MR, Medeiros F, Saleemuddin A, *et al.* A candidate precursor to serous carcinoma that originates in the distal fallopian tube. *J Pathol* 2007;211:26–35.
31. Herrington CS, McCluggage WG. The emerging role of the distal fallopian tube and p53 in pelvic serous carcinogenesis. *J Pathol* 2010;220:5–6.
32. Malpica A, Deavers MT, Lu K, Bodurka DC, Atkinson EN, Gershenson DM, *et al.* Grading ovarian serous carcinoma using a two-tier system. *Am J Surg Pathol* 2004;28:496–504.
33. Dehari R, Kurman RJ, Logani S, Shih IeM. The development of high-grade serous carcinoma from atypical proliferative (borderline) serous tumors and low-grade micropapillary serous carcinoma: a morphologic and molecular genetic analysis. *Am J Surg Pathol* 2007;31:1007–12.
34. Ahmed AA, Etemadmoghadam D, Temple J, Lynch AG, Riad M, Sharma R, *et al.* Driver mutations in *TP53* are ubiquitous in high grade serous carcinomas of the ovary. *J Pathol* 2010;221:49–56.
35. Vang R, Shih IeM, Kurman RJ. Ovarian low-grade and high-grade serous carcinoma: pathogenesis, clinicopathologic and molecular biologic features, and diagnostic problems. *Adv Anat Pathol* 2009;16:267–82.
36. Hart WR. Mucinous tumors of the ovary: a review. *Int J Gynecol Pathol* 2005;24:4–25.
37. Lerwill MF, Young RH. Mucinous tumours of the ovary. *Diagn Histopathol* 2008;14:366–87.
38. Ronnett BM, Kajdacsy-Balla A, Gilks CB, Merino MJ, Silva E, Werness BA, *et al.* Mucinous borderline ovarian tumors: points of general agreement and persistent controversies regarding nomenculature, diagnostic criteria, and behaviour. *Hum Pathol* 2004;35:959–60.
39. Lee KR, Young RH. The distinction between primary and secondary mucinous carcinomas of the ovary: gross and histologic findings in 50 cases. *Am J Surg Pathol* 2003;27:281–92.
40. Seidman JD, Kurman RJ, Ronnett BM. Primary and metastatic mucinous adenocarcinomas in the ovary: incidence in routine practice with a new approach to improve intraoperative diagnosis. *Am J Surg Pathol* 2003;27:985–93.
41. Lewis MR, Deavers MT, Silva EG, Malpica A. Ovarian involvement by metastatic colorectal adenocarcinoma: still a diagnostic challenge. *Am J Surg Pathol* 2006;30:177–84.
42. McCluggage WG, Wilkinson N. Metastatic neoplasms involving the ovary: a review with an emphasis on morphological and immunohistochemical features. *Histopathology* 2005;47:231–47.
43. Berezowski K, Stasny JF, Kornstein MJ. Cytokeratins 7 and 20 and carcinoembryonic antigen in ovarian and colonic carcinoma. *Mod Pathol* 1996;9: 1040–4.
44. Lagendijk JH, Mullink H, van Diest PJ, Meijer GA, Meijer CJ. Immunohistochemical differentiation between primary adenocarcinomas of the ovary and ovarian metastases of colon and breast origin. Comparison between a statistical and intuitive approach. *J Clin Pathol* 1999;52:283–90.
45. Park SO, Kim HS, Hong EK, Kim WH. Expression of cytokeratins 7 and 20 in primary carcinomas of the stomach and colorectum and their value in the differential diagnosis of metastatic carcinomas to the ovary. *Hum Pathol* 2002;33:1078–85.

46. Vang R, Gown AM, Wu LS, Barry TS, Wheeler DT, Yemelyanova A, *et al.* Immunohistochemical expression of CDX2 in primary ovarian mucinous tumors and metastatic mucinous carcinomas involving the ovary: comparison with CK20 and correlation with coordinate expression of CK7. *Mod Pathol* 2006;19:1421–8.
47. Vang R, Gown AM, Barry TS, Wheeler DT, Yemelyanova A, Seidman JD, *et al.* Cytokeratins 7 and 20 in primary and secondary mucinous tumors of the ovary: analysis of coordinate immunohistochemical expression profiles and staining distribution in 179 cases. *Am J Surg Pathol* 2006;30:1130–9.
48. Fragetta F, Pelosi G, Cafici A, Scollo P, Nuciforo P, Viale G. CDX2 immunoreactivity in primary and metastatic ovarian mucinous tumours. *Virchows Arch* 2003;443:782–6.
49. Logani S, Oliva E, Arnell PM, Amin MB, Young RH. Use of novel immunohistochemical markers expressed in colonic adenocarcinoma to distinguish primary ovarian tumors from metastatic colorectal carcinoma. *Mod Pathol* 2005;18:19–25.
50. Raspollini MR, Amunni G, Villanucci A, Baroni G, Taddei A, Taddei GL. Utility of CDX-2 in distinguishing between primary and secondary (intestinal) mucinous ovarian carcinoma: an immunohistochemical comparison of 43 cases. *Appl Immunohistochem Mol Morphol* 2004;12:127–31.
51. Ronnett BM, Zahn CM, Kurman RJ, Kass ME, Sugarbaker PH, Shmookler BM. Disseminated peritoneal adenomucinosis and peritoneal mucinous carcinomatosis: a clinicopathologic analysis of 109 cases with emphasis on distinguishing pathologic features, site of origin, prognosis and relationship to "pseudomyxoma peritonei". *Am J Surg Pathol* 1995;19:1390–408.
52. Guerrieri C, Franlund B, Boeryd B. Expression of cytokeratin 7 in simultaneous mucinous tumors of the ovary and appendix. *Mod Pathol* 1995;8:573–6.
53. Ronnett BM, Shmookler BM, Diener-West M, Sugarbaker PH, Kurman RJ. Immunohistochemical evidence supporting the appendiceal origin of pseudomyxoma peritonei in women. *Int J Gynecol Pathol* 1997;16:1–9.
54. Vang R, Gown AM, Zhao C, Barry TS, Isacson C, Richardson MS, *et al.* Ovarian mucinous tumors associated with mature cystic teratomas: morphologic and immunohistochemical analysis identifies a subset of potential teratomatous origin that shares features of lower gastrointestinal tract mucinous tumors more commonly encountered as secondary tumors in the ovary. *Am J Surg Pathol* 2007;31:854–69.
55. Tabrizi AD, Kalloger SE, Kobel M, Cipollone J, Roskelley CD, Mehl E, *et al.* Primary ovarian mucinous carcinoma of intestinal type: significance of pattern of invasion and immunohistochemical expression profile in a series of 31 cases. *Int J Gynecol Pathol* 2010;29:99–107.
56. Chiesa AG, Deavers MT, Veras E, Silva EG, Gershenson D, Malpica A. Ovarian intestinal type mucinous borderline tumors: are we ready for a nomenculature change? *Int J Gynecol Pathol* 2010;29:108–12.
57. Rodriguez IM, Irving JA, Prat J. Endocervical-like mucinous borderline tumors of the ovary: a clinicopathologic analysis of 31 cases. *Am J Surg Pathol* 2004;28:1311–18.
58. Lee KR, Nucci MR. Ovarian mucinous and mixed epithelial carcinomas of mullerian (endocervical-like) type: a clinicopathologic analysis of four cases of an uncommon variant associated with endometriosis. *Int J Gynecol Pathol* 2003;22:42–51.
59. Scott M, McCluggage WG. Current concepts in ovarian epithelial tumorigenesis: correlation between morphological and molecular data. *Histol Histopathol* 2006;21:81–92.
60. Cantrecasas M, Villaneuva A, Matias-Guiu X, Prat J. *K-ras* mutations in mucinous ovarian tumors: a clinicopathologic and molecular study of 95 cases. *Cancer* 1997;70:1581–6.
61. Gemignani ML, Schlaerth AC, Bogomolnly F, Barakat RR, Lin O, Soslow R, *et al.* Role of *KRAS* and *BRAF* gene mutations in mucinous ovarian carcinoma. *Gynecol Oncol* 2003;90:378–81.
62. Tenti P, Aguzzi A, Riva C, Usellini L, Zappatore R, Bara J, *et al.* Ovarian mucinous tumors frequently express markers of gastric, intestinal and pancreaticobiliary epithelial cells. *Cancer* 1992;69:2131–42.
63. Vang R, Gown AM, Barry TS, Wheeler DT, Ronnett BM. Ovarian atypical proliferative (borderline) mucinous tumors: gastrointestinal and seromucinous (endocervical-like) types are immunophenotypically distinctive. *Int J Gynecol Pathol* 2006;25:83–9.

64. Vang R, Gown AM, Barry TS, Wheeler DT, Ronnett BM. Immunohistochemistry for estrogen and progesterone receptors in the distinction of primary and metastatic mucinous tumors in the ovary: an analysis of 124 cases. *Mod Pathol* 2006;19:97–105.
65. Kelly P, Archbold P, Price JH, Cardwell C, McCluggage WG. Serum CA19.9 levels are commonly elevated in primary ovarian mucinous tumours but cannot be used to predict the histological subtype. *J Clin Pathol* 2010;63:169–73.
66. Stern RC, Dash R, Bentley RC, Snyder MJ, Haney AF, Robboy SJ. Malignancy in endometriosis: frequency and comparison of ovarian and extraovarian types. *Int J Gynecol Pathol* 2001;20:133–9.
67. Bell KA, Kurman RJ. A clinicopathologic analysis of atypical proliferative (borderline) tumors and well-differentiated endometrioid adenocarcinomas of the ovary. *Am J Surg Pathol* 2000; 24:1465–79.
68. Zaino RJ. Synchronous carcinomas of the uterine corpus and ovary. *Gynecol Oncol* 1984;19:329–35.
69. Catasus L, Bussaglia E, Rodriguez I, Gallardo A, Pons C, Irving JA, *et al.* Molecular genetic alterations in endometrioid carcinomas of the ovary: similar frequency of beta-catenin abnormalities but lower rate of microsatellite instability and *PTEN* alterations than in uterine endometrioid carcinomas. *Hum Pathol* 2004;35:1360–8.
70. Tan DS, Kaye S. Ovarian clear cell carcinoma: a continuing enigma. *J Clin Pathol* 2007;60:355–60.
71. Wiegand KC, Shah SP, Al-Agha OM, Zhao Y, Tse K, Zeng T, *et al.* *ARID1A* mutations in endometriosis-associated ovarian carcinomas. *N Engl J Med* 2010;363:1532–43.
72. Eichhorn JH, Young RH. Transitional cell carcinoma of the ovary: a morphologic study with emphasis on differential diagnosis. *Am J Surg Pathol* 2004;28:453–63.
73. Logani S, Oliva E, Amin MB, Folpe AL, Cohen C, Young RH. Immunoprofile of ovarian tumors with putative transitional cell (urothelial) differentiation using novel urothelial markers: histogenetic and diagnostic implications. *Am J Surg Pathol* 2003;27:1434–41.
74. Silva EG, Deavers MT, Malpica A. Undifferentiated carcinoma of the endometrium: a review. *Pathology* 2007;39:134–8.
75. McCluggage WG. WT1 is of value in ascertaining the site of origin of serous carcinomas within the female genital tract. *Int J Gynecol Pathol* 2004;23:97–9.
76. Shimizu M, Toki T, Takagi Y, Konishi I, Fujii S. Immunohistochemical detection of the Wilms' tumor gene (WT1) in epithelial ovarian tumors. *Int J Gynecol Pathol* 2000;19:158–63.
77. Al-Hussaini M, Stockman A, Foster H, McCluggage WG. WT-1 assists in distinguishing ovarian from uterine serous carcinoma and in distinguishing between serous and endometrioid ovarian carcinoma. *Histopathology* 2004;44:109–15.
78. Goldstein NS, Uzieblo A. WT-1 immunoreactivity in uterine papillary serous carcinomas is different from ovarian serous carcinomas. *Am J Clin Pathol* 2002;117:541–5.

Chapter 2

Novel treatment strategies for targeting genetic changes in endometrial cancer

Susana Banerjee

Introduction

Endometrial cancer is the most common gynaecological malignancy in Europe and the USA and the fourth most common cancer in women in the UK. In 2007, 7536 cases of endometrial cancer were diagnosed (approximately 5% of all female cancers) and 1741 deaths in 2008 were attributed to the disease, accounting for 2.3% of all deaths from malignancy in women.[1] In the USA, approximately 42 200 cases are diagnosed annually and 7780 deaths occur.[2] The incidence of endometrial cancer increases with age and over 90% of women are diagnosed above the age of 50 years (median age 63 years). Most of these women (approximately 75%) are diagnosed at an early stage (stage I/II) and are potentially cured by surgery with or without adjuvant radiotherapy, resulting in a 5 year survival rate of 75–91%.[3] However, the prognosis for women with recurrent or advanced endometrial cancer is poor, with a median overall survival of 9–10 months.[4,5]

Current treatments for advanced endometrial cancer are chemotherapy or hormonal therapy. Doxorubicin, cisplatin, carboplatin, docetaxel, topotecan and paclitaxel have all shown activity as monotherapy, with response rates in the range 17–37%.[6] Various combination regimens that include doxorubicin and/or a platinum have been investigated. However, randomised trials have failed to show any survival benefit of combinations of doxorubicin plus either cyclophosphamide or cisplatin compared with single-agent doxorubicin.[5,7] Although the addition of paclitaxel to doxorubicin in combination with cisplatin was found to be superior in terms of response rate, progression-free survival (PFS) and overall survival (OS) compared with doxorubicin combined with cisplatin, this was associated with increased toxicities including neurotoxicity, myelosuppression and vomiting.[8] Hormonal therapy is a particularly attractive option for the treatment of advanced endometrial cancer because it is well tolerated and lacks the toxicities associated with cytotoxic chemotherapy. However, phase II studies indicate that response rates and PFS with progestins or tamoxifen are modest (response rate 10–15%; PFS 1.9–3.2 months).[4,9] Randomised phase II trials of tamoxifen and progestins in combination have shown response rates of 27–33% and PFS of 2.7–3.0 months.[10,11] So far, aromatase inhibitors have shown limited activity in advanced endometrial cancer (response rate 9%).[12,13]

Despite advances in radiotherapy, surgery and chemotherapeutic strategies, these approaches have only led to small improvements in outcome for advanced endometrial cancer. A considerable risk of recurrence and resistance to therapy remains and there is, therefore, a need to improve current treatment options. Advances in tumour biology have fuelled enthusiasm for the development of novel cancer treatments. There is increasing appreciation that endometrial cancer is a heterogeneous disease and that histological sub-types are associated with distinct molecular genetic alterations. Understanding the molecular genetics of endometrial cancer is critical in choosing appropriate candidate drugs and for the success of these agents in improving clinical outcome.

This chapter describes the molecular genetic alterations associated with hereditary and sporadic endometrial carcinomas and explores potential treatment strategies arising from this knowledge.

Inherited endometrial cancer

In approximately 5–10% of endometrial carcinoma cases there is an inherited predisposition to cancer.[14,15] A family history of endometrial cancer in first-degree relatives is reported to be associated with an increased risk of endometrial cancer (relative risk 1.3–2.8).[14,16] In addition, endometrial cancer can occur as part of inherited syndromes. Lynch syndrome, also known as hereditary non-polyposis colorectal cancer, is linked with the majority of inherited endometrial cancers.[17] This is an autosomal dominant condition caused by germline mutations in DNA mismatch repair (MMR) genes (*MLH1, MSH2, MSH6, PMS1, PMS2*) that predispose carriers to cancers, in particular colorectal and endometrial carcinomas. Women with Lynch syndrome inherit a germline DNA mutation in one allele of an MMR gene. Loss of the corresponding normal allele in the tumour leads to impaired DNA MMR, DNA microsatellite instability (MSI) and subsequent tumour development. The lifetime risk of endometrial cancer in women with *MLH2* and *MSH2* germline mutations is 40–60%[18,19] and may be even higher in women with *MSH6* mutations (71% by age 70 years).[20] Moreover, women with Lynch syndrome-associated endometrial cancer present approximately 10–20 years earlier than the general population. The risk of endometrial cancer in women with Lynch syndrome is at least as great as for colorectal cancer and women usually present with a gynaecological malignancy (endometrial or ovarian) as their first cancer.[19] However, so far, reports suggest that the prognosis for women with Lynch syndrome-associated endometrial cancer does not differ from the prognosis for those with sporadic cancers.[17]

Other inherited syndromes associated with endometrial cancer are familial site-specific endometrial carcinoma, in which 8% of women are reported to have a germline MMR mutation,[21] and Cowden syndrome. Cowden syndrome is an autosomal dominant disorder caused by a germline mutation in the *PTEN* gene that leads to a high risk of breast, thyroid and endometrial cancers . The lifetime risk for endometrial carcinoma in women with Cowden syndrome is 5–10%.

Type I and type II endometrial cancer

Classically, endometrial cancer has been categorised into two groups based on clinical and histopathological features:[22] type I (endometrioid) and type II (non-endometrioid) endometrial carcinomas (Table 2.1).

Table 2.1 Clinical and histological features of type I and type II endometrial carcinomas

	Type I (endometrioid)	Type II (non-endometrioid)
Histological features		
Background endometrium	Hyperplasia	Atrophy
Tumour grade	Low	High
Hormone receptors	ER/PgR+	ER/PgR–
Depth of myometrial invasion	Superficial	Deep
Clinical features		
Menstrual status	Pre- and perimenopausal	Postmenopausal
Endocrine-metabolic disturbance	Present	Absent
Estrogen-associated	Yes	No
Clinical behaviour	Indolent	Aggressive
Prognosis	More favourable (86% 5 year survival)	Poor (59% 5 year survival)

Type I (endometrioid) endometrial cancer

Type I endometrial cancers account for over 80% of sporadic cases, are typically of endometrioid histological sub-type, are low grade, exhibit superficial invasion of the myometrium and express estrogen (ER) and/or progesterone (PR) receptors. They often arise on the background of hyperplasia and are associated with estrogen exposure. Risk factors include obesity, hyperlipidaemia, nulliparity and late onset of menopause.[22] Type I endometrial carcinomas are reported to predominantly affect pre- and perimenopausal women. Generally, the clinical course has been considered relatively indolent, with low rates of local or distant metastases. In a series of 355 women with stage I–III endometrioid endometrial cancers who underwent radical treatment, the recurrence rate was 9%.[23] The majority of women with type I cancers are diagnosed at an early stage (86% at stage I–II) and the prognosis is relatively favourable: the 5 year survival is more than 90% for stage I and approximately 80% for stage II disease. However, the 5 year survival for stage III and IV disease is 68% and 25%, respectively.[3] Type I cancers are often hormone sensitive and respond to hormonal treatments such as progestins and tamoxifen.

Type II (non-endometrioid) endometrial cancer

Type II carcinomas represent 10–20% of endometrial carcinomas and include papillary serous and clear cell histological sub-types. They are usually high grade, invade deep into the myometrium and lack hormone receptors. In contrast to type I carcinomas, they arise in an atrophic endometrium, do not appear to be estrogen dependent and they affect older, postmenopausal women.[22] The clinical course for type II cancers is aggressive and often associated with distant metastases. Many women present with stage III or IV disease (41% papillary serous, 33% clear cell).[3] Reflecting this, although the prevalence of type I cancer is much higher than that of type II, non-endometrioid cancers accounts for over 45% of endometrial cancer-related deaths.[24] The 5 year survival rates for papillary serous (41%) and clear cell carcinomas (63%) are lower than for the endometrioid sub-type (80%) (type I). The prognosis is very poor for women with stage IV papillary serous or clear cell carcinomas (6–8% 4 year survival).[3]

Genetic alterations in endometrial cancer

There is accumulating evidence that, in addition to the morphological and clinical differences between type I and II endometrial cancers, these tumours are also characterised by a distinct constellation of genetic alterations that can lead to distinct aberrations in cell signalling and different mechanisms of tumorigenesis (Table 2.2).

PI3K/PTEN/AKT pathway

The most frequently dysregulated signalling pathway in endometroid endometrial carcinoma is the PI3K (phosphatidylinositol 3-kinase)-PTEN (phosphatase and tensin homolog deleted on chromosome 10)-AKT pathway.

PTEN, a tumour suppressor gene located on chromosome 10q23.3, encodes a lipid phosphatase that dephosphorylates PIP3 at the plasma membrane and thereby inhibits PI3K-mediated signals for growth, proliferation and survival. PTEN inactivation may be caused by mechanisms such as mutations, loss of heterozygosity and promoter hypermethylation and is reported in up to 83%[25] of endometrioid carcinomas compared with only 5% in type II endometrial cancers.[26] PTEN loss leads to activation of the PI3K/AKT-mTOR pathway resulting in processes such as cell proliferation, cell migration, invasion, angiogenesis, apoptotic escape and cell survival.

In addition to the established role of PTEN outlined above, more recent evidence suggests that PTEN may also have an important role in maintaining genomic integrity. PTEN-deficient cells were reported to exhibit genomic instability, which may be explained by either impaired RAD51-mediated DNA double-strand break repair[27] or defects in cell cycle checkpoints.[28]

Table 2.2 Molecular alterations in type I and type II endometrial cancer

Alteration	Prevalence in endometrial cancer (%)	
	Type I	Type II
TP53 mutation[31,39,48]	17	54–96
Microsatellite instability[36,37]	20–45	0–5
PIK3CA mutation[29–32]	30	20
exon 9	7–15.5	0
exon 20	10–34	21
PIK3CA amplification[33,34]	2–14	44–46
AKT mutation[35]	2	0
PTEN loss of function[25,26]	37–83	5
KRAS mutation[39]	26	2
FGFR2 mutation[40]	16	2
β-catenin nuclear accumulation[44,45]	31–47	0–3
HER2 (*ERBB2*) overexpression[41]	8	31
HER2 (*ERBB2*) amplification[41,42]	1	17–18
EGFR overexpression[42]	46	34
E-cadherin loss[46,47]	5–57	62–87
p16 loss of function[49]	8	45

Activating mutations in *PIK3CA*, the gene encoding the catalytic subunit of PI3K (p110), have been reported in 30–36% of type I and in 15–21% of type II endometrial carcinomas.[29–31] *PIK3CA* mutations mostly occur in exon 9 (helical domain) or exon 20 (kinase domain). In type I endometrial carcinoma, exon 9 and exon 20 mutations have been reported in 7–15.5% and 10–34% of the disease, respectively.[29,32,33] However, for type II cancers, exon 9 mutations have not been found but exon 20 mutations have been reported in 21% of cases.[31] Amplification of the chromosomal region harbouring *PIK3CA* (3q26) has also been reported in 2–14% of type I and in 46% of type II endometrial cancers.[33,34] Mutations of *AKT* appear to be very rare in type I (2.5%) and absent in type II cancers.[35]

Microsatellite instability

The term microsatellite instability describes the propensity to develop changes in the number of nucleotide repeat elements in microsatellites (short segments of repetitive DNA found in coding and non-coding elements) compared with normal tissue. MSI is caused by the inactivation of DNA repair genes such as *MLH1*, *MSH2*, *MSH6* and *PMS2*, which leads to loss of expression of functional proteins that repair nucleotide mismatches, insertions and deletions produced during DNA replication. MSI has been reported in 20–45% of sporadic type I endometrial cancers but is much rarer in type II tumours (0–5%).[36,37] Higher rates of *PTEN* mutation have been observed in cancers with MSI (59%) than in those without MSI (30%).[38]

KRAS

Activating mutations of *KRAS* have been found in 26% of endometroid carcinomas but are almost completely absent in type II (2%).[39]

FGFR2

Activating mutations of the tyrosine kinase receptor *FGFR2* have been reported in 16% and 2% of type I and type II endometrial cancer, respectively, and appear to be mutually exclusive with *KRAS* mutations, but not *PTEN* abrogation.[40]

HER2/neu (*ERBB2*) and EGFR

Overexpression of HER2 (*ERBB2*), a member of the EGFR family of receptor tyrosine kinases, has been found in 3–10% of type I endometrial cancers and in approximately 30% of endometrial serous carcinoma.[41] HER2 gene amplification has been reported to be present in 1% of type I and 17% of type II endometrial cancers.[42]

Although neither *EGFR*-activating gene mutations nor amplification have been recorded in endometrial cancers, EGFR expression is reported in 35–56% of type II cancers (serous sub-type).[30,42,43]

β-catenin (Wnt signalling)

Alterations in components of the Wnt signalling pathway have been described in endometrial cancer. Similar to the PI3K/AKT pathway, these molecular aberrations differ between the two types of endometrial cancer. β-catenin acts as a downstream transcriptional activator in the Wnt signal transduction pathway. Nuclear accumulation of β-catenin has been reported in 31–47% of type I endometrial carcinomas and in

0–3% of type II tumours.[44,45] Loss of E-cadherin expression has been reported in 5–57% and 62–87% of type I and type II endometrial cancers, respectively.[46,47]

p53

The most common genetic alteration in type II endometrial cancers is mutation of the tumour suppressor p53 (*TP53*). Over 90% of type II serous carcinomas harbour mutant *TP53*, whereas only 17% of type I endometrial cancers are associated with this abnormality.[31,39,48] Type II cancers also display changes in the pRb-cyclinD1-cdk4/6-p16 pathway. Loss of p16 (*CDKN2A*) nuclear accumulation is seen in 44.8% of type II cancers compared with 8.2% of type I cancers.[49] p16 plays an important function in cell cycle regulation and inactivation results in uncontrolled cell growth. Loss of p16 expression appears to be correlated with *KRAS* and *TP53* mutations, and is associated with high stage, high grade and poor survival.

In view of the complexity of genetic aberrations in different sub-types of endometrial cancer, it is unlikely that the 'one treatment fits all' approach is optimal. The clinical relevance of the two types of endometrial cancer, in terms of management, has not previously been exploited. Most clinical trials so far have included both endometrioid and non-endometrioid cancers and have not stratified patients according to type. In current practice, endometrial carcinomas are treated similarly, regardless of histological type. However, as described, endometrial cancer is clearly a heterogeneous disease in terms of clinical behaviour, and genetic alterations and treatments targeted at these differences may improve clinical outcome. Recognition of these key differences is a step towards tailoring future clinical trials and selecting patients according to the molecular abnormalities driving sub-types of endometrial cancer.

Novel targeted agents

Novel biologically targeted agents have proved successful in a variety of malignancies such as breast, colon and renal cancers. The promise of targeted therapy is to selectively exploit molecules that are aberrant in cancers so sparing normal cells, thus potentially providing anti-tumour effects without the toxicity associated with traditional modalities such as chemotherapy. Novel agents such as EGFR inhibitors, anti-angiogenesis agents and mTOR inhibitors are currently being tested in recurrent or metastatic endometrial cancer (Table 2.3).

HER2 and EGFR inhibitors

Given the success of trastuzumab in HER2-positive breast cancer, it was hoped that targeting HER2 might be a worthwhile approach in endometrial cancer. Although *HER2* gene amplification was observed in 11.5% of all endometrial carcinomas (28–38% in type II; 7% in type I), trastuzumab as a single agent did not demonstrate activity against endometrial carcinomas with HER2 overexpression or *HER2* amplification in the phase II Gynecologic Oncology Group study.[50] Furthermore, although EGFR overexpression is common in endometrial cancer (36–87%), the activity of EGFR inhibitors reported so far is modest (response rate 12.5%).[51]

Angiogenesis inhibitors

Angiogenesis is a critical component of cancer growth and metastasis. Results from phase III trials of bevacizumab, a monoclonal antibody against vascular endothelial

Table 2.3 Phase II trials of targeted therapies for recurrent or metastatic endometrial cancer

Molecular target	Drug	Evaluable patients (*n*)	Prior chemotherapy	Partial response	Stable disease[a]	6 month progression-free survival
mTOR	Everolimus[61]	28	≤2	0%	43%	–
	Temsirolimus[62]	19	None	26%	63%	–
	Temsirolimus[64]	27	Yes	7%	44%	–
	Ridaforolimus[63]	27	≤2	7%	26%[b]	–
HER2	Trastuzumab[50]	23	Median 1	0%	9%	–
EGFR	Erlotinib[51]	32	No	13%	47%	9.3%
VEGF	Bevacizumab[60]	53	≤2	15%[c]	–	36%
	Thalidomide[56]	24	≤1	13%	8%	8%
VEGFR	Sunitinib[57]	16	≤1	13%	13%	19%
	Sunitinib[58]	20	≤1	15%	25%	20%
	Sorafenib[59]	39	≤1	5%	49%	13%

[a] at 8 weeks unless specified otherwise

[b] at 16 weeks

[c] 2% had complete response

growth factor (VEGF), suggest that targeting this process is a promising strategy in colorectal, breast, renal and ovarian cancers.[52–55]

A phase II trial of thalidomide, which has anti-angiogenic properties, demonstrated limited activity in chemo-refractory endometrial cancer (response rate 13%; 8% 6 month PFS).[56] Results from phase II trials of the VEGF receptor tyrosine kinase inhibitors sunitinib and sorafenib are slightly more encouraging. Response rates of 5–15% and 6 month PFS rates of 13–20% have been reported in previously treated patients with recurrent or metastatic endometrial cancer.[57–59] Preliminary data for bevacizumab are promising: the response rate was 15%, PFS 4.2 months, 6 month PFS 36% and median OS 10.5 months in previously treated recurrent or persistent endometrial cancer.[60] Bevacizumab is under further investigation in combination with chemotherapy in endometrial cancer and aflibercept (VEGF-Trap) has also entered clinical trials in endometrial cancer.

mTOR inhibitors

There has been much interest in the use of mTOR inhibitors in endometrial cancer owing to the high prevalence of PTEN loss of function and PI3K mutations and amplifications resulting in activation of the mTOR pathway. A phase II study of everolimus in endometrioid endometrial cancer reported disease stabilisation in 43% of patients but no responses.[61] Preliminary phase II results of the intravenous mTOR inhibitor temsirolimus (CCI-779) in women who had not received prior chemotherapy showed a response rate of 26%.[62] In contrast, for women who had previously received chemotherapy, the response rate was minimal (temsirolimus 7%; ridaforolimus 7.5%).[63,64] Interestingly, efficacy of temsirolimus appeared to be independent of PTEN expression.[62] This raises the possibility that mTOR inhibitors may exert their effects through additional mechanisms such as inhibition of mTOR-activated HIF-induced angiogenesis.

Future approaches

FGFR2 inhibitors

The identification of activating mutations in *FGFR2* in endometrioid endometrial cancers provides a potential theraputic target. Pre-clinical studies have shown that endometrial cancer cell lines with activating *FGFR2* mutations are selectively sensitive to the pan-FGFR inhibitor PD173074.[65] Further investigation of agents that target FGFR2 in patients with endometrial cancers harbouring *FGFR2* gene mutations or amplification are warranted.

PARP inhibitors

There has been much enthusiasm surrounding targeting the base excision repair pathway with polyadenosine diphosphate-ribose polymerase (PARP) inhibitors in *BRCA* mutation-associated breast and ovarian cancer.[66,67] This approach utilises the concept of synthetic lethality: two repair pathway defects alone are ineffective, but when combined they become lethal.[68] PARP inhibitors work by generating specific DNA lesions that require functional *BRCA1* and *BRCA2* for DNA repair. However, tumours arising in carriers of *BRCA* mutations are unable to efficiently perform homologous recombination (HR). People with *BRCA* mutation-associated cancers lack wild-type *BRCA1* or *BRCA2* in tumour cells but normal cells retain a single wild-type copy of the relevant gene. This difference between tumour and normal cells means that PARP inhibitors can kill tumour cells while sparing normal cells and thus this approach is likely to have a better toxicity profile than chemotherapy. The profound sensitivity of *BRCA*-mutant cells to PARP inhibitors is most likely explained by an HR defect.[69] It has been proposed that PARP inhibitors may be more widely applicable in the treatment of sporadic cancers with impaired DNA repair mechanisms.

As discussed earlier, PTEN loss of function may contribute to genomic instability as a result of defects in RAD51-mediated DNA double-strand break repair (HR).[27] Pre-clinical studies have demonstrated that PTEN deficiency causes an HR defect rendering cancer cells profoundly sensitive to PARP inhibitors.[70] In view of the fact that endometrioid endometrial cancers commonly have PTEN loss of function (55–83%), these data provide a rationale for testing PARP inhibitors in these cancers (Figure 2.1). Results from pre-clinical studies provide evidence for such an approach.[71] Endometrioid endometrial carcinoma (ECC) cells lacking PTEN expression were unable to elicit HR DNA repair. PTEN-deficient EEC cells showed a significantly greater sensitivity to the PARP inhibitor KU0058948 than PTEN wild-type EEC cells. PTEN silencing in PTEN-expressing EEC cells resulted in reduced formation of RAD51 foci (indicating defective HR) and increased sensitivity to PARP inhibition. PTEN re-expression in PTEN-deficient EEC cells resulted in enhanced formation of RAD51 foci and in a lower sensitivity to KU0058948.

A strong rationale thus exists to perform a clinical trial evaluating the efficacy of PARP inhibition in the treatment of advanced endometrioid endometrial cancer. The POEM study is a randomised, placebo-controlled phase II trial of the PARP inhibitor olaparib versus best supportive care or progestogen in advanced endometrial cancer. A further treatment arm compares the addition of olaparib with the combination of weekly carboplatin and paclitaxel. Retrospective PTEN analysis will be performed. This study is planned to open for recruitment in the UK in 2011.

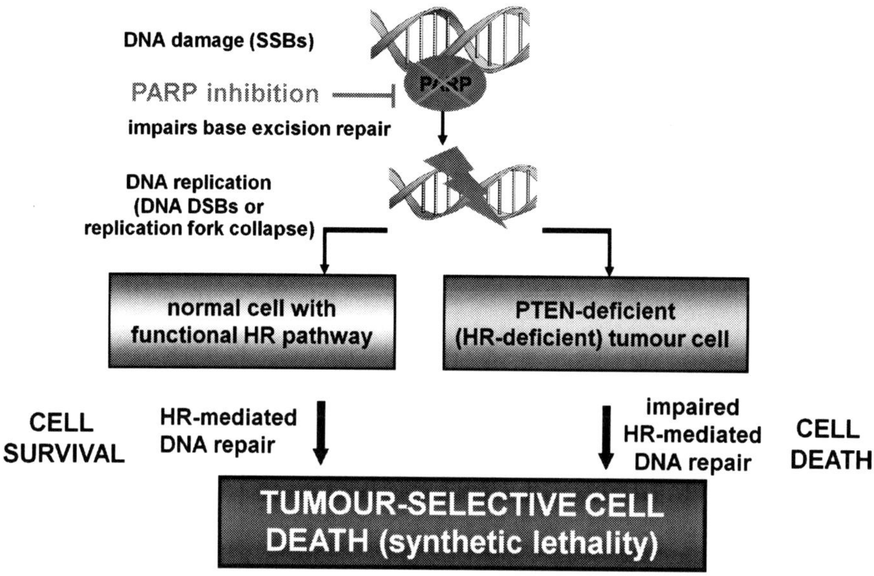

Figure 2.1 Proposed mechanism of PTEN as a synthetic lethal target in endometrial cancer. PARP inhibition leads to persistence of SSBs. A replication fork may encounter a persistent SSB during DNA replication, which causes collapse of the replication fork or the formation of a DSB. In the absence of functional HR, for example through PTEN loss, the DNA cannot be repaired, or is repaired by alternative pathways that are highly error prone, which results in genomic instability and cell death. DSB = double-strand break; HR = homologous recombination; PARP = polyadenosine diphosphate-ribose polymerase; SSB = single-strand break.

Conclusion

The treatment of recurrent or metastatic endometrial cancer is a challenge. Advances in molecular targeted therapies have led to these agents being tested in endometrial cancer, though, overall, early results of clinical trials are relatively disappointing. However, it is noteworthy that many patients enrolled in clinical trials so far had been heavily pretreated. Furthermore, most clinical trials have not used stratification based on molecular sub-type or biomarker. The recognition that endometrial cancer is a heterogeneous disease characterised by distinct molecular aberrations provides a strong rationale for patient selection into clinical trials, rather than a 'one treatment fits all' approach. The future of successful treatment strategies for advanced endometrial cancer is dependent on individualisation of treatments based on molecular genetics that characterise the tumour biology. The identification of robust molecular markers that predict sensitivity to targeted therapies is paramount. Success in the field of endometrial cancer will depend on the integration of translational biomarker studies within clinical trial design.

Future clinical trials should explore the role of PTEN as a synthetic lethality target for PARP inhibitors in endometrial cancer. Other potential strategies include targeting FGFR2 and MSI.

References

1. Cancer Research UK. *Ovarian cancer – UK incidence statistics* [info.cancerresearchuk.org/cancerstats/types/ovary/incidence].
2. Jemal A, Siegel R, Ward E, Hao Y, Xu J, Thun MJ. Cancer statistics, 2009. *CA Cancer J Clin* 2009;59:225–49.
3. Creasman WT, Odicino F, Maisonneuve P, Quinn MA, Beller U, Benedet JL, *et al.* Carcinoma of the corpus uteri. FIGO 6th Annual Report on the Results of Treatment in Gynecological Cancer. *Int J Gynaecol Obstet* 2006;95 Suppl 1:S105–43.
4. Thigpen T, Brady MF, Homesley HD, Soper JT, Bell J. Tamoxifen in the treatment of advanced or recurrent endometrial carcinoma: a Gynecologic Oncology Group study. *J Clin Oncol* 2001;19:364–7.
5. Thigpen JT, Brady MF, Homesley HD, Malfetano J, DuBeshter B, Burger RA, *et al.* Phase III trial of doxorubicin with or without cisplatin in advanced endometrial carcinoma: a gynecologic oncology group study. *J Clin Oncol* 2004;22:3902–8.
6. Fleming GF. Systemic chemotherapy for uterine carcinoma: metastatic and adjuvant. *J Clin Oncol* 2007;25:2983–90.
7. Thigpen JT, Blessing JA, DiSaia PJ, Yordan E, Carson LF, Evers C. A randomized comparison of doxorubicin alone versus doxorubicin plus cyclophosphamide in the management of advanced or recurrent endometrial carcinoma: A Gynecologic Oncology Group study. *J Clin Oncol* 1994;12:1408–14..
8. Fleming GF, Brunetto VL, Cella D, Look KY, Reid GC, Munkarah AR, *et al.* Phase III trial of doxorubicin plus cisplatin with or without paclitaxel plus filgrastim in advanced endometrial carcinoma: a Gynecologic Oncology Group Study. *J Clin Oncol* 2004;22:2159–66..
9. Thigpen JT, Brady MF, Alvarez RD, Adelson MD, Homesley HD, Manetta A, *et al.* Oral medroxyprogesterone acetate in the treatment of advanced or recurrent endometrial carcinoma: a dose–response study by the Gynecologic Oncology Group. *J Clin Oncol* 1999;17:1736–44.
10. Fiorica JV, Brunetto VL, Hanjani P, Lentz SS, Mannel R, Andersen W. Phase II trial of alternating courses of megestrol acetate and tamoxifen in advanced endometrial carcinoma: a Gynecologic Oncology Group study. *Gynecol Oncol* 2004;92:10–14.
11. Whitney CW, Brunetto VL, Zaino RJ, Lentz SS, Sorosky J, Armstrong DK, *et al.* Phase II study of medroxyprogesterone acetate plus tamoxifen in advanced endometrial carcinoma: a Gynecologic Oncology Group study. *Gynecol Oncol* 2004;92:4–9.
12. Rose PG, Brunetto VL, VanLe L, Bell J, Walker JL, Lee RB. A phase II trial of anastrozole in advanced recurrent or persistent endometrial carcinoma: a Gynecologic Oncology Group study. *Gynecol Oncol* 2000;78:212–16.
13. Ma BB, Oza A, Eisenhauer E, Stanimir G, Carey M, Chapman W, *et al.* The activity of letrozole in patients with advanced or recurrent endometrial cancer and correlation with biological markers: a study of the National Cancer Institute of Canada Clinical Trials Group. *Int J Gynecol Cancer* 2004;14:650–8.
14. Gruber SB, Thompson WD. A population-based study of endometrial cancer and familial risk in younger women. Cancer and Steroid Hormone Study Group. *Cancer Epidemiol Biomarkers Prev* 1996;5:411–17.
15. Okuda T, Sekizawa A, Purwosunu Y, Nagatsuka M, Morioka M, Hayashi M, *et al.* Genetics of endometrial cancers. *Obstet Gynecol Int* 2010; 2010: 984013.
16. Lucenteforte E, Talamini R, Montella M, Dal Maso L, Pelucchi C, Franceschi S, *et al.* Family history of cancer and the risk of endometrial cancer. *Eur J Cancer Prev* 2009;18:95–9.
17. Meyer LA, Broaddus RR, Lu KH. Endometrial cancer and Lynch syndrome: clinical and pathologic considerations. *Cancer Control* 2009;16:14–22.
18. Dunlop MG, Farrington SM, Carothers AD, Wyllie AH, Sharp L, Burn J, *et al.* Cancer risk associated with germline DNA mismatch repair gene mutations. *Hum Mol Genet* 1997:6:105–10.
19. Aarnio M, Sankila R, Pukkala E, Salovaara R, Aaltonen LA, de la Chapelle A, *et al.* Cancer risk in mutation carriers of DNA-mismatch-repair genes. *Int J Cancer* 1999;81:214–18.
20. Hendriks YM, Wagner A, Morreau H, Menko F, Stormorken A, Quehenberger F, *et al.* Cancer risk in hereditary nonpolyposis colorectal cancer due to *MSH6* mutations: impact on counseling and surveillance. *Gastroenterology* 2004;127:17–25.

21. Ollikainen M, Abdel-Rahman WM, Moisio AL, Lindroos A, Kariola R, Järvelä I, *et al.* Molecular analysis of familial endometrial carcinoma: a manifestation of hereditary nonpolyposis colorectal cancer or a separate syndrome? *J Clin Oncol* 2005;23:4609–16.
22. Bokhman JV. Two pathogenetic types of endometrial carcinoma. *Gynecol Oncol* 1983;15:10–17.
23. Fujimoto T, Nanjyo H, Fukuda J, Nakamura A, Mizunuma H, Yaegashi N, *et al.* Endometrioid uterine cancer: histopathological risk factors of local and distant recurrence. *Gynecol Oncol* 2009;112:342–7.
24. Hamilton CA, Cheung MK, Osann K, Chen L, Teng NN, Longacre TA, *et al.* Uterine papillary serous and clear cell carcinomas predict for poorer survival compared to grade 3 endometrioid corpus cancers. *Br J Cancer* 2006;94:642–6.
25. Mutter GL, Lin MC, Fitzgerald JT, Kum JB, Baak JP, Lees JA, *et al.* Altered PTEN expression as a diagnostic marker for the earliest endometrial precancers. *J Natl Cancer Inst* 2000;92:924–30.
26. Risinger JI, Hayes K, Maxwell GL, Carney ME, Dodge RK, Barrett JC, *et al. PTEN* mutation in endometrial cancers is associated with favorable clinical and pathologic characteristics. *Clin Cancer Res* 1998;4:3005–10.
27. Shen WH, Balajee AS, Wang J, Wu H, Eng C, Pandolfi PP, Yin Y, *et al.* Essential role for nuclear PTEN in maintaining chromosomal integrity. *Cell* 2007;128:157–70.
28. Gupta A, Yang Q, Pandita RK, Hunt CR, Xiang T, Misri S, *et al.* Cell cycle checkpoint defects contribute to genomic instability in PTEN deficient cells independent of DNA DSB repair. *Cell Cycle* 2009;8:2198–210.
29. Oda K, Stokoe D, Taketani Y, McCormick F. High frequency of coexistent mutations of *PIK3CA* and *PTEN* genes in endometrial carcinoma. *Cancer Res* 2005;65:10669–73.
30. Hayes MP, Douglas W, Ellenson LH. Molecular alterations of *EGFR* and *PIK3CA* in uterine serous carcinoma. *Gynecol Oncol* 2009;113:370–3.
31. Catasus L, Gallardo A, Cuatrecasas M, Prat J. Concomitant PI3K-AKT and p53 alterations in endometrial carcinomas are associated with poor prognosis. *Mod Pathol* 2009;22:522–9.
32. Catasus L, Gallardo A, Cuatrecasas M, Prat J. *PIK3CA* mutations in the kinase domain (exon 20) of uterine endometrial adenocarcinomas are associated with adverse prognostic parameters. *Mod Pathol* 2008;21:131–9.
33. Miyake T, Yoshino K, Enomoto T, Takata T, Ugaki H, Kim A, *et al. PIK3CA* gene mutations and amplifications in uterine cancers, identified by methods that avoid confounding by *PIK3CA* pseudogene sequences. *Cancer Lett* 2008;261:120–6.
34. Salvesen HB, Carter SL, Mannelqvist M, Dutt A, Getz G, Stefansson IM, *et al.* Integrated genomic profiling of endometrial carcinoma associates aggressive tumors with indicators of PI3 kinase activation. *Proc Natl Acad Sci U S A* 2009;106:4834–9.
35. Shoji K, Oda K, Nakagawa S, Hosokawa S, Nagae G, Uehara Y, *et al.* The oncogenic mutation in the pleckstrin homology domain of AKT1 in endometrial carcinomas. *Br J Cancer* 2009;101:145–8.
36. MacDonald ND, Salvesen HB, Ryan A, Iversen OE, Akslen LA, Jacobs IJ. Frequency and prognostic impact of microsatellite instability in a large population-based study of endometrial carcinomas. *Cancer Res* 2000;60:1750–2.
37. Basil JB, Goodfellow PJ, Rader JS, Mutch DG, Herzog TJ. Clinical significance of microsatellite instability in endometrial carcinoma. *Cancer* 2000;89:1758–64.
38. Bilbao C, Rodríguez G, Ramírez R, Falcón O, León L, Chirino R, *et al.* The relationship between microsatellite instability and PTEN gene mutations in endometrial cancer. *Int J Cancer* 2006;119:563–70.
39. Lax SF, Kendall B, Tashiro H, Slebos RJ, Hedrick L. The frequency of p53, K-*ras* mutations, and microsatellite instability differs in uterine endometrioid and serous carcinoma: evidence of distinct molecular genetic pathways. *Cancer* 2000;88:814–24.
40. Pollock PM, Gartside MG, Dejeza LC, Powell MA, Mallon MA, Davies H, *et al.* Frequent activating FGFR2 mutations in endometrial carcinomas parallel germline mutations associated with craniosynostosis and skeletal dysplasia syndromes. *Oncogene* 2007;26:7158–62.
41. Morrison C, Zanagnolo V, Ramirez N, Cohn DE, Kelbick N, Copeland L, *et al.* HER-2 is an independent prognostic factor in endometrial cancer: association with outcome in a large cohort of surgically staged patients. *J Clin Oncol* 2006;24:2376–85.

42. Konecny GE, Santos L, Winterhoff B, Hatmal M, Keeney GL, Mariani A, *et al.* HER2 gene amplification and EGFR expression in a large cohort of surgically staged patients with nonendometrioid (type II) endometrial cancer. *Br J Cancer* 2009;100:89–95.
43. Khalifa MA, Mannel RS, Haraway SD, Walker J, Min KW. Expression of EGFR, HER-2/*neu*, p53, and PCNA in endometrioid, serous papillary, and clear cell endometrial adenocarcinomas. *Gynecol Oncol* 1994;53:84–92.
44. Moreno-Bueno G, Hardisson D, Sánchez C, Sarrió D, Cassia R, García-Rostán G, *et al.* Abnormalities of the APC/beta-catenin pathway in endometrial cancer. *Oncogene* 2002;21:7981–90.
45. Schlosshauer PW, Ellenson LH, Soslow RA. Beta-catenin and E-cadherin expression patterns in high-grade endometrial carcinoma are associated with histological subtype. *Mod Pathol* 2002;15:1032–7.
46. Moreno-Bueno G, Hardisson D, Sarrió D, Sánchez C, Cassia R, Prat J, *et al.* Abnormalities of E- and P-cadherin and catenin (beta-, gamma-catenin, and p120ctn) expression in endometrial cancer and endometrial atypical hyperplasia. *J Pathol* 2003;199:471–8.
47. Holcomb K, Delatorre R, Pedemonte B, McLeod C, Anderson L, Chambers J. E-cadherin expression in endometrioid, papillary serous, and clear cell carcinoma of the endometrium. *Obstet Gynecol* 2002;100:1290–5.
48. Jia L, Liu Y, Yi X, Miron A, Crum CP, Kong B, *et al.* Endometrial glandular dysplasia with frequent p53 gene mutation: a genetic evidence supporting its precancer nature for endometrial serous carcinoma. *Clin Cancer Res* 2008;14:2263–9.
49. Salvesen HB, Das S, Akslen LA. Loss of nuclear p16 protein expression is not associated with promoter methylation but defines a subgroup of aggressive endometrial carcinomas with poor prognosis. *Clin Cancer Res* 2000;6:153–9.
50. Fleming GF, Sill MW, Darcy KM, McMeekin DS, Thigpen JT, Adler LM, *et al.* Phase II trial of trastuzumab in women with advanced or recurrent, HER2-positive endometrial carcinoma: a Gynecologic Oncology Group study. *Gynecol Oncol* 2010;116:15–20.
51. Oza AM, Eisenhauer EA, Elit L, Cutz JC, Sakurada A, Tsao MS, *et al.* Phase II study of erlotinib in recurrent or metastatic endometrial cancer: NCIC IND-148. *J Clin Oncol* 2008;26:4319–25.
52. Hurwitz H, Fehrenbacher L, Novotny W, Cartwright T, Hainsworth J, Heim W, *et al.* Bevacizumab plus irinotecan, fluorouracil, and leucovorin for metastatic colorectal cancer. *N Engl J Med* 2004;350:2335–42.
53. Miller K, Wang M, Gralow J, Dickler M, Cobleigh M, Perez EA, *et al.* Paclitaxel plus bevacizumab versus paclitaxel alone for metastatic breast cancer. *N Engl J Med* 2007;357:2666–76.
54. Burger RA, Brady MF, Bookman MA, Walker JL, Homesley HD, Fowler J, *et al.* Phase III trial of bevacizumab (BEV) in the primary treatment of advanced epithelial ovarian cancer (EOC), primary peritoneal cancer (PPC), or fallopian tube cancer (FTC): A Gynecologic Oncology Group study. *J Clin Oncol* 2010;28(18s):abstr LBA1.
55. Escudier B, Pluzanska A, Koralewski P, Ravaud A, Bracarda S, Szczylik C, *et al.* Bevacizumab plus interferon alfa-2a for treatment of metastatic renal cell carcinoma: a randomised, double-blind phase III trial. *Lancet* 2007;370:2103–11.
56. McMeekin DS, Sill MW, Benbrook D, Darcy KM, Stearns-Kurosawa DJ, Eaton L, *et al.* A phase II trial of thalidomide in patients with refractory endometrial cancer and correlation with angiogenesis biomarkers: a Gynecologic Oncology Group study. *Gynecol Oncol* 2007;105:508–16.
57. Welch S, Mackay HJ, Hirte H, Fleming GF, Morgan R, Wang L, *et al.* A phase II study of sunitinib in recurrent or metastatic endometrial carcinoma: A trial of the PMH Phase II Consortium. *J Clin Oncol* 2009;27(15s):abstr 5576.
58. Correa R, Mackay H, Hirte HW, Morgan R, Welch S, Fleming GF, *et al.* A phase II study of sunitinib in recurrent or metastatic endometrial carcinoma: A trial of the Princess Margaret Hospital, The University of Chicago, and California Cancer Phase II Consortia. *J Clin Oncol* 2010;28(15s):abstr 5038.
59. Nimeiri HS, Oza AM, Morgan RJ, Huo D, Elit L, Knost J, *et al.* Sorafenib (SOR) in patients (pts) with advanced/recurrent uterine carcinoma (UCA) or carcinosarcoma (CS): A phase II trial of the University of Chicago, PMH, and California Phase II Consortia. *J Clin Oncol* 2008;26(15s):abstr 5585.

60. Aghajanian C, Sill MW, Darcy K, Greer B, McMeekin DS, Rose PG, *et al.* A phase II evaluation of bevacizumab in the treatment of recurrent or persistent endometrial cancer: A Gynecologic Oncology Group (GOG) Study. *J Clin Oncol* 2009;27(15s):abstr 5531.
61. Slomovitz BM, Lu KH, Johnston T, Coleman RL, Munsell M, Broaddus RR, *et al.* A phase 2 study of the oral mammalian target of rapamycin inhibitor, everolimus, in patients with recurrent endometrial carcinoma. *Cancer* 2010;116:5415–19.
62. Oza AM, Elit L, Biagi J, Chapman W, Tsao M, Hedley D, *et al.* Molecular correlates associated with a phase II study of temsirolimus (CCI-779) in patients with metastatic or recurrent endometrial cancer–NCIC IND 160. *J Clin Oncol* 2006;24(18s):abstr 3003.
63. Colombo N, McMeekin S, Schwartz P, Kostka J, Sessa C, Gehrig P, *et al.* A phase II trial of the mTOR inhibitor AP23573 as a single agent in advanced endometrial cancer. *J Clin Oncol* 2007;25(18s):abstr 5516.
64. Oza AM, Elit L, Provencher D, Biagi JJ, Panasci L, Sederias J, *et al.* A phase II study of temsirolimus (CCI-779) in patients with metastatic and/or locally advanced recurrent endometrial cancer previously treated with chemotherapy: NCIC CTG IND 160b. *J Clin Oncol* 2008;26(15s):abstr 5516.
65. Byron SA, Gartside MG, Wellens CL, Mallon MA, Keenan JB, Powell MA, *et al.* Inhibition of activated fibroblast growth factor receptor 2 in endometrial cancer cells induces cell death despite PTEN abrogation. *Cancer Res* 2008;68:6902–7. Erratum in: *Cancer Res* 2008;68:10005.
66. Fong PC, Boss DS, Yap TA, Tutt A, Wu P, Mergui-Roelvink M, *et al.* Inhibition of poly(ADP-ribose) polymerase in tumors from *BRCA* mutation carriers. *N Engl J Med* 2009;361:123–34.
67. Banerjee S, Kaye SB, Ashworth A. Making the best of PARP inhibitors in ovarian cancer. *Nat Rev Clin Oncol* 2010;7:508–19.
68. Ashworth A. A synthetic lethal therapeutic approach: poly(ADP) ribose polymerase inhibitors for the treatment of cancers deficient in DNA double-strand break repair. *J Clin Oncol* 2008;26:3785–90.
69. Farmer H, McCabe N, Lord CJ, Tutt AN, Johnson DA, Richardson TB, *et al.* Targeting the DNA repair defect in *BRCA* mutant cells as a therapeutic strategy. *Nature* 2005;434:917–21.
70. Mendes-Pereira AM, Martin SA, Brough R, McCarthy A, Taylor JR, Kim JS, *et al.* Synthetic lethal targeting of PTEN mutant cells with PARP inhibitors. *EMBO Mol Med* 2009;1:315–22.
71. Dedes KJ, Wetterskog D, Mendes-Pereira AM, Natrajan R, Lambros MB, Geyer FC, *et al.* PTEN deficiency in endometrioid endometrial adenocarcinomas predicts sensitivity to PARP inhibitors. *Sci Transl Med* 2010;2:53ra75.

3

Chapter 3

Epigenetic biomarkers in ovarian cancer

Robert Brown and Janet Graham

Introduction

In addition to genomic changes in cancer, there is also selection for aberrant epigenetic changes that do not involve an alteration in DNA sequence but result in a stable alteration in gene expression. Indeed, epigenetic, rather than genetic, changes may be a more prevalent driver of tumour development and progression. Such epigenetic mechanisms include DNA methylation, post-translational modifications of histones, nucleosomal positioning and non-coding RNAs. All types of gynaecological cancer show widespread aberrant epigenetic changes, leading to changes in expression of genes involved in all the hallmarks of cancer and of genes involved in how tumours will respond to chemotherapy. Such epimutations can be reversed using small-molecule inhibitors of maintenance of the epigenetic state. Tumour biomarkers and an understanding of the mechanisms of epigenetic regulation will be key to identifying novel epigenetic therapies, and epigenetic biomarkers also have potential to impact on clinical management in gynaecological cancer. Currently, there is much interest in the potential to target epigenetic mechanisms in tumour stem cells as a means of eradicating subpopulations of cells that may lead to tumour recurrence and drug resistance. However, there remain many obstacles to the implementation of these epigenetic approaches in clinical practice.

DNA methylation and gene transcription

One of the most widely studied epigenetic changes is DNA methylation occurring in mammalian DNA at CpG dinucleotides where the hydrogen bond at the 5 position of cytosine becomes methylated (Figure 3.1). DNA methylation is catalysed by a group of enzymes called the DNA methyltransferases (DNMTs).[1,2] CpG dinucleotides are under-represented in the genome but there are CpG-rich regions (CpG islands) that generally remain unmethylated and are located in the promoter or first exon regions of approximately 70% of genes.[3] The definition of a CpG island is inevitably arbitrary and perhaps should be more based on its functional effect on gene transcription. Nevertheless, one widely used definition of a CpG island is based on DNA sequence: a region of at least 200 base pairs, with a guanine-cytosine (GC) percentage greater than 50% and with an observed/expected CpG ratio greater than 60%.[4] CpG islands at gene transcription start sites in normal cells are usually unmethylated, while CpG sites elsewhere in the genome and particularly in the

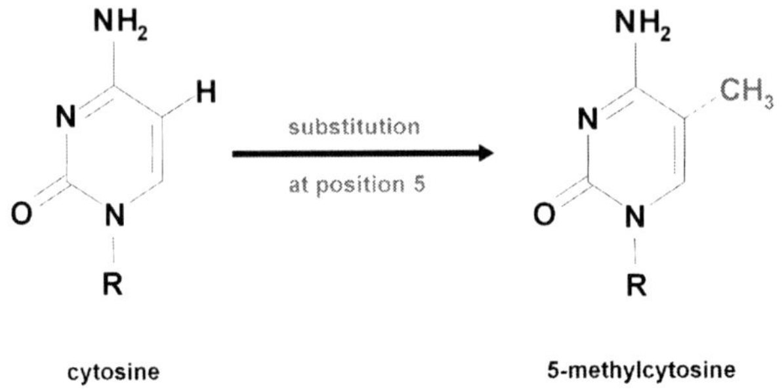

Figure 3.1 Methylation of the base cytosine to 5-methylcytosine following enzymatic transfer of a methyl (CH_3) group

coding sequence are relatively more methylated. In ageing and cancer, these contrasting states of methylation tend to reverse,[5,6] with non-CpG island CpG sites becoming hypomethylated while many hundreds of CpG islands become hypermethylated (Figure 3.2). Aberrant hypermethylation of CpG islands occurs in all tumour types and is strongly correlated to transcriptional gene silencing and epigenetic maintenance of the silenced state.[7] Repetitive genomic sequences are heavily methylated and this may have a role in the protection of chromosome integrity, by preventing chromosome instability, translocations and gene disruption.[6,7] Thus, the global demethylation observed in tumour cells may contribute to genomic instability and chromosomal aberrations during cancer development.[8]

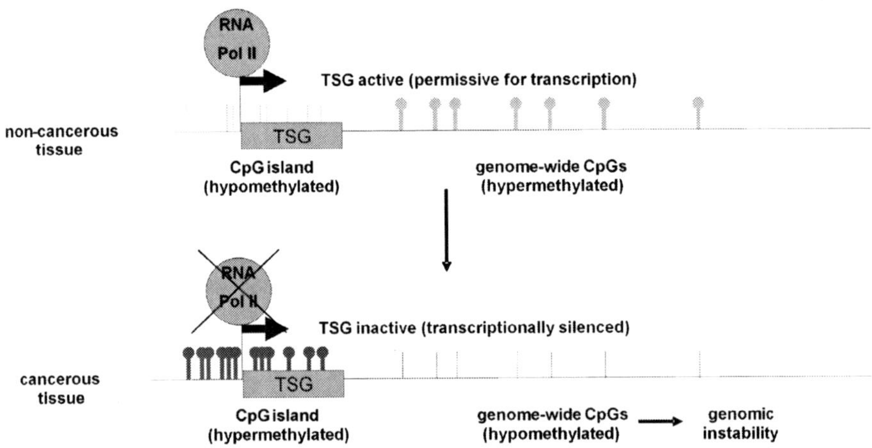

Figure 3.2 DNA methylation and transcriptional silencing – a representation of a region of DNA in non-cancerous and cancerous tissues showing the differences in DNA methylation in the two phenotypes: in non-cancerous tissue, genome-wide hypermethylation of CpGs (light grey circles) and an actively transcribed tumour suppressor gene (TSG) is associated with a hypomethylated CpG island (light grey lines); in cancerous tissue, the opposite is seen with genome-wide hypomethylation (dark grey lines) leading to genomic instability, and CpG island hypermethylation (dark grey circles) contributing to transcriptional silencing of a TSG;[53] RNA Pol II = RNA polymerase II

DNA methylation at CpG islands is associated with chromatin being in a repressive state for gene transcription.[7,9,10] In general, condensed chromatin mediates transcriptional repression, whereas transcriptionally active genes are in areas of open chromatin. DNA wraps around histone proteins forming nucleosomes and extending out of the nucleosome are charged amino-terminal histone tails, which are subject to post-translational modification such as acetylation, phosphorylation and methylation.[11] As an example, the lysine on histone 3 at amino acid 9 (H3-K9) is a site of both acetylation and methylation. H3-K9 acetylation is associated with chromatin being in a permissive state for gene transcription. Deacetylation of H3-K9 is required for methylation to occur, which is then a repressive epigenetic mark associated with gene silencing. Trimethylation of H3-K9 results in the recruitment and binding of the transcriptional repressor heterochromatin protein HP1. HP1 binding to the methylated H3 forms a positive feedback loop, mediating the propagation of repressive chromatin over wide chromosomal ranges. Thus, covalent modification of the histone tails directly affects higher order chromatin structure and thereby offers a mechanism of epigenetic gene activation or silencing.

A crucial aspect of both DNA methylation and histone acetylation is that they are reversible.[2,12] Epigenetic change in gene expression is maintained during cell division and requires active maintenance of the epigenetic signature. Enzymes such as DNMTs are required to maintain this epigenetic signature at each cell division and this can therefore be manipulated using small molecules that have the potential to be developed into epigenetic drugs. The most investigated epigenetic therapies to date are the DNMT inhibitors and histone deacetylase (HDAC) inhibitors.[2,12]

DNA methylation as a biomarker in ovarian cancer

A biomarker can be defined as a characteristic that is objectively measured and evaluated as an indicator of normal biological processes, pathological processes, or responses (pharmacological or otherwise) to a therapeutic intervention.[13] DNA methylation has many potential advantages as a cancer biomarker since it is stable, provides a binary read-out and is frequently aberrant in cancer. DNA methylation-mediated epigenetic silencing can occur at many genes in a given tumour and has the potential to influence the activity of multiple biochemical pathways in a tumour cell.[6] Highly sensitive polymerase chain reaction (PCR)-based assays can accurately quantify the level of CpG island methylation at a given locus.[14] These assays are mainly based on resistance of methylated cytosines to chemical modification to uracil by sodium bisulphite treatment of DNA. Unmethylated cytosines are converted to uracil whereas methylated cytosines are not, resulting in a DNA base sequence difference depending on methylation status, which can then by assayed using PCR-specific primers (for example, methylation-specific PCR; MSP) or by DNA sequencing. However, the highly sensitive nature of these assays can lead to false positives, especially due to incomplete bisulphite modification of DNA.

As well as approaches to examining methylation at individual loci, there are now a variety of methods for examining global changes in DNA methylation in the genome by hibridisation to microarrays or DNA sequencing.[14] These are based on bisulphite modification of DNA, restriction enzyme digestion of DNA using enzymes that cut DNA only when given sequences are methylated and pull-down of methylated DNA using methyl-binding domain proteins or antibodies to methylated DNA.

Although there are many advantages to using DNA methylation as a biomarker, there are two major disadvantages. Firstly, there are currently no simple methods for examining heterogeneity of DNA methylation in tumours and thus there are no *in situ* methods of detecting DNA methylation in tumour sections. Secondly, there remains uncertainty about what level of methylation will affect gene expression. DNA methylation is thus only an indication of gene activity, and the relationship between methylation and expression, especially at non-CpG island loci, remains uncertain. This is further compounded by potential variability in methylation of normal cells.

Predisposition epigenetic biomarkers

In addition to the DNA methylation changes that can occur during tumour initiation and progression, studies have shown significant DNA methylation variation in non-cancerous cells across unrelated individuals that may be associated with cancer risk. Examples include methylation of intragenic element within the *ATM* gene in bilateral breast cancer cases[15] and germline DNA methylation at CpG islands of cancer susceptibility loci, such as *MLH1*, in people with hereditary nonpolyposis colorectal cancer.[16] This raises the possibility that DNA methylation quantified in, for instance, blood cells could be used as a biomarker of cancer risk or prognosis, analogously to how single-nucleotide polymorphisms are currently used.[17] However, this is still a relatively unexplored area in ovarian cancer.

Diagnostic epigenetic biomarkers

DNA methylation changes are widespread in various gynaecological cancers.[18,19] While there are significant associations of particular methylation events with histological sub-types or stage of disease, so far there are no specific patterns of methylation that are diagnostic for different histological sub-types or stage of ovarian cancer with sufficient specificity to be of clinical value. The Cancer Genome Atlas (TCGA; cancergenome.nih.gov) project has recently completed a methylation analysis of high-grade serous ovarian cancer using an Illumina 27K methylation bead array and this may identify biomarkers of serous ovarian cancer that are highly methylated that would have potential as markers for early diagnosis of ovarian cancer. Indeed, it has previously been suggested that a small panel of loci would have potential for detection of tumour DNA in plasma from women with ovarian cancer.[20,21] The problem with this approach is the high sensitivity and specificity that will be required for an early detection test. This will be further confounded by the limited amounts of tumour DNA released into body fluids in those with early-stage disease. However, ultra-deep bisulphite sequencing may allow sufficient sensitivity and specificity, even for detection of early-stage disease.

Prognostic epigenetic biomarkers

Identifying robust prognostic markers following conventional treatment of epithelial ovarian cancer will provide a solid basis for characterising potential predictive biomarkers for novel treatment strategies and hence for stratification of patients for targeted care in clinical practice. In unpublished results, we have shown that hypermethylation of multiple CpG islands in the Wnt signalling pathway is frequently observed in epithelial ovarian cancer and we have identified methylation of key loci as significantly associated with poor progression-free survival independent from clinical parameters. Reduced expression of *FZD4* and *DVL1* correlates with increased methylation and low expression of these two genes correlates with poor progression-free survival in an independent tumour set. It remains to be established exactly how methylation of these loci affects function of different Wnt pathways. However, since Wnt pathways control a variety of biological processes including cell proliferation, differentiation, migration and tissue homeostatis, they can clearly impact not just on tumour progression but also on regrowth of cancer following treatment.[22] This will be relevant for patient stratification in future clinical trials of ovarian cancer, and particularly for novel drugs targeting the Wnt pathway.[23]

Predictive epigenetic biomarkers

Methylation profiling of tumours has allowed the identification of genome-wide DNA methylation patterns as well as the identification of loci that are associated with response or survival of women with ovarian cancer following chemotherapy.[19,24] For instance, *BRCA1* has a role in homologous recombination and its methylation is associated with an enhanced response to platinum chemotherapy in ovarian cancer.[25] In contrast, the DNA mismatch repair gene *MLH1* is required for engaging an apoptotic response to platinum drugs and methylation of *MLH1* is associated with poor patient survival.[26] Examples such as these highlight the importance of patient selection for future epigenetic treatments and the need for patient stratification based on methylation profiling within clinical trials.

Changes in DNA methylation occur during tumour development as part of the selection for malignant transformation but methylation changes can also occur during chemotherapy. In ovarian cell line models of cisplatin resistance, acquired hypermethylation of loci is much more frequent than hypomethylation.[27] Acquired methylation of *MLH1* has been observed in ovarian tumours at relapse compared with at presentation and this is associated with poor patient survival.[26] This gives rise to the hypothesis that acquired resistance to platinum agents may be due at least in part to hypermethylation of genes involved in platinum sensitivity. If this is the case then such resistance might be reversed by demethylating agents. Consistent with this hypothesis, treatment of platinum-resistant tumour xenografts with the demethylating agent decitabine (2-deoxy-5′-azacytidine) leads to increased inhibition of growth by cisplatin and carboplatin.[28] However, in these studies not all xenograft models were sensitised to chemotherapy by demethylation, again stressing the potential importance of stratifying patients on the basis of methylation profile in clinical trials of epigenetic chemo-sensitisers.

Pharmacodynamic epigenetic biomarkers

Pharmacodynamic biomarkers of demethylation such as levels of DNA demethylation in surrogate and tumour tissue can be used to identify maximal biological effect rather than maximum tolerated dose. Appleton *et al.*[29] have reported the results of a phase I trial of carboplatin and the demethylating agent decitabine in patients with solid tumours. Decitabine was found to induce dose-dependent reversible demethylation in peripheral blood mononuclear cells (PBMCs) maximally at day 10. Furthermore, decitabine induced demethylation of CpG islands at gene promoters in PBMCs, buccal cells and tumour biopsies, as well as elevation of epigenetically regulated gene expression. The conclusions from this phase I trial were that decitabine could be combined safely with carboplatin at a dose and schedule that caused epigenetic changes equivalent to or greater than that observed in mice with carboplatin-sensitised xenografts.[29]

Two other phase I studies have investigated the combination of a demethylating agent and carboplatin in women with ovarian cancer. Both studies included women with disease relapsing within 6 months of their last carboplatin treatment and both used 5 day schedules for the demethylating agent. Fang *et al.*[30] proposed a recommended dose of 10 mg/m^2 of decitabine on days 1–5 with carboplatin (AUC = 5) on day 8, while Fu *et al.*[31] used azacitidine (75 mg/m^2 subcutaneously) on days 1–5 with carboplatin (AUC = 4 or 5) on day 2. Despite the relatively low dose intensity of carboplatin and the more platinum-resistant populations, both studies saw responses (11% and 13.8%, respectively).

Based on the dose and schedule of decitabine combined with carboplatin that had shown epigenetic pharmacodynamic responses,[29] a randomised phase II trial was started in women with recurrent ovarian cancer.[32] Women with advanced ovarian cancer, progressing 6–12 months after response to previous platinum therapy, were randomised to decitabine on day 1 and carboplatin (AUC = 6) on day 8 of a 28 day cycle or to carboplatin alone. Based on previous studies showing acquired methylation of *MLH1* following platinum treatment,[26] it was hypothesised that those women with methylation of specific genes within their tumours would have a greater chance of benefiting from the combined decitabine/carboplatin treatment. The study was thus powered to contain a sufficient number of patients to allow the primary endpoint to be a comparison of response to carboplatin with and without decitabine in those with methylated *MLH1*. However, the starting dose of decitabine was reduced from 90 to 45 mg/m^2 after the first four women in the combination arm had a 1–2 week delay owing to neutropenia between cycles 1 and 2, and the study was stopped early after 15 women had been treated with decitabine and carboplatin, owing to lack of efficacy and poor treatment deliverability.[32] Possible reasons for the lack of efficacy seen in this phase II trial may have been the reduced dose intensity of the carboplatin or the additional myelosuppression associated with the decitabine treatment. In order for these agents to progress as potential treatments within the solid tumour setting, it will be important to develop ones that are less myelosuppressive or to optimise schedules that are less toxic while retaining demethylating activity. Clinical activity of decitabine has been observed in studies of haematological malignancies using a 1 hour infusion of decitabine over 5 or 10 days.[33] In ovarian cancer, studies are currently under way combining platinum chemotherapy with similar schedules.[34] Another feasible explanation may have been that the demethylation of certain genes including *BRCA* led to an adverse affect counteracting the carboplatin-sensitising effect of demethylated *MLH1*. This again highlights the importance of patient selection based on their tumour methylation profile for treatments and future studies.

Ovarian tumour stem cells

It has been proposed that subpopulations of tumour cells with stem cell-like properties, such as the so-called side populations that overexpress ABC drug transporters, can sustain the growth of drug-resistant tumour cells, leading to tumour recurrence following chemotherapy.[35] In support of the existence of tumour stem cell-like cells in ovarian tumours, subpopulations of tumour-initiating or -sustaining cells have been identified that grow more readily in an anchorage-independent manner and as tumours in xenogeneic mice.[36–41] These subpopulations can be shown to overexpress stem cell-associated markers and to be more resistant to drugs used in the treatment of ovarian cancer.[40,41] We have identified a subpopulation of cells from ovarian cell lines that have a more aggressive phenotype, as defined by anchorage-independent growth and tumour formation in NOD/SCID mice, and are resistant to carboplatin and paclitaxel.[42] Consistent with the *in vitro* observation of a survival advantage of these side populations following exposure to carboplatin and hence potential drug selection, we observed increased side population in tumour cells isolated from ovarian cancer patient ascites following chemotherapy and at relapse compared with chemo-naïve patients.[42]

We have shown that side populations isolated from IGROV1 ovarian tumour cells overexpress PRC2 genes, while, consistent with this, PRC2-repressed targets are underexpressed. PRC2 contains the histone methyltransferase EZH2, which, together with EED and SUZ12, trimethylates histone H3 on lysine 27 (H3K27me3) and is associated with a repressive chromatin state.[43] Many genes in cancer, including tumour suppressor genes, are epigenetically silenced by mechanisms associated with H3K27me3 that can be independent of DNA methylation.[10] Since H3K27me3 is somatically inherited during cell division,[44] this argues that it truly is an epigenetic mark that is maintained and as such is a key target for reversing aberrant epigenetic silencing. Consistent with the data presented in our current study in ovarian cancer, EZH2 has been shown to be essential for glioblastoma cancer stem cell maintenance.[45] EZH2 is overexpressed in many cancers and levels of EZH2 correlate with poor prognosis in various cancers, including ovarian cancer.[46–49]

EZH2 knockdown in ovarian cell lines has been shown to lead to reduced cell growth/proliferation, as well as cell migration and/or invasion *in vitro*.[49] It has also led to the re-sensitisation of drug-resistant ovarian cancer cells to cisplatin.[50] This drug-resistant subpopulation will be important to eradicate if we are to improve the treatment of ovarian cancer. Catalytic site inhibitors of histone methyltransferase have been reported,[51] as has indirect pharmacological inhibition of PRC2,[52] but so far no specific EZH2 inhibitor has been described. Development of specific inhibitors of EZH2 will have potential as drugs that target this key subpopulation of drug-resistant tumour-sustaining cells.

Conclusion

It is now clear that normal differentiation control breaks down during tumour development and that all tumour types show aberrant regulation of the epigenetic code, including changes in DNA methylation, histone modification and microRNAs. This has led to much interest in the development of epigenetic cancer therapies to target this aberrant epigenetic regulation. HDAC and DNMT inhibitors are now used in the treatment of certain haematological malignancies. However, their more general applicability to solid tumours such as ovarian cancer will be limited by lack of specificity and by delivery challenges. Novel approaches to overcome these limitations and to develop more specific drugs are required. In addition, tumour biomarkers and an increased understanding of the biology will be key to improved epigenetic therapy approaches. As cancer results from a combination of epigenetic and genetic aberrations, it is anticipated that having both 'epigenetic' and 'genetic' therapy/ standard cytotoxics available will be important. This raises additional challenges of optimising the dose and schedule of these agents when given in combination and personalising therapies depending on the molecular characteristics of the patient's tumours. Defining the epigenetic and genetic landscape for individual patients may allow epigenetic therapies to be targeted to groups of patients who will particularly benefit from these therapies.

References

1. Li E, Bestor TH, Jaenisch R. Targeted mutation of the DNA methyltransferase gene results in embryonic lethality. *Cell* 1992;69:915–26.
2. Issa JP, Kantarjian HM. Targeting DNA methylation. *Clin Cancer Res* 2009;15:3938–46.
3. Saxonov S, Berg P, Brutlag DL. A genome-wide analysis of CpG dinucleotides in the human genome distinguishes two distinct classes of promoters. *Proc Natl Acad Sci U S A* 2006;103:1412–17.
4. Gardiner-Garden M, Frommer M. CpG islands in vertebrate genomes. *J Mol Biol* 1987;196:261–82.
5. Maegawa S, Hinkal G, Kim HS, Shen L, Zhang L, Zhang J, *et al.* Widespread and tissue specific age-related DNA methylation changes in mice. *Genome Res* 2010;20:332–40.
6. Esteller M. Cancer epigenomics: DNA methylomes and histone-modification maps. *Nat Rev Genet* 2007;8:286–98.
7. Jones PA, Baylin SB. The epigenomics of cancer. *Cell* 2007;128:683–92.
8. McCabe MT, Brandes JC, Vertino PM. Cancer DNA methylation: molecular mechanisms and clinical implications. *Clin Cancer Res* 2009;15:3927–37.
9. Jorgensen HF, Bird A. MeCP2 and other methyl-CpG binding proteins. *Ment Retard Dev Disabil Res Rev* 2002;8:87–93.
10. Kondo Y, Shen L, Cheng AS, Ahmed S, Boumber Y, Charo C, *et al.* Gene silencing in cancer by histone H3 lysine 27 trimethylation independent of promoter DNA methylation. *Nat Genet* 2008;40:741–50.
11. Kouzarides T. Chromatin modifications and their function. *Cell* 2007;128:693–705.
12. Chapman-Rothe N, Brown R. Approaches to target the genome and its epigenome in cancer. *Future Med Chem* 2009;1:1481–95.
13. Biomarkers Definitions Working Group. Biomarkers and surrogate endpoints: preferred definitions and conceptual framework. *Clin Pharmacol Ther* 2001;69:89–95.
14. Estecio MR, Issa JP. Tackling the methylome: recent methodological advances in genome-wide methylation profiling. *Genome Med* 2009;1:106.
15. Flanagan JM, Munoz-Alegre M, Henderson S, Tang T, Sun P, Johnson N, *et al.* Gene-body hypermethylation of ATM in peripheral blood DNA of bilateral breast cancer patients. *Hum Mol Genet* 2009;18:1332–42.
16. Hitchins MP, Wong JJ, Suthers G, Suter CM, Martin DI, Hawkins NJ, *et al.* Inheritance of a cancer-associated MLH1 germ-line epimutation. *N Engl J Med* 2007;356:697–705.
17. Paige AJ, Brown R. Pharmaco(epi)genomics in ovarian cancer. *Pharmacogenomics* 2008;9:1825–34.
18. Asadollahi R, Hyde CA, Zhong XY. Epigenetics of ovarian cancer: from the lab to the clinic. *Gynecol Oncol* 2010;118:81–7.
19. Glasspool RM, Teodoridis JM, Brown R. Epigenetics as a mechanism driving polygenic clinical drug resistance. *Br J Cancer* 2006;94:1087–92.
20. Liggett TE, Melnikov A, Yi Q, Replogle C, Hu W, Rotmensch J, *et al.* Distinctive DNA methylation patterns of cell-free plasma DNA in women with malignant ovarian tumors. *Gynecol Oncol* 2010;120: 113–20.
21. Ibanez de Caceres I, Battagli C, Esteller M, Herman JG, Dulaimi E, Edelson MI, *et al.* Tumor cell-specific *BRCA1* and *RASSF1A* hypermethylation in serum, plasma, and peritoneal fluid from ovarian cancer patients. *Cancer Res* 2004;64:6476–81.
22. Boyer A, Goff AK, Boerboom D. WNT signaling in ovarian follicle biology and tumorigenesis. *Trends Endocrinol Metab* 2010;21:25–32.
23. Luu HH, Zhang R, Haydon RC, Rayburn E, Kang Q, Si W, *et al.* Wnt/beta-catenin signaling pathway as a novel cancer drug target. *Curr Cancer Drug Targets* 2004;4:653–71.
24. Wei SH, Balch C, Paik HH, Kim YS, Baldwin RL, Liyanarachchi S, *et al.* Prognostic DNA methylation biomarkers in ovarian cancer. *Clin Cancer Res* 2006;12:2788–94.
25. Teodoridis JM, Hall J, Marsh S, Kannall HD, Smyth C, Curto J, *et al.* CpG island methylation of DNA damage response genes in advanced ovarian cancer. *Cancer Res* 2005;65:8961–7.
26. Gifford G, Paul J, Vasey PA, Kaye SB, Brown R. The acquisition of *hMLH1* methylation in plasma DNA after chemotherapy predicts poor survival for ovarian cancer patients. *Clin Cancer Res* 2004;10:4420–6.

27. Dai W, Teodoridis JM, Graham J, Zeller C, Huang TH, Yan P, *et al.* Methylation linear discriminant analysis (MLDA) for identifying differentially methylated CpG islands. *BMC Bioinformatics* 2008;9:337.
28. Plumb JA, Strathdee G, Sludden J, Kaye SB, Brown R. Reversal of drug resistance in human tumor xenografts by 2′-deoxy-5-azacytidine-induced demethylation of the *hMLH1* gene promoter. *Cancer Res* 2000;60:6039–44.
29. Appleton K, Mackay HJ, Judson I, Plumb JA, McCormick C, Strathdee G, *et al.* Phase I and pharmacodynamic trial of the DNA methyltransferase inhibitor decitabine and carboplatin in solid tumors. *J Clin Oncol* 2007;25:4603–9.
30. Fang F, Balch C, Schilder J, Breen T, Zhang S, Shen C, *et al.* A phase 1 and pharmacodynamic study of decitabine in combination with carboplatin in patients with recurrent, platinum-resistant, epithelial ovarian cancer. *Cancer* 2010;116:4043–53.
31. Fu S, Hu W, Iyer R, Kavanagh JJ, Coleman RL, Levenback CF, *et al.* Phase 1b-2a study to reverse platinum resistance through use of a hypomethylating agent, azacitidine, in patients with platinum-resistant or platinum-refractory epithelial ovarian cancer. *Cancer* 2010 Nov 8. [Epub ahead of print]
32. Glasspool RM, Gore M, Rustin G, McNeish I, Wilson R, Pledge S, *et al.* Randomized phase II study of decitabine in combination with carboplatin compared with carboplatin alone in patients with recurrent advanced ovarian cancer. *J Clin Oncol* 2009;27:15S.
33. Issa JP, Garcia-Manero G, Giles FJ, Mannari R, Thomas D, Faderl S, *et al.* Phase 1 study of low-dose prolonged exposure schedules of the hypomethylating agent 5-aza-2′-deoxycytidine (decitabine) in hematopoietic malignancies. *Blood* 2004;103:1635–40.
34. Matei DE, Nephew KP. Epigenetic therapies for chemoresensitization of epithelial ovarian cancer. *Gynecol Oncol* 2010;116:195–201.
35. Dean M. ABC transporters, drug resistance, and cancer stem cells. *J Mammary Gland Biol Neoplasia* 2009;14:3–9.
36. Ferrandina G, Bonanno G, Pierelli L, Perillo A, Procoli A, Mariotti A, *et al.* Expression of *CD133-1* and *CD133-2* in ovarian cancer. *Int J Gynecol Cancer* 2008;18:506–14.
37. Bapat SA, Mali AM, Koppikar CB, Kurrey NK. Stem and progenitor-like cells contribute to the aggressive behavior of human epithelial ovarian cancer. *Cancer Res* 2005;65:3025–9.
38. Szotek PP, Pieretti-Vanmarcke R, Masiakos PT, Dinulescu DM, Connolly D, Foster R, *et al.* Ovarian cancer side population defines cells with stem cell-like characteristics and Mullerian Inhibiting Substance responsiveness. *Proc Natl Acad Sci U S A* 2006;103:11154–9.
39. Moserle L, Indraccolo S, Ghisi M, Frasson C, Fortunato E, Canevari S, *et al.* The side population of ovarian cancer cells is a primary target of IFN-alpha antitumor effects. *Cancer Res* 2008;68:5658–68.
40. Zhang S, Balch C, Chan MW, Lai HC, Matei D, Schilder JM, *et al.* Identification and characterization of ovarian cancer-initiating cells from primary human tumors. *Cancer Res* 2008;68:4311–20.
41. Hu L, McArthur C, Jaffe RB. Ovarian cancer stem-like side-population cells are tumourigenic and chemoresistant. *Br J Cancer* 2010;102:1276–83.
42. Rizzo S, Hersey JM, Mellor P, Dai W, Santos-Silva A, Liber D, *et al.* Ovarian cancer stem cell-like side populations are enriched following chemotherapy and overexpress EZH2. *Mol Cancer Ther* 2011;10:325–35.
43. Cao R, Zhang Y. The functions of E(Z)/EZH2-mediated methylation of lysine 27 in histone H3. *Curr Opin Genet Dev* 2004;14:155–64.
44. Margueron R, Justin N, Ohno K, Sharpe ML, Son J, Drury WJ 3rd, *et al.* Role of the polycomb protein EED in the propagation of repressive histone marks. *Nature* 2009;461:762–7.
45. Suva ML, Riggi N, Janiszewska M, Radovanovic I, Provero P, Stehle JC, *et al.* EZH2 is essential for glioblastoma cancer stem cell maintenance. *Cancer Res* 2009;69:9211–18.
46. Matsukawa Y, Semba S, Kato H, Ito A, Yanagihara K, Yokozaki H. Expression of the enhancer of zeste homolog 2 is correlated with poor prognosis in human gastric cancer. *Cancer Sci* 2006;97:484–91.
47. Collett K, Eide GE, Arnes J, Stefansson IM, Eide J, Braaten A, *et al.* Expression of enhancer of zeste homologue 2 is significantly associated with increased tumor cell proliferation and is a marker of aggressive breast cancer. *Clin Cancer Res* 2006;12:1168–74.
48. Bryant RJ, Cross NA, Eaton CL, Hamdy FC, Cunliffe VT. *EZH2* promotes proliferation and invasiveness of prostate cancer cells. *Prostate* 2007;67:547–56.

49. Rao ZY, Cai MY, Yang GF, He LR, Mai SJ, Hua WF, *et al.* EZH2 supports ovarian carcinoma cell invasion and/or metastasis via regulation of TGF-beta1 and is a predictor of outcome in ovarian carcinoma patients. *Carcinogenesis* 2010;31:1576–83.
50. Hu S, Yu L, Li Z, Shen Y, Wang J, Cai J, *et al.* Overexpression of *EZH2* contributes to acquired cisplatin resistance in ovarian cancer cells *in vitro* and *in vivo*. *Cancer Biol Ther* 2010;10:788–95.
51. Chang Y, Zhang X, Horton JR, Upadhyay AK, Spannhoff A, Liu J, *et al.* Structural basis for G9a-like protein lysine methyltransferase inhibition by BIX-01294. *Nat Struct Mol Biol* 2009;16:312–17.
52. Tan J, Yang X, Zhuang L, Jiang X, Chen W, Lee PL, *et al.* Pharmacologic disruption of Polycomb-repressive complex 2-mediated gene repression selectively induces apoptosis in cancer cells. *Genes Dev* 2007;21:1050–63.
53. Graham JS, Kaye SB, Brown R. The promises and pitfalls of epigenetic therapies in solid tumours. *Eur J Cancer* 2009;45:1129–36.

4

Chapter 4
Predictive biology of ovarian cancer

Christine A Parkinson and James D Brenton

Introduction

Over the past 5 years, new insights into the molecular basis of epithelial ovarian cancer (EOC) have brought about rapid change in our understanding of the disease. However, survival rates for women with advanced EOC have not changed significantly over the past two decades and fewer than 30% remain alive 5 years after diagnosis despite multiple clinical trials of novel chemotherapy combinations.[1–3] The most important clinical question for the management of EOC is how to identify individuals with different risks of response or relapse, and how to implement personalised selection of optimum systemic therapies. Since 1999 there have been extensive efforts to use new genomic tools, particularly expression microarrays, to identify better biomarkers for ovarian cancer treatment. This chapter concentrates on recent robust advances that are likely to affect clinical care over the short to medium term.

The phrase 'stratified medicine' describes the use of better classifiers, both clinical and molecular, to separate patients into defined groups for the selection of optimum treatment. With the rapid reduction in cost of DNA sequencing, there is now a strong scientific justification to use next-generation sequencing technologies to discover a more detailed molecular stratification. 'Personalised' medicine describes the ability to choose a specific treatment for an individual patient and requires biomarkers with high predictive value. The terms 'predictive' and 'prognostic' are often used imprecisely to describe biomarkers. In this chapter we use the term 'predictive' to refer to biomarkers that choose therapy for patients. Prognostic markers are informative for an outcome (usually death or progression) within a population of patients.

Biomarkers are specific to EOC sub-types

To develop reliable biomarkers for a disease, it is critically important to use homogeneous data sets that are representative of the population at risk.[4] Although traditionally treated as one disease, EOCs have considerable morphological heterogeneity and their pathological classification encompasses high-grade serous (HGSOC), clear-cell, endometrioid and mucinous sub-types. However, these classifications have shown poor reproducibility between pathologists, despite each major sub-type having different risk, epidemiological and molecular factors.[5] Particular areas of difficulty include the distinction between serous and endometrioid carcinoma, mixed versus pure cell types, and poorly differentiated tumours. In a seminal study examining the classification of ovarian cancer sub-types, the expression of 21 immunohistochemical markers was examined across a population-based cohort of 500 ovarian carcinomas using tissue microarrays.[6] Strikingly, the expression of 20 of the 21 biomarkers showed significant differences between sub-types, but were relatively invariant by stage within each sub-type. Nine of the 21 biomarkers had prognostic value when applied across the entire cohort but only three remained informative when analysed by sub-type-specific expression. For example, the proliferation marker Ki-67 appeared to be a poor prognostic marker across the entire cohort but its expression level was highest in HGSOC and it was not prognostic within any of the subgroups. In effect, Ki-67 is a surrogate marker for HGSOC and therefore has an apparent prognostic effect across all sub-types, owing to the poorer outcomes of HGSOC cases. Similarly, the HGSOC-specific marker WT1 was a poor prognostic factor overall but was a favourable marker within the HGSOC cases. These findings emphasise the wide biological and survival differences between high-grade serous neoplasms and lower grade endometrioid and clear-cell sub-types. This important study demonstrated for the first time that the association between ovarian biomarkers and survival was highly variable between different sub-types and that stratification by sub-type is needed to interpret biomarker data in EOC.

Stage remains an important prognostic factor in all cancers but the distribution of stage at diagnosis is also different between ovarian sub-types. A comprehensive pathology review of 1009 cases using modern criteria for EOC classification showed that HGSOC accounted for 87.7% of stage III/IV cancers and 35.5% of stage I/II cancers.[5,7] In contrast, low-stage EOCs were significantly enriched for endometrioid (26.6% versus 2.5%) and clear-cell (26.2% versus 4.5%) sub-types as compared with stage III/IV disease, and similar results were confirmed in a validation set of 410 consecutive cases. This shows that low-stage EOC is not an 'earlier' or anatomically restricted version of high-stage disease. Instead, the differences in stage at diagnosis are determined by the underlying biology of the sub-types.

Grade is another important prognostic factor in many cancers but assessment of grade in EOC is poorly reproducible.[7–9] In a study of 605 stage I/II EOC cases, tumour sub-type and sub-stage (stage IA or IB) had more prognostic value than grade and it was not possible to identify a subset of HGSOC with excellent outcome.[10] This work shows that with current clinical variables it is difficult, even within low-stage endometrioid and mucinous cases, to identify women who could be excluded from adjuvant chemotherapy treatment because of a high likelihood of cure. It also demonstrates that histological grade and sub-type are covariates, and, although grade is a surrogate for sub-type, it cannot reproduce the biological variability within or between sub-types. For example, HGSOC is always grade 2 or 3 but there are no differences for outcome within HGSOC by grade.[11] Although mucinous or clear-cell sub-type have a comparatively good prognosis when diagnosed with stage I/II disease, this is reversed in women with high-stage disease. In a Gynecologic Cancer InterGroup (GCIG) study of 8704 women with stage III/IV disease, mucinous and clear-cell tumours had shorter times to progression and this effect remained after controlling for age and residual disease.[12] Median overall survival in this study for serous, clear-cell, mucinous and endometrioid histology was 40.8, 21.3 14.6 and 50.9 months, respectively, reflecting the low effectiveness of treatment for advanced non-HGSOC sub-types.

Previous models of ovarian carcinogenesis have suggested that the earliest steps in the development of EOC involve metaplastic change in the normal ovarian epithelium (NOE), and that this is related to structural epithelial abnormalities on the surface of the ovary, such as clefts and inclusion cysts.[13] The HGSOC, mucinous and endometrioid sub-types were thought to arise from trans-differentiation of the NOE via pathways recapitulating Müllerian development of the fallopian tube, endocervix and endometrium, respectively. These models were first questioned by Dubeau,[13] who suggested that 'ovarian' cancers might arise from the secondary Müllerian system, including endosalpingiosis, endometriosis and para-ovarian and para-tubal cysts. Evidence that dysplastic lesions could be found in the distal fallopian tube was demonstrated by careful pathological studies on the fimbria of women with *BRCA1* or *BRCA2* mutations undergoing risk-reducing surgery.[14–20] Subsequent studies on fimbria of sporadic HGSOC cases showed that tubal intraepithelial carcinomas (TICs) were present in 75% of cases and that fallopian tube lesions were under-diagnosed by standard histopathological examination.[21] Identical *TP53* mutations were found between TIC and ovarian metastases, which is consistent with a single clonal origin for HGSOC arising in the tubal epithelium.[18,21] These studies now strongly implicate TIC, or similar changes in endosalpingiosis tissues, as the cell of origin for HGSOC. In contrast, endometrioid and clear-cell ovarian cancers are strongly epidemiologically linked to endometriosis.[22,23] Next-generation sequencing of RNA and DNA of clear-cell ovarian cancers has shown that inactivating mutations in *ARID1A* were present in 46–57% and 30% of clear-cell and endometrioid sub-types, respectively.[24,25] In two cases, it was possible to demonstrate that the contiguous atypical endometriosis tissue had also lost ARID1A expression and had the same *ARID1A* mutation that was present in the adjacent clear-cell cancer.[24] These studies have established *ARID1A* as a tumour suppressor gene in clear-cell and endometrioid ovarian cancer, and provide molecular evidence for endometriosis tissue being the cell of origin for these sub-types.

These data show that the various sub-types of EOC differ in cell of origin, epidemiology, natural history and biology. Logically, they are different diseases, and the term 'sub-type' is misleading as it implies a common tissue of origin. Although these differences provide compelling reasons to treat women in a disease-specific manner, targeted therapies for endometrioid and clear-cell ovarian cancer do not currently exist.

The remainder of this chapter discusses potential biomarkers for stratified treatment of HGSOC and their relationship with platinum sensitivity and resistance. The accurate diagnosis of sub-type before chemotherapy treatment is vital as it provides strong prognostic and biological information. This is particularly important when neoadjuvant treatment is considered before definitive surgery, as chemotherapy may alter histological appearances and it may be challenging to exclude a non-EOC diagnosis or to identify the type of EOC reliably, when only a small sample is available from an image-guided core biopsy.[26] Refinement of immunohistochemical markers for ovarian cancer sub-type was carried out using nominal logistic regression to assign the probability of correct classification.[27] Based on expression patterns from 744 EOC cases, nine markers (CDKN2A, DKK1, HNF1B, MDM2, PGR, TFF3, TP53, VIM and WT1) were the most predictive of ovarian cancer sub-type in both the training set and an independent test cohort of 81 cases ($\kappa = 0.85$ and 0.78, respectively).[27] These markers should now replace the use of the inferior CK7 and CK20 markers for EOC diagnosis, as these have low specificity and cannot assign sub-type.

Molecular classification of HGSOC

HGSOC is the most common EOC sub-type, comprising about 70% of all invasive cases, and represents the majority of the treatment burden and mortality.[28] In contrast to other common epithelial cancers, HGSOC rarely metastasises to organs outside the abdomen and is characterised by local spread onto peritoneal surfaces and subsequent local invasion. The 'seeding' hypothesis proposes that metastatic cells are carried to other sites in the abdomen as tumour spheroids in ascites fluid.[29] HGSOC usually presents with high stage, has frequent *TP53* mutation and may, even in sporadic cases, have loss of BRCA1 and BRCA2 function.[30] This results in a neoplasm with a high proliferation rate and chromosomal instability. Common oncogene mutations have not been identified (for example, *ERBB2*, *EGFR* or *BRAF*) and this has limited targeted therapeutic approaches.[31] Despite multiple phase III studies of many combinations of cytotoxic chemotherapy, the standard of care remains treatment with carboplatin and paclitaxel but no biomarkers for individualisation of these treatments are in use in clinical practice.[1–3] The major barrier for improving treatment strategies for HGSOC remains the lack of understanding of the molecular basis for clinical drug resistance, compounded by the molecular heterogeneity of the disease.

Many expression microarray studies have attempted to define prognostic and predictive signatures for chemoresistance in EOC.[32–42] The major limitation of these studies has been small sample size, poor internal and external validation, and variability in clinicopathological factors in the study sets. These factors may partly explain the lack of success in identifying widely applicable expression biomarkers.[43–45] It has also been suggested that prognostic stratification may have limited utility when only a few therapeutic alternatives exist for women with advanced stage HGSOC.[44] This lack of success is in marked contrast to similar efforts in breast cancer, where profiling of a relatively small numbers of cases quickly identified a new molecular classification that was consistent with existing knowledge about the biology of the disease and had prognostic value.[46,47]

Expression profiling of a large series of 285 serous and endometrioid cases has defined four main molecular sub-types, described as C1 (high stromal response), C2 (high immune signature), C4 (low stromal response) and C5 (mesenchymal, low immune signature).[42] Cases classified as high stromal response sub-type C1 had early relapse and worse survival, with strong enrichment of extracellular matrix (ECM) components such as SPARC and MMP2. Other microarray studies have also shown that ECM-enriched signatures indicate poor prognosis in EOC.[32,38–40] Tissues from the C1 sub-type also showed extensive desmoplasia that was consistent with earlier reports showing that an enhanced stromal response may reduce the effectiveness of chemotherapy and overall survival.[48–51] These classifications are now being tested as part of the Cancer Genome Atlas (TCGA) project, which is carrying out a comprehensive genomic analysis of approximately 400 HGSOC cases.[52] The TCGA ovarian project is expected to publish initial findings from this work in 2011. If the results from this study are confirmatory, further refinement of the signatures will need to be carried out (together with additional validation) to produce discrete antibody or RNA assays that are suitable for routine use in pathology laboratories.

DNA copy number analysis has also been investigated as a predictive marker. The largest series to date studied 118 HGSOC cases and showed that amplification of chromosome 20q11 is a strongly adverse prognostic factor that is correlated with platinum resistance, consistent with genomic data from previous publications.[53–55] This region includes *CCNE1*, encoding the cell cycle checkpoint protein cyclin E, and the anti-apoptotic oncogene *C19orf2* (also known as *URI*). Knockdown of *CCNE1* in EOC cell lines with 20q11 amplification did not reverse cisplatin resistance in short-term assays (resistance actually increased), although it did result in reduced clonogenic survival, suggesting an oncogenic effect.[56] Amplification or overexpression of *C19orf2* resulted in cisplatin resistance both *in vitro* and *in vivo*, mediated by increased S6K1-BAD survival signalling.[57] Given the strong prognostic effect of 20q11 amplification, it is important that future clinical trials consider stratifying for this marker using assays to test for amplification of the region. However, determining which is the most important driver oncogene (and therefore therapeutic target) will require highly specific pharmacological inhibitors and biomarker-driven clinical trials.

TP53 is a driver mutation in HGSOC

The gene *TP53* that encodes the p53 tumour suppressor protein is among the most commonly mutated genes in human cancer.[58,59] *TP53* mutations are common in EOC and over the past two decades over 70 publications have tested associations between *TP53* mutation in tumour tissue and clinical outcome.[60–62] However, many reports are contradictory, suggesting both good and poor prognostic effects of *TP53* mutation.[63,64] The predictive value of *TP53* mutations has also been unclear, with reports suggesting better response to platinum-based treatment or increased treatment failure.[65,66]

A meta-analysis of 64 publications examining *TP53* mutation and clinical outcome showed that only six studies fulfilled minimum expected quality criteria for mutation detection or assignment of clinical response.[67] A common limitation of p53 biomarker studies is the use of immunostaining as a surrogate marker for *TP53* mutation, even though this results in a high rate of misclassification.[62,68] Strong positive immunostaining may suggest mutations that cause accumulation of p53 by preventing interaction with its negative regulator MDM2. However, high levels of wild-type protein can also occur following stress or DNA damage (as is seen in the normal fallopian tube). A negative staining pattern cannot exclude frame-shift mutations and intragenic deletions that produce truncated p53 protein, and these types of mutation are unreliably identified by immunohistochemistry.[63,69] It is likely that previous studies using p53 immunostaining under-report the true frequency of *TP53* mutations and have significantly biased outcomes.[67]

Sequencing of *TP53* in tumour DNA is the most reliable method to detect mutation and should be used for any prognostic or predictive study. Despite this, there has been considerable variation in the reported mutation rate, with 12 publications reporting frequencies in the range 15–80%.[67] These discrepancies may be explained by the fact that only limited sequencing of the *TP53* coding region was performed and the analyses included variable numbers of EOC sub-types in the analysis. The frequency of *TP53* mutation is markedly different between EOC sub-types and, as discussed earlier, it is critical that biomarkers are stratified by sub-type.[62,70–72] The first comprehensive mapping of *TP53* mutation in HGSOC was performed by sequencing exons 2–11 in tumour DNA from 145 women with serous neoplasms.[73] Pathogenic mutations were identified in 119 of 123 HGSOC cases (96.7%) and mutation-negative cases had evidence of altered p53 pathway function from MDM2/MDM4 dysfunction. Taken together, this study showed for the first time that *TP53* mutation in HGSOC approaches 100%, establishing *TP53* as an essential driver mutation for the disease. The very high prevalence of mutation is consistent with the findings of p53 accumulation and mutation in fallopian tube p53 signature foci and TICs.[20] Early loss of p53 function may be required in HGSOC to create a permissive environment for subsequent loss of BRCA1 or BRCA2 function, which would otherwise result in apoptosis from checkpoint activation.[74] However, the fact that signature foci in the fallopian tube have *TP53* mutation but do not develop into TICs suggests that loss of p53 is required but not sufficient for the development of HGSOC.

Given its extremely high prevalence, the presence of *TP53* mutation per se cannot be prognostic or predictive of outcome in HGSOC. The most common type of mutation found are missense mutations, occurring in about 50% of cases, with null mutations (including nonsense, frame-shift and splice site mutations) accounting for about 30%.[73] The presence of a null mutation may be a poor prognostic factor, as compared with missense mutations, which have a reduced risk of recurrence (HR 0.71; 95% CI 0.51–0.99).[75] Although this result was suggested by an earlier study, larger cohorts are needed to show definite adverse prognostic effect.[75,76] The type of mutation is not predictive for platinum chemotherapy.[73] However, this does not exclude the possibility that mutation-specific therapy will become available for HGSOC.[77,78]

Platinum sensitivity in HGSOC

HGSOC is initially extremely sensitive to platinum-based chemotherapy, with response rates of up to 70–80% after initial chemotherapy and surgery. In comparison with common epithelial cancers, HGSOC is relatively hypersensitive to carboplatin but, despite this, 5 year survival for stage III HGSOC is less than 30%. The importance of platinum chemotherapy in EOC is further emphasised by the fact that relapsed disease is classified by its likely response to further treatment with platinum-based chemotherapy (Figure 4.1).[79]

The hypersensitivity to platinum chemotherapy in HGSOC is likely to be because of high rates of intrinsic homologous recombination deficiency (HRD). Carboplatin is a DNA damaging agent that induces inter- and intra-strand cross-linking that results in both single- and double-strand DNA breaks. In normal cells, both types of damage can be repaired by either error-free homologous recombination (HR) or by the error-prone non-homologous end joining (NHEJ) pathway. Cancer cells that lack BRCA1 or BRCA2 function cannot carry out HR repair and are therefore very sensitive to platinum-induced DNA damage which induces apoptotic death (discussed in detail in

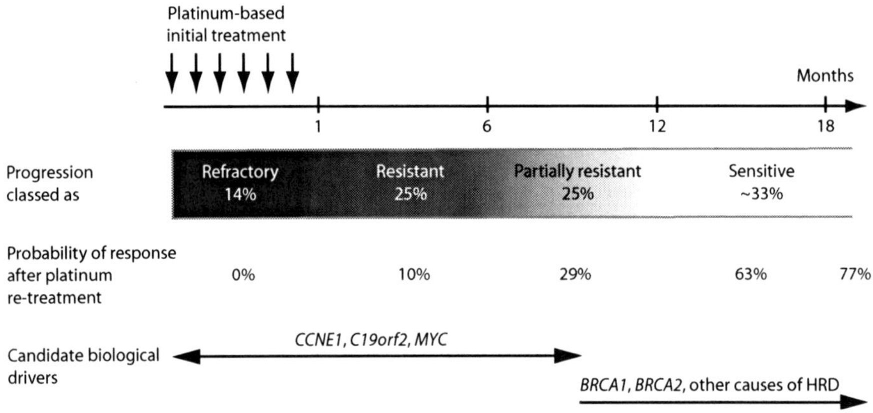

Figure 4.1 The biology of platinum resistance in high-grade serous ovarian cancer. The shaded horizontal bar indicates the clinical definitions for platinum-relapsed disease and the proportion of women in each category. Women who have progressive disease during initial treatment (including 1 month after completion of chemotherapy) are classed as refractory. Those relapsing within 6 months of completing initial treatment are classed as platinum resistant and those relapsing more than 12 months later are defined as platinum sensitive. The probability of response to re-treatment with platinum-based chemotherapy is shown below, together with candidate molecular drivers for the refractory/resistant and sensitive categories. HRD = homologous recombination deficiency.

Chapter 6). This is correlated with significantly longer survival in EOC patients with *BRCA1* or *BRCA2* germline mutations as compared with non-mutated cases.[80–82] HRD has been exploited for synthetic lethal therapy with polyadenosine diphosphate-ribose polymerase (PARP) inhibitors in early-phase clinical trials in women with known *BRCA1* and *BRCA2* mutations (discussed in detail in Chapter 7).[83,84]

Recent data suggest that the proportion of HGSOC patients with HRD may be higher than previously believed. Firstly, *BRCA1* and *BRCA2* mutation carriers predominantly develop HGSOC and not other ovarian cancer sub-types, suggesting that there is some sub-type specificity. Secondly, mutation studies of *BRCA1* and *BRCA2* in unselected HGSOC patients have shown combined mutation rates of 3–17%, and additional pathogenic somatic mutations can be shown in cancer tissue.[82,85] Thirdly, functional HR assays on ascites cells taken from women with HGSOC at primary surgery show that HRD occurs in approximately 50% of cases.[86] Unpublished analyses from TCGA, based on mutation and expression data, also predict HRD in up to 50% of women with HGSOC. These additional cases may arise from other mechanisms that can directly alter BRCA1 and BRCA2 function, including silencing by promoter methylation of *BRCA1* and loss of *BRCA2* expression by methylation-independent means.[87–89] Altered BRCA2 function can also occur from methylation silencing of its upstream regulator *FANCF* or by amplification and overexpression of *C11orf30* (also known as *EMSY*).[90,91] Further clinical studies are needed to determine whether these alternative mechanisms of HRD can confer the same degree of platinum sensitivity and survival advantages as seen in *BRCA1* or *BRCA2* mutation carriers. However, it is clear that much wider access to *BRCA1* and *BRCA2* testing is needed. Genetic counselling and testing should be considered for all women with HGSOC, even if they do not have a family history of breast or ovarian cancer. Specific features that can be used to target testing include young age at diagnosis (less than 50 years), HGSOC histology and ethnicity suggesting increased risk of founder mutations.[82] Given the greatly improved prognosis for carriers, these women need to be identified prospectively and separate stratification for *BRCA1* and *BRCA2* status may be required in clinical trials.[92] Testing for *BRCA1* status may have additional predictive benefit, as there are strong pre-clinical data showing that loss of BRCA1 function results in reduced response to microtubule-targeted therapy such as paclitaxel.[93,94]

These findings have important implications for clinical models of relapsed platinum-sensitive and platinum-resistant disease (Figure 4.1). In stage III/IV HGSOC cases in the SCOTROC1 trial, in which all women underwent primary surgery and adjuvant carboplatin/taxane chemotherapy, 14% were platinum refractory, 25% were platinum resistant and 25% had progressive disease 6–12 months after treatment (Figure 4.1).[95] The proportion of women with platinum-sensitive relapse was approximately 33%. Response rates to re-treatment with carboplatin in this group are typically 50–60%, consistent with significant enrichment for cases with intrinsic HRD. Similar time-to-progression data are not available for *BRCA1* and *BRCA2* mutation carriers but, in a large retrospective study, 1 year survival for carriers with stage III/IV disease was approximately 97% and overall survival was significantly longer than for non-carriers.[80] In addition, a case–control study of 22 *BRCA1* or *BRCA2* mutation carriers showed that carriers had higher partial and complete response rates and two- to three-fold longer median survival than matched controls.[81] Carriers also had significantly longer treatment-free interval. This suggests that HRD may be an important predictive factor for platinum response and that women with platinum-refractory or platinum-resistant disease may constitute a different non-HRD sub-type of HGSOC with differing molecular classification (Figure 4.1).

Although platinum sensitivity has been intensively studied using *in vitro* models, the clinical evidence for involvement of apoptosis pathways, drug excretion and tolerance to DNA adducts is very limited.[96] Recent publications have shown that platinum resistance in women with germline mutation in *BRCA1* or *BRCA2* can develop by secondary mutations that restore hypomorphic BRCA1 or BRCA2 protein function.[97,98] In addition, mouse cells engineered to have a large *BRCA1* deletion (and therefore not vulnerable to revertant events) do not develop platinum resistance despite repeated exposure.[99] This indicates the genetic dominance of *BRCA1* in determining sensitivity and suggests that other acquired mechanisms of resistance cannot overcome it (note that these cells are able to develop resistance to other drugs). This has important clinical implications for women with HGSOC and *BRCA1* or *BRCA2* mutations, as the most likely cause of resistance may be a secondary mutation. However, the number of cases studied to date are very few as the identification of secondary mutations requires re-biopsy of tumour material. It is also unknown whether other mechanisms that induce HRD are subject to reversion in a similar manner.

The challenge now is to define clinically what other pathways are responsible for intrinsic HRD in the platinum-sensitive HGSOC population, and how platinum sensitivity is lost in relapsed disease. It is important to distinguish this conceptually from previous models that aimed to understand how platinum resistance was acquired across all sub-types of EOC, potentially including very diverse mechanisms. These efforts will require sequential collection of tissue from women with HGSOC, both at diagnosis and at relapse. Ultrasound- or computed tomography (CT)-guided biopsy is safe and feasible, and is the standard of care for initial diagnosis of women with suspected ovarian cancer.[100] However, re-biopsy of recurrent disease is not routinely performed before treatment and has significant cost. Although studies on malignant cells from abdominal ascites can offer a less morbid approach to assaying cancer cells, only a small proportion of women with relapsed disease will have ascites that can be aspirated. Efforts to build these longitudinal cohorts have started within large international collaboratives as part of TCGA and the International Cancer Genome Consortium (ICGC).

Genetic heterogeneity and evolution of resistance

Carcinogenesis is an evolutionary process that selects advantageous mutations from genetic variation that is generated by underlying genomic instability during tumour development.[101] The existence of intratumoral genetic heterogeneity was first demonstrated in a mouse mammary tumour model when multiple cell lines were isolated from a single tumour and showed divergent karyotypes and differing cellular characteristics.[102] However, it was not possible to test the hypothesis that pre-existing resistant clones could be selected by therapy in solid tumours until technologies such as array comparative genomic hybridisation (aCGH) and next-generation sequencing allowed changes to be identified at high resolution. There is now renewed interest in the existence and role of rare genetic subpopulations within cancers, particular as an explanation for the development of resistance to systemic therapies.[103–106]

There is strong evidence that selective effects can explain drug resistance in haematological cancers.[107,108] Point mutations conferring resistance to imatinib have been shown to be present at low frequency before treatment in both acute lymphocytic leukaemia and chronic myeloid leukaemia. At relapse, these mutations are present in high frequency in the leukaemic blasts.[109–111] In acute lymphocytic leukaemia, a higher frequency of resistant mutations in the initial presenting disease is directly correlated with shorter remission.[111] Similar changes have been shown in breast cancer using next-generation sequencing of primary and relapsed disease in a single case of lobular breast cancer. Relapse-specific mutations could be detected at a frequency of 1–13% in the primary tumour 7 years before disease recurrence.[112]

Intratumoral genetic heterogeneity in HGSOC has been demonstrated both within a region of tumour and between different metastatic sites.[113–115] These genetic differences could be expected to alter chemosensitivity. Consistent with this, variable *in vitro* responses to a variety of chemotherapeutic agents were observed in primary EOC cells obtained from different metastatic sites from the same individual, suggesting the existence of genetically or epigenetically diverse subpopulations.[116] Similar differential effects have also been shown in women during chemoradiation of advanced cervical cancer.[105] In three out of ten cases there were distinct genetic subpopulations before treatment and these regions showed differential responses to chemo-radiotherapy, leading to mixed response and selection of resistant disease. Studies of cell lines derived before and after relapse in three cases of HGSOC have found that presentation and resistant disease are not linearly genetically related, showing that the relapsed genotype cannot have arisen by direct descent from a dominant clone at disease presentation.[104] These studies suggest a hypothesis for platinum-resistant disease in HGSOC where strong selection for a minor resistant clonal population occurs, rather than genetic progression from presentation disease. These models may also be relevant in platinum-sensitive disease as it will be important to determine whether revertant mutations in *BRCA1* and *BRCA2* exist before treatment, as is seen for *ABL* mutations in chronic myeloid leukaemia.

Summary

The emerging molecular data indicate that EOC is a group of distinct diseases, each with different clinical and epidemiological characteristics. Previous work to identify predictive and prognostic biomarkers has been greatly weakened by the inclusion of different ovarian sub-types. Platinum resistance in HGSOC may represent a distinct molecular sub-type, but further work is required to define the driver mutations in this disease and the mechanisms of intrinsic resistance. As discussed in Chapter 7, the use of PARP inhibitors in platinum-sensitive HGSOC heralds the real possibility of curative strategies based on maintenance treatment. However, understanding how platinum sensitivity may be lost in HGSOC will require genomic comparison of sequential tissues taken at diagnosis and at time of relapse. Stratified medicine for EOC, particularly for platinum-sensitive disease, is now feasible but will require much wider access to *BRCA1* and *BRCA2* testing for women with HGSOC and genomic tests of HRD in tumour tissue.

References

1. Bookman MA, Brady MF, McGuire WP, Harper PG, Alberts DS, Friedlander M, *et al.* Evaluation of new platinum-based treatment regimens in advanced-stage ovarian cancer: a Phase III Trial of the Gynecologic Cancer Intergroup. *J Clin Oncol* 2009;27:1419–25.
2. du Bois A, Weber B, Rochon J, Meier W, Goupil A, Olbricht S, *et al.* Addition of epirubicin as a third drug to carboplatin-paclitaxel in first-line treatment of advanced ovarian cancer: a prospectively randomized gynecologic cancer intergroup trial by the Arbeitsgemeinschaft Gynaekologische Onkologie Ovarian Cancer Study Group and the Groupe d'Investigateurs Nationaux pour l'Etude des Cancers Ovariens. *J Clin Oncol* 2006;24:1127–35.
3. du Bois A, Herrstedt J, Hardy-Bessard AC, Müller HH, Harter P, Kristensen G, *et al.* Phase III trial of carboplatin plus paclitaxel with or without gemcitabine in first-line treatment of epithelial ovarian cancer. *J Clin Oncol* 2010;28:4162–9.

4. Simon R. Development and validation of therapeutically relevant multi-gene biomarker classifiers. *J Natl Cancer Inst* 2005;97:866–7.
5. Köbel M, Kalloger SE, Baker PM, Ewanowich CA, Arseneau J, Zherebitskiy V, *et al.* Diagnosis of ovarian carcinoma cell type is highly reproducible: a transcanadian study. *Am J Surg Pathol* 2010;34:984–93.
6. Köbel M, Kalloger SE, Boyd N, McKinney S, Mehl E, Palmer C, *et al.* Ovarian carcinoma subtypes are different diseases: implications for biomarker studies. *PLoS Med* 2008;5:e232.
7. Gilks CB, Ionescu DN, Kalloger SE, Köbel M, Irving J, Clarke B, *et al.* Tumor cell type can be reproducibly diagnosed and is of independent prognostic significance in patients with maximally debulked ovarian carcinoma. *Hum Pathol* 2008;39:1239–51.
8. Singh N, Ayhan A, Menon U, Chin Aleong JA, Faruqi AZ, Gayther SA, *et al.* Grading of serous ovarian carcinoma: further evidence of a lack of agreement between conventional grading systems. *Histopathology* 2008;52:393–5.
9. Kommoss S, Schmidt D, Kommoss F, Hedderich J, Harter P, Pfisterer J, *et al.* Histological grading in a large series of advanced stage ovarian carcinomas by three widely used grading systems: consistent lack of prognostic significance. A translational research subprotocol of a prospective randomized phase III study (AGO-OVAR 3 protocol). *Virchows Arch* 2009;454:249–56.
10. Köbel M, Kalloger SE, Santos JL, Huntsman DG, Gilks CB, Swenerton KD. Tumor type and substage predict survival in stage I and II ovarian carcinoma: insights and implications. *Gynecol Oncol* 2010;116:50–6.
11. Bell J, Brady MF, Young RC, Lage J, Walker JL, Look KY, *et al.* Randomized phase III trial of three versus six cycles of adjuvant carboplatin and paclitaxel in early stage epithelial ovarian carcinoma: a Gynecologic Oncology Group study. *Gynecol Oncol* 2006;102:432–9.
12. Mackay HJ, Brady MF, Oza AM, Reuss A, Pujade-Lauraine E, Swart AM, *et al.* Prognostic relevance of uncommon ovarian histology in women with stage III/IV epithelial ovarian cancer. *Int J Gynecol Cancer* 2010;20:945–52.
13. Dubeau L. The cell of origin of ovarian epithelial tumors and the ovarian surface epithelium dogma: does the emperor have no clothes? *Gynecol Oncol* 1999;72:437–42.
14. Piek JM, van Diest PJ, Zweemer RP, Kenemans P, Verheijen RH. Tubal ligation and risk of ovarian cancer. *Lancet* 2001;358:844.
15. Piek JM, van Diest PJ, Zweemer RP, Jansen JW, Poort-Keesom RJ, Menko FH, *et al.* Dysplastic changes in prophylactically removed Fallopian tubes of women predisposed to developing ovarian cancer. *J Pathol* 2001;195:451–6.
16. Leeper K, Garcia R, Swisher E, Goff B, Greer B, Paley P. Pathologic findings in prophylactic oophorectomy specimens in high-risk women. *Gynecol Oncol* 2002;87:52–6.
17. Piek JM, Verheijen RH, Kenemans P, Massuger LF, Bulten H, van Diest PJ. *BRCA1/2*-related ovarian cancers are of tubal origin: a hypothesis. *Gynecol Oncol* 2003;90:491.
18. Lee Y, Miron A, Drapkin R, Nucci MR, Medeiros F, Saleemuddin A, *et al.* A candidate precursor to serous carcinoma that originates in the distal fallopian tube. *J Pathol* 2007;211:26–35.
19. Crum CP, Drapkin R, Kindelberger D, Medeiros F, Miron A, Lee Y. Lessons from *BRCA*: the tubal fimbria emerges as an origin for pelvic serous cancer. *Clin Med Res* 2007;5:35–44.
20. Callahan MJ, Crum CP, Medeiros F, Kindelberger DW, Elvin JA, Garber JE, *et al.* Primary fallopian tube malignancies in *BRCA*-positive women undergoing surgery for ovarian cancer risk reduction. *J Clin Oncol* 2007;25:3985–90.
21. Kindelberger DW, Lee Y, Miron A, Hirsch MS, Feltmate C, Medeiros F, *et al.* Intraepithelial carcinoma of the fimbria and pelvic serous carcinoma: Evidence for a causal relationship. *Am J Surg Pathol* 2007;31:161–9.
22. Viganó P, Somigliana E, Chiodo I, Abbiati A, Vercellini P. Molecular mechanisms and biological plausibility underlying the malignant transformation of endometriosis: a critical analysis. *Hum Reprod Update* 2006;12:77–89.
23. Ness RB. Endometriosis and ovarian cancer: thoughts on shared pathophysiology. *Am J Obstet Gynecol* 2003;189:280–94.
24. Wiegand KC, Shah SP, Al-Agha OM, Zhao Y, Tse K, Zeng T, *et al.* *ARID1A* mutations in endometriosis-associated ovarian carcinomas. *N Engl J Med* 2010;363:1532–43.

25. Jones S, Wang TL, Shih IM, Mao TL, Nakayama K, Roden R, *et al.* Frequent mutations of chromatin remodelling gene *ARID1A* in ovarian clear cell carcinoma. *Science* 2010;330:228–31.
26. McCluggage WG, Lyness RW, Atkinson RJ, Dobbs SP, Harley I, McClelland HR, *et al.* Morphological effects of chemotherapy on ovarian carcinoma. *J Clin Pathol* 2002;55:27–31.
27. Kalloger SE, Köbel M, Leung S, Mehl E, Gao D, Marcon KM, *et al.* Calculator for ovarian carcinoma sub-type prediction. *Mod Pathol* 2011;24:512–21.
28. Salvador S, Rempel A, Soslow RA, Gilks B, Huntsman D, Miller D. Chromosomal instability in fallopian tube precursor lesions of serous carcinoma and frequent monoclonality of synchronous ovarian and fallopian tube mucosal serous carcinoma. *Gynecol Oncol* 2008;110:408–17.
29. Naora H, Montell DJ. Ovarian cancer metastasis: integrating insights from disparate model organisms. *Nat Rev Cancer* 2005;5:355–66.
30. Press JZ, De Luca A, Boyd N, Young S, Troussard A, Ridge Y, *et al.* Ovarian carcinomas with genetic and epigenetic *BRCA1* loss have distinct molecular abnormalities. *BMC Cancer* 2008;8:17.
31. Bast RC Jr, Hennessy B, Mills GB. The biology of ovarian cancer: new opportunities for translation. *Nat Rev Cancer* 2009;9:415–28.
32. Spentzos D, Levine DA, Ramoni MF, Joseph M, Gu X, Boyd J, *et al.* Gene expression signature with independent prognostic significance in epithelial ovarian cancer. *J Clin Oncol* 2004;22:4700–10.
33. Selvanayagam ZE, Cheung TH, Wei N, Vittal R, Lo KW, Yeo W, *et al.* Prediction of chemotherapeutic response in ovarian cancer with DNA microarray expression profiling. *Cancer Genet Cytogenet* 2004;154:63–6.
34. Spentzos D, Levine DA, Kolia S, Otu H, Boyd J, Libermann TA, *et al.* Unique gene expression profile based on pathologic response in epithelial ovarian cancer. *J Clin Oncol* 2005;23:7911–18.
35. Berchuck A, Iversen ES, Lancaster JM, Pittman J, Luo J, Lee P, *et al.* Patterns of gene expression that characterize long-term survival in advanced stage serous ovarian cancers. *Clin Cancer Res* 2005;11:3686–96.
36. Hartmann LC, Lu KH, Linette GP, Cliby WA, Kalli KR, Gershenson D, *et al.* Gene expression profiles predict early relapse in ovarian cancer after platinum-paclitaxel chemotherapy. *Clin Cancer Res* 2005;11:2149–55.
37. Bernardini M, Lee CH, Beheshti B, Prasad M, Albert M, Marrano P, *et al.* High-resolution mapping of genomic imbalance and identification of gene expression profiles associated with differential chemotherapy response in serous epithelial ovarian cancer. *Neoplasia* 2005;7:603–13.
38. Jazaeri AA, Awtrey CS, Chandramouli GV, Chuang YE, Khan J, Sotiriou C, *et al.* Gene expression profiles associated with response to chemotherapy in epithelial ovarian cancers. *Clin Cancer Res* 2005;11:6300–10.
39. Helleman J, Jansen MP, Span PN, van Staveren IL, Massuger LF, Meijer-van Gelder ME, *et al.* Molecular profiling of platinum resistant ovarian cancer. *Int J Cancer* 2006;118:1963–71.
40. Dressman HK, Berchuck A, Chan G, Zhai J, Bild A, Sayer R, *et al.* An integrated genomic-based approach to individualized treatment of patients with advanced-stage ovarian cancer. *J Clin Oncol* 2007;25:517–25.
41. Crijns AP, Fehrmann RS, de Jong S, Gerbens F, Meersma GJ, Klip HG, *et al.* Survival-related profile, pathways, and transcription factors in ovarian cancer. *PLoS Med* 2009;6:e24.
42. Tothill RW, Tinker AV, George J, Brown R, Fox SB, Lade S, *et al.* Novel molecular subtypes of serous and endometrioid ovarian cancer linked to clinical outcome. *Clin Cancer Res* 2008;14:5198–208.
43. Fehrmann RS, Li XY, van der Zee AG, de Jong S, Te Meerman GJ, de Vries EG, *et al.* Profiling studies in ovarian cancer: a review. *Oncologist* 2007;12:960–6.
44. Agarwal R, Kaye SB. Expression profiling and individualisation of treatment for ovarian cancer. *Curr Opin Pharmacol* 2006;6:345–9.
45. Na YJ, Farley J, Zeh A, del Carmen M, Penson R, Birrer MJ. Ovarian cancer: markers of response. *Int J Gynecol Cancer* 2009;19 Suppl 2:S21–9.
46. Sorlie T, Perou CM, Tibshirani R, Aas T, Geisler S, Johnsen H, *et al.* Gene expression patterns of breast carcinomas distinguish tumor subclasses with clinical implications. *Proc Natl Acad Sci U S A* 2001;98:10869–74.
47. Sotiriou C, Neo SY, McShane LM, Korn EL, Long PM, Jazaeri A, *et al.* Breast cancer classification and prognosis based on gene expression profiles from a population-based study. *Proc Natl Acad Sci U S A* 2003;100:10393–8.

48. Sethi T, Rintoul RC, Moore SM, MacKinnon AC, Salter D, Choo C, *et al.* Extracellular matrix proteins protect small cell lung cancer cells against apoptosis: a mechanism for small cell lung cancer growth and drug resistance *in vivo*. *Nat Med* 1999;5:662–8.
49. Finak G, Bertos N, Pepin F, Sadekova S, Souleimanova M, Zhao H, *et al.* Stromal gene expression predicts clinical outcome in breast cancer. *Nat Med* 2008;14:518–27.
50. Bergamaschi A, Tagliabue E, Sørlie T, Naume B, Triulzi T, Orlandi R, *et al.* Extracellular matrix signature identifies breast cancer subgroups with different clinical outcome. *J Pathol* 2008;214:357–67.
51. Olive KP, Jacobetz MA, Davidson CJ, Gopinathan A, McIntyre D, Honess D, *et al.* Inhibition of Hedgehog signaling enhances delivery of chemotherapy in a mouse model of pancreatic cancer. *Science* 2009;324:1457–61.
52. Kaiser J. National Institutes of Health. NCI gears up for cancer genome project. *Science* 2005;307:1182.
53. Nakayama K, Nakayama N, Jinawath N, Salani R, Kurman RJ, Shih IM, *et al.* Amplicon profiles in ovarian serous carcinomas. *Int J Cancer* 2007;120:2613–17.
54. Farley J, Smith LM, Darcy KM, Sobel E, O'Connor D, Henderson B, *et al.* Cyclin E expression is a significant predictor of survival in advanced, suboptimally debulked ovarian epithelial cancers: a Gynecologic Oncology Group study. *Cancer Res* 2003;63:1235–41.
55. Etemadmoghadam D, deFazio A, Beroukhim R, Mermel C, George J, Getz G, *et al.* Integrated genome-wide DNA copy number and expression analysis identifies distinct mechanisms of primary chemoresistance in ovarian carcinomas. *Clin Cancer Res* 2009;15:1417–27.
56. Etemadmoghadam D, George J, Cowin PA, Cullinane C, Kansara M, Australian Ovarian Cancer Study Group, *et al.* Amplicon-dependent *CCNE1* expression is critical for clonogenic survival after cisplatin treatment and is correlated with 20q11 gain in ovarian cancer. *PLoS One* 2010;5:e15498.
57. Theurillat JP, Metzler SC, Henzi N, Djouder N, Helbling M, Zimmermann AK, *et al.* *URI* is an oncogene amplified in ovarian cancer cells and is required for their survival. *Cancer Cell* 2011;19:317–32.
58. Nigro JM, Baker SJ, Preisinger AC, Jessup JM, Hostetter R, Cleary K, *et al.* Mutations in the p53 gene occur in diverse human tumour types. *Nature* 1989;342:705–8.
59. Vogelstein B, Kinzler KW. Cancer genes and the pathways they control. *Nat Med* 2004;10:789–99.
60. Marks JR, Davidoff AM, Kerns BJ, Humphrey PA, Pence JC, Dodge RK, *et al.* Overexpression and mutation of p53 in epithelial ovarian cancer. *Cancer Res* 1991;51:2979–84.
61. Okamoto A, Sameshima Y, Yokoyama S, Terashima Y, Sugimura T, Terada M, *et al.* Frequent allelic losses and mutations of the p53 gene in human ovarian cancer. *Cancer Res* 1991;51:5171–6.
62. de Graeff P, Crijns AP, de Jong S, Boezen M, Post WJ, de Vries EG, *et al.* Modest effect of p53, EGFR and HER-2/neu on prognosis in epithelial ovarian cancer: a meta-analysis. *Br J Cancer* 2009;101:149–59.
63. Reles A, Wen WH, Schmider A, Gee C, Runnebaum IB, Kilian U, *et al.* Correlation of p53 mutations with resistance to platinum-based chemotherapy and shortened survival in ovarian cancer. *Clin Cancer Res* 2001;7:2984–97.
64. Galic V, Willner J, Wollan M, Garg R, Garcia R, Goff BA, *et al.* Common polymorphisms in *TP53* and *MDM2* and the relationship to *TP53* mutations and clinical outcomes in women with ovarian and peritoneal carcinomas. *Genes Chromosomes Cancer* 2007;46:239–47.
65. Havrilesky L, Darcy KM, Hamdan H, Priore RL, Leon J, Bell J, *et al.* Prognostic significance of p53 mutation and p53 overexpression in advanced epithelial ovarian cancer: a Gynecologic Oncology Group study. *J Clin Oncol* 2003;21:3814–25.
66. Bartel F, Jung J, Böhnke A, Gradhand E, Zeng K, Thomssen C, *et al.* Both germ line and somatic genetics of the p53 pathway affect ovarian cancer incidence and survival. *Clin Cancer Res* 2008;14:89–96.
67. Hall J, Paul J, Brown R. Critical evaluation of p53 as a prognostic marker in ovarian cancer. *Expert Rev Mol Med* 2004;6:1–20.
68. Soussi T, Ishioka C, Claustres M, Béroud C. Locus-specific mutation databases: pitfalls and good practice based on the p53 experience. *Nat Rev Cancer* 2006;6:83–90.
69. Soussi T, Béroud C. Assessing *TP53* status in human tumours to evaluate clinical outcome. *Nat Rev Cancer* 2001;1:233–40.
70. Stewart RL, Royds JA, Burton JL, Heatley MK, Wells M. Direct sequencing of the p53 gene shows absence of mutations in endometrioid endometrial adenocarcinomas expressing p53 protein. *Histopathology* 1998;33:440–5.

71. Singer G, Stöhr R, Cope L, Dehari R, Hartmann A, Cao DF, *et al.* Patterns of p53 mutations separate ovarian serous borderline tumors and low- and high-grade carcinomas and provide support for a new model of ovarian carcinogenesis: a mutational analysis with immunohistochemical correlation. *Am J Surg Pathol* 2005;29:218–24.
72. Kuo KT, Mao TL, Jones S, Veras E, Ayhan A, Wang TL, *et al.* Frequent activating mutations of *PIK3CA* in ovarian clear cell carcinoma. *Am J Pathol* 2009;174:1597–601.
73. Ahmed AA, Etemadmoghadam D, Temple J, Lynch AG, Riad M, Sharma R, *et al.* Driver mutations in *TP53* are ubiquitous in high grade serous carcinoma of the ovary. *J Pathol* 2010;221:49–56.
74. Venkitaraman AR. Cancer susceptibility and the functions of *BRCA1* and *BRCA2*. *Cell* 2002;108:171–82.
75. Köbel M, Reuss A, Bois Ad, Kommoss S, Kommoss F, Gao D, *et al.* The biological and clinical value of p53 expression in pelvic high-grade serous carcinomas. *J Pathol* 2010;222:191–8.
76. Shahin MS, Hughes JH, Sood AK, Buller RE. The prognostic significance of p53 tumor suppressor gene alterations in ovarian carcinoma. *Cancer* 2000;89:2006–17.
77. Brown CJ, Lain S, Verma CS, Fersht AR, Lane DP. Awakening guardian angels: drugging the p53 pathway. *Nat Rev Cancer* 2009;9:862–73.
78. Cheok CF, Verma CS, Baselga J, Lane DP. Translating p53 into the clinic. *Nat Rev Clin Oncol* 2011;8:25–37.
79. Markman M, Rothman R, Hakes T, Reichman B, Hoskins W, Rubin S, *et al.* Second-line platinum therapy in patients with ovarian cancer previously treated with cisplatin. *J Clin Oncol* 1991;9:389–93.
80. Chetrit A, Hirsh-Yechezkel G, Ben-David Y, Lubin F, Friedman E, Sadetzki S. Effect of *BRCA1/2* mutations on long-term survival of patients with invasive ovarian cancer: the national Israeli study of ovarian cancer. *J Clin Oncol* 2008;26:20–5.
81. Tan DS, Rothermundt C, Thomas K, Bancroft E, Eeles R, Shanley S, *et al.* "BRCAness" syndrome in ovarian cancer: a case–control study describing the clinical features and outcome of patients with epithelial ovarian cancer associated with *BRCA1* and *BRCA2* mutations. *J Clin Oncol* 2008;26:5530–6.
82. Trainer AH, Meiser B, Watts K, Mitchell G, Tucker K, Friedlander M. Moving toward personalized medicine: treatment-focused genetic testing of women newly diagnosed with ovarian cancer. *Int J Gynecol Cancer* 2010;20:704–16.
83. Fong PC, Yap TA, Boss DS, Carden CP, Mergui-Roelvink M, Gourley C, *et al.* Poly(ADP)-ribose polymerase inhibition: frequent durable responses in *BRCA* carrier ovarian cancer correlating with platinum-free interval. *J Clin Oncol* 2010;28:2512–19.
84. Audeh MW, Carmichael J, Penson RT, Friedlander M, Powell B, Bell-McGuinn KM, *et al.* Oral poly(ADP-ribose) polymerase inhibitor olaparib in patients with *BRCA1* or *BRCA2* mutations and recurrent ovarian cancer: a proof-of-concept trial. *Lancet* 2010;376:245–51.
85. Hennessy BT, Timms KM, Carey MS, Gutin A, Meyer LA, Flake DD 2nd, *et al.* Somatic mutations in *BRCA1* and *BRCA2* could expand the number of patients that benefit from poly (ADP ribose) polymerase inhibitors in ovarian cancer. *J Clin Oncol* 2010;28:3570–6.
86. Mukhopadhyay A, Elattar A, Cerbinskaite A, Wilkinson SJ, Drew Y, Kyle S, *et al.* Development of a functional assay for homologous recombination status in primary cultures of epithelial ovarian tumor and correlation with sensitivity to poly(ADP-ribose) polymerase inhibitors. *Clin Cancer Res* 2010;16:2344–51.
87. Geisler JP, Hatterman-Zogg MA, Rathe JA, Buller RE. Frequency of BRCA1 dysfunction in ovarian cancer. *J Natl Cancer Inst* 2002;94:61–7.
88. Esteller M, Silva JM, Dominguez G, Bonilla F, Matias-Guiu X, Lerma E, *et al.* Promoter hypermethylation and BRCA1 inactivation in sporadic breast and ovarian tumors. *J Natl Cancer Inst* 2000;92:564–9.
89. Hilton JL, Geisler JP, Rathe JA, Hattermann-Zogg MA, DeYoung B, Buller RE. Inactivation of BRCA1 and BRCA2 in ovarian cancer. *J Natl Cancer Inst* 2002;94:1396–406.
90. Hughes-Davies L, Huntsman D, Ruas M, Fuks F, Bye J, Chin SF, *et al.* *EMSY* links the BRCA2 pathway to sporadic breast and ovarian cancer. *Cell* 2003;115:523–35.
91. Taniguchi T, Tischkowitz M, Ameziane N, Hodgson SV, Mathew CG, Joenje H, *et al.* Disruption of the Fanconi anemia-BRCA pathway in cisplatin-sensitive ovarian tumors. *Nat Med* 2003;9:568–74.
92. Kauff ND. Is It time to stratify for *BRCA* mutation status in therapeutic trials in ovarian cancer? *J Clin Oncol* 2008;26:9–10.

93. Quinn JE, Carser JE, James CR, Kennedy RD, Harkin DP. BRCA1 and implications for response to chemotherapy in ovarian cancer. *Gynecol Oncol* 2009;113:134–42.
94. De Ligio JT, Velkova A, Zorio DA, Monteiro AN. Can the status of the breast and ovarian cancer susceptibility gene 1 product (BRCA1) predict response to taxane-based cancer therapy? *Anticancer Agents Med Chem* 2009;9:543–9.
95. Vasey PA, Jayson GC, Gordon A, Gabra H, Coleman R, Atkinson R, *et al.* Phase III randomized trial of docetaxel-carboplatin versus paclitaxel-carboplatin as first-line chemotherapy for ovarian carcinoma. *J Natl Cancer Inst* 2004;96:1682–91.
96. Borst P, Rottenberg S, Jonkers J. How do real tumors become resistant to cisplatin? *Cell Cycle* 2008;7:1353–9.
97. Sakai W, Swisher EM, Karlan BY, Agarwal MK, Higgins J, Friedman C, *et al.* Secondary mutations as a mechanism of cisplatin resistance in *BRCA2*-mutated cancers. *Nature* 2008;451:1116–20.
98. Swisher EM, Sakai W, Karlan BY, Wurz K, Urban N, Taniguchi T. Secondary *BRCA1* mutations in *BRCA1*-mutated ovarian carcinomas with platinum resistance. *Cancer Res* 2008;68:2581–6.
99. Rottenberg S, Jonkers J. Modeling therapy resistance in genetically engineered mouse cancer models. *Drug Resist Updat* 2008;11:51–60.
100. Spencer JA, Weston MJ, Saidi SA, Wilkinson N, Hall GD. Clinical utility of image-guided peritoneal and omental biopsy. *Nat Rev Clin Oncol* 2010;7:623–31.
101. Nowell PC. The clonal evolution of tumor cell populations. *Science* 1976;194:23–8.
102. Dexter DL, Kowalski HM, Blazar BA, Fligiel Z, Vogel R, Heppner GH. Heterogeneity of tumor cells from a single mouse mammary tumor. *Cancer Res* 1978;38:3174–81.
103. Navin N, Krasnitz A, Rodgers L, Cook K, Meth J, Kendall J, *et al.* Inferring tumor progression from genomic heterogeneity. *Genome Res* 2010;20:68–80.
104. Cooke SL, Ng CK, Melnyk N, Garcia MJ, Hardcastle T, Temple J, *et al.* Genomic analysis of genetic heterogeneity and evolution in high-grade serous ovarian carcinoma. *Oncogene* 2010;29:4905–13.
105. Cooke SL, Temple J, Macarthur S, Zahra MA, Tan LT, Crawford RA, *et al.* Intra-tumour genetic heterogeneity and poor chemoradiotherapy response in cervical cancer. *Br J Cancer* 2011;104:361–8.
106. Navin NE, Hicks J. Tracing the tumor lineage. *Mol Oncol* 2010;4:267–83.
107. Shipitsin M, Campbell LL, Argani P, Weremowicz S, Bloushtain-Qimron N, Yao J, *et al.* Molecular definition of breast tumor heterogeneity. *Cancer Cell* 2007;11:259–273.
108. Mullighan CG, Phillips LA, Su X, Ma J, Miller CB, Shurtleff SA, *et al.* Genomic analysis of the clonal origins of relapsed acute lymphoblastic leukemia. *Science* 2008;322:1377–80.
109. Roche-Lestienne C, Soenen-Cornu V, Grardel-Duflos N, Laï JL, Philippe N, Facon T, *et al.* Several types of mutations of the *Abl* gene can be found in chronic myeloid leukemia patients resistant to STI571, and they can pre-exist to the onset of treatment. *Blood* 2002;100:1014–18.
110. Shah NP, Nicoll JM, Nagar B, Gorre ME, Paquette RL, Kuriyan J, *et al.* Multiple *BCR-ABL* kinase domain mutations confer polyclonal resistance to the tyrosine kinase inhibitor imatinib (STI571) in chronic phase and blast crisis chronic myeloid leukemia. *Cancer Cell* 2002;2:117–25.
111. Choi S, Henderson MJ, Kwan E, Beesley AH, Sutton R, Bahar AY, *et al.* Relapse in children with acute lymphoblastic leukemia involving selection of a pre-existing drug-resistant subclone. *Blood* 2007;110:632–9.
112. Shah SP, Morin RD, Khattra J, Prentice L, Pugh T, Burleigh A, *et al.* Mutational evolution in a lobular breast tumour profiled at single nucleotide resolution. *Nature* 2009;461:809–13.
113. Khalique L, Ayhan A, Weale ME, Jacobs IJ, Ramus SJ, Gayther SA. Genetic intra-tumour heterogeneity in epithelial ovarian cancer and its implications for molecular diagnosis of tumours. *J Pathol* 2007;211:286–95.
114. Khalique L, Ayhan A, Whittaker JC, Singh N, Jacobs IJ, Gayther SA, *et al.* The clonal evolution of metastases from primary serous epithelial ovarian cancers. *Int J Cancer* 2009;124:1579–86.
115. Micci F, Haugom L, Ahlquist T, Abeler VM, Trope CG, Lothe RA, *et al.* Tumor spreading to the contralateral ovary in bilateral ovarian carcinoma is a late event in clonal evolution. *J Oncol* 2010;2010:646340.
116. McAlpine JN, Eisenkop SM, Spirtos NM. Tumor heterogeneity in ovarian cancer as demonstrated by *in vitro* chemoresistance assays. *Gynecol Oncol* 2008;110:360–4.

Section 2

The translation of biology to the clinic

Chapter 5

Biology of *BRCA1* and *BRCA2* genes and implications for cancer management

Timothy A Yap, Yvette Drew and Susan Shanley

Introduction

Approximately 5% of breast cancers and up to 10% of epithelial ovarian cancers may be attributed to mutations (errors) in high-risk susceptibility genes.[1,2] These genes include *BRCA1* and *BRCA2*, which are mutated in about 15% of site-specific breast cancer families and in up to 80% of families with multiple cases of both ovarian and breast cancer.[3] The importance of *BRCA1* and *BRCA2* genes stems from the fact that they are 'caretaker' cancer-susceptibility genes, which encode molecules that act as sensors of DNA defects and participate in the repair process.[4] Deficiencies in such caretaker genes permit other genetic defects to accumulate and this ultimately results in genetic instability.

The *BRCA1* and *BRCA2* tumour suppressor genes

The *BRCA1* gene locus was first identified by Hall and colleagues at University of California, Berkeley, in 1990[5] and was subsequently cloned in 1994 (Figure 5.1).[6] At the same time in 1994, the *BRCA2* gene was discovered by Stratton and Wooster at The Institute of Cancer Research, UK.[7] The identification of *BRCA1* and *BRCA2* were significant milestones in the management of families with breast and ovarian cancers, facilitating the subsequent incorporation of these genes into familial risk assessment, genetic counselling and mutational analysis.

The *BRCA1* gene, located on chromosome 17q21, encodes a large, predominantly nuclear 1863 amino acid protein with an estimated molecular weight of 220 kDa.[8] It consists of multiple functional domains, including an N-terminal RING, two nuclear localisation signals and two C-terminal BRCT domains of approximately 110 residues. The *BRCA2* gene, located on chromosome 13q12.3, encodes a larger 3418 amino acid protein with an estimated molecular weight of 384 kDa.[8] An important feature of the BRCA2 protein is the eight copies of the 30–80 amino acid BRC repeats, which are thought to be the main binding sites for RAD51.[9]

Although the BRCA1 and BRCA2 proteins have different functions involving multiple cellular pathways, both share important regulatory roles in coordinating the response to and repair of DNA damage. As a result, loss of BRCA1 or BRCA2

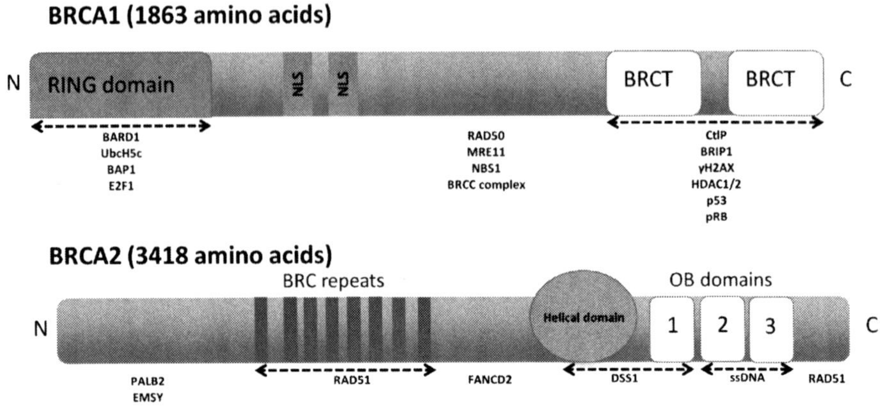

Figure 5.1 Schematic representation of the human BRCA1 and BRCA2 proteins; some of the proteins that interact with BRCA1 or BRCA2 are indicated below the site of interaction; NLS = nuclear localisation signal

function leads to genomic instability and increased risk of oncogenesis, as seen in carriers of germline *BRCA1/2* mutations.[10]

Functions of BRCA1

BRCA1, predominantly a nuclear protein, is able to shuttle between the nucleus and cytoplasm[11] to fulfil its multiple cellular functions, which include DNA damage signalling response, DNA damage repair, transcriptional regulation and cell cycle checkpoint control.[12]

BRCA1 and DNA damage response and repair

The first evidence to suggest a role for BRCA1 in DNA damage response was the observation that it co-localises with the nuclear foci of the recombinase protein RAD51 and the phosphorylated histone H2AX (γH2AX), a marker of DNA double-strand breaks (DSBs).[13] Studies have since shown that BRCA1 acts within a large protein complex known as the BRCA1-associated genome surveillance complex (BASC) as a sensor of DNA damage. This complex includes the MRN proteins RAD50, MRE11 and Nijmegen breakage syndrome 1, the mismatch repair proteins MSH2, MSH6 and MLH1, the Bloom syndrome helicase (BLS) and the ataxia telangiectasia mutated (ATM) kinase.[14] Once a DNA DSB is detected, ATM or ATM and RAD3-related (ATR) kinase can activate BRCA1 by phosphorylation. It is now known that phosphorylated BRCA1 has a major role in DNA DSB repair via the error-free homologous recombination (HR) DNA repair pathway. Moynahan *et al.*[15] were the first to link BRCA1 with HR by observing that Brca1-deficient mouse embryonic stem cells have impaired HR repair of chromosomal DSBs. It has since been proposed that phosphorylated BRCA1 acts together with the phosphorylated MRN protein complex to resect the sequence of DNA damage, exposing single strands of DNA at the 3′ ends on either side of the DSB allowing subsequent repair.[16]

A role for BRCA1 is also emerging in the repair of DBSs via the non-homologous end joining (NHEJ) DNA repair pathway. NHEJ is the dominant DNA DSB repair pathway in mammalian cells as, unlike HR which requires the availability of a homologous DNA sequence for repair, it can occur at any stage in the cell cycle. It consists of two sub-pathways: the conservative NHEJ (C-NHEJ) pathway and the alternative NHEJ (A-NHEJ) pathway.[17] C-NHEJ is a process dependent on the DNA-PK, Ku70/80, XRCC4 (X-ray cross-complementation group 4) and ligase IV proteins. The A-NHEJ pathway acts independently of DNA-PK/Ku70/80 and it rejoins chromosomal DNA ends with imperfect microhomology creating non-random deletions of up to 300 base pairs. This alternative pathway is dependent on MRE11 and could be highly mutagenic.[18] It has been reported that BRCA1 can suppress the A-NHEJ pathway by inhibiting MRE11 activity.[17] This proposal is supported by the observation that the less error-prone C-NHEJ requires BRCA1 and that BRCA1-deficient cells demonstrate an increased tendency to generate large deletions during NHEJ repair.[19]

In addition to DNA DSB repair pathways, BRCA1 has been reported to play a role in the DNA nucleotide excision repair (NER) pathway. NER repairs damage that disrupts both the DNA helical structure and DNA chemistry, for example adducts induced by cisplatin chemotherapy. It is proposed that BRCA1 regulates the global genomic repair sub-pathway of NER via its direct transcriptional control of the NER genes *XPC*, *DDB2* and *GADD45*.[20]

BRCA1 and cell cycle checkpoint control

The ability to control the timing and sequence of cell cycle events following DNA damage is essential for maintaining genome stability. This function is governed by a family of cyclin-dependent kinases acting at cell cycle checkpoints. BRCA1 is rapidly phosphorylated after DNA damage and plays a number of key roles in cell cycle regulation.[12] Firstly, BRCA1 has been shown, via a number of p53 dependent/independent pathways, to stimulate the transcription of the $p21^{WAF1/CIP1}$ promoter of the p21 gene, leading to G_1/S checkpoint cycle arrest,[21] a process that is dependent on the phosphorylation status of BRCA1.

Secondly, BRCA1 is thought to be involved in intra-S phase checkpoint activation. Following DNA damage by ionising radiation, activation of the intra-S phase checkpoint requires the phosphorylation of BRCA1 by ATR.[22] BRCA1 has also been reported to upregulate the expression of the cyclin-dependent kinase inhibitor $p27^{Kip1}$, which results in intra-S phase arrest.[23]

Thirdly, the CHK1 and CHK2 kinases, which act downstream of ATM and ATR, are responsible for maintaining the G_2/M checkpoint. BRCA1 is phosphorylated by CHK2 in response to ionising radiation, while BRCA1-deficient cell lines have been shown to be unable to activate G_2/M arrest following ionising radiation-induced DNA damage.[24] Finally, BRCA1 is also known to be a transcriptional regulator of genes involved in the G_2/M checkpoint. The strongest evidence for this comes from the regulation of GADD45 by BRCA1, which activates the G_2/M checkpoint by inhibiting the activity of cyclin B-cdc2 complex.[25]

BRCA1 and transcriptional regulation

BRCA1 can regulate transcription by its direct interaction with the core component of transcription – RNA polymerase II and its co-activation or co-repression of a number of known transcription factors.[26] One such factor is the estrogen receptor-alpha (ERα) and, given the fact that carriers of *BRCA* mutations have a high lifetime risk of developing cancers in estrogen-responsive tissues such as breast and ovary, the relationship of the *BRCA1* gene to the ERα has been the focus of much research.[27] Studies have revealed that BRCA1 can both induce ERα mRNA expression and negatively regulate ERα signalling.[28] BRCA1 has also been reported to inhibit the induction of over 90% of known estrogen-inducible genes.[29] For example, the transcriptional activation of vascular endothelial growth factor (VEGF), an important protein for tumour growth and angiogenesis, is severely impaired by the presence of exogenous, wild-type *BRCA1*.[30] These data suggest that BRCA1 may function to 'protect' the cell against ERα-driven cell proliferation and that this is lost in *BRCA*-mutated cells.

BRCA1 has also been shown to stimulate the transcriptional activity of the tumour suppressor protein p53 by interacting with its C-terminus, resulting in tumour suppression.[21,31] Interestingly, mutations in *TP53* are commonly found in cancers from *BRCA* mutation carriers and this loss of function may be important in tumorigenesis.[32]

Functions of BRCA2

The main function of BRCA2 is its role in HR-mediated DNA DSB repair through its direct interaction with RAD51.[12] BRCA2 binds directly to RAD51 via its BRC repeat zone, transporting it into the nucleus and the site of DSBs. This BRCA2-RAD51 complex binds to the exposed single-stranded DNA, enabling the loading of RAD51 onto the break and the formation of the pre-synaptic filament.[33] It has been suggested that BRCA2 also has a role in regulating the DNA-binding activity of RAD51, holding it in an inactive state when it is not required for repair.[34] Loss of BRCA2 results in the repair of DSBs through the preferential use of error-prone mechanisms, potentially resulting in chromosomal instability.[35] BRCA2-deficient cells have also been shown to have impaired formation of RAD51 foci in response to DNA damage.[36]

In addition to its role in HR DNA DSB repair, BRCA2 may have a role as a regulator of cell cycle progression at the mitotic checkpoint. BRCA2 associates with the DNA-binding protein BRAF35 and both proteins co-localise on mitotic chromosomes. Injections of antibodies that block either BRCA2 or BRAF35 into cells have been shown to block progression through mitosis.[37]

In summary, the BRCA1 and BRCA2 proteins play major roles in the maintenance of genomic stability. They are essential cogs of the error-free HR DNA repair pathway. Cells deficient in either BRCA1 or BRCA2 function demonstrate a high degree of chromosome instability, including chromosome breaks and aberrations, such as quadri-radial and tri-radial chromosomes.[35,38,39] This observation, in part, explains the high lifetime risk of the development of cancer in *BRCA1* and *BRCA2* mutation carriers.

Likelihood of a *BRCA* mutation in ovarian and/or breast cancer families

Most ovarian cancers occur sporadically, although approximately 10% of patients will report an associated family history of the disease.[40,41] In unselected series, about 6–15% of ovarian cancers have been found to be due to *BRCA* mutations.[42] Other rarer inherited causes of ovarian cancer include Lynch syndrome due to defects in mismatch repair genes, which may account for about 2% of unselected ovarian cancers.[43]

Fifteen percent of familial breast cancers are associated with germline *BRCA1/2* mutations, while an additional 10% are associated with other known susceptibility genes, including some high-risk genes such as *TP53* and *PTEN* and other moderate-risk genes such as *ATM* and *CHEK2*. The remaining 75% of breast cancer familial risk is attributed to a combination of variants in a large number of genes, each conferring a small excess of risk.[44] Genome-wide scans continue to seek further such variants in large collaborative consortia.[45]

The likelihood of a *BRCA* mutation being present in a family can be gauged by predictors such as the number of individuals affected with ovarian and/or breast cancer, the ages at diagnosis, histological features and the ancestry of the individual. Founder mutations (mutations that have been concentrated in certain populations over generations) are relevant to consider as they influence the likelihood of a mutation being present and the practicalities of genetic testing (see later section on genetic testing).

Lifetime breast and ovarian cancer risk in *BRCA* mutation carriers

The average cumulative risk of developing ovarian cancer in a *BRCA* mutation carrier by the age of 70 years has been estimated in a meta-analysis at 30–40% for *BRCA1* and 10–15% for *BRCA2*,[46] but is higher in some families where presumably other modifier genes and environmental effects add to the risk. Maximal lifetime *BRCA*-related ovarian risks are up to 60% for *BRCA1* and 30% for *BRCA2* and are thought to be most applicable to families where multiple cases of ovarian cancer have already occurred.[47,48]

The average cumulative lifetime risk of developing breast cancer is estimated at 50–70% in *BRCA1* mutation carriers and 40–50% in *BRCA2* mutation carriers.[46] Maximal breast cancer risks are up to 90% for *BRCA1* and up to 85% for *BRCA2*[47,48] and, as with ovarian cancer risk figures, these are thought most applicable to families where there is already evidence of multiple affected individuals.

Modifying factors can also affect the age of onset of hereditary *BRCA*-associated cancers. Onset is generally much earlier than in sporadic tumours, being up to 20 years earlier for breast cancer in *BRCA* mutation carriers than in individuals with sporadic disease.[49] The actual age of onset in any individual is variable, with some carriers presenting in their third decade and others beyond their seventh decade, or not at all.

The ability to predict an individual's cancer risk accurately is thus currently limited by the influence of factors other than whether a *BRCA1* or *BRCA2* mutation has been inherited. The nature and location of the mutation in the gene may affect its impact on risk,[41] but other modifier genetic variants and environmental factors are also important.[50–52] An example of such a potential modifier is a single-nucleotide polymorphism (a single base change) in the non-coding region of the *RAD51* gene, whose protein binds to the BRCA2 protein and increases the risk of breast cancer.[51] Also, common single-nucleotide polymorphisms in genes such as *FGFR2* or *MAP3K1* that influence risk in the general population also increase breast cancer risk in *BRCA1/2* mutation carriers, suggesting a common polygenic component in such people.[52]

In practice, ranges of cumulative risk may be quoted and the context of the strength of the family history used to comment on whether an individual is likely to be at either end of the risk spectrum. Genetic modifier variants highlight the polygenic nature of cancer susceptibility and will be useful in future risk assessment but their interactions are not yet sufficiently characterised for application in the clinical setting at present.

Histology of *BRCA*-related cancers

The histology of *BRCA1/2*-associated ovarian tumours tends to be high-grade, poorly differentiated, serous adenocarcinomas, while the stage at first presentation is similar to that of the general population, with approximately 70% of patients presenting with stage III or IV disease.[53] *BRCA* mutations are very rare in non-epithelial ovarian tumours or in mucinous or borderline tumours.[54] It has also been reported that p53 abnormalities are common in *BRCA*-mutated ovarian cancers, in line with the hypothesis that the p53 gatekeeper function has to be altered so that *BRCA1/2*-deficient tumours are able to proliferate.[40]

BRCA1-deficient breast cancers generally exhibit features of the basal-like breast cancer subgroup, unlike *BRCA2* tumours. These characteristics include negativity for estrogen receptor (ER) expression, staining for cytokeratins typical of basal myoepithelial cells and characteristic histopathological appearances. This is in contrast to *BRCA2* tumours, which show a pattern of ER expression similar to those of sporadic breast cancers, and have no distinct histopathological features, although they may be distinguished from sporadic cancers by gene expression profiling.

Other cancer risks in *BRCA* mutation carriers

Aside from the risk of a first breast cancer, the risk of a contralateral primary breast cancer is increased in *BRCA* mutation carriers. The overall cumulative risk is estimated at 50%[55] but varies between studies depending on how individuals are selected. Adjuvant treatment for the first breast cancer is thought to reduce contralateral risk. The contralateral risk is an important consideration for some women in deciding whether to have their initial breast cancer treated with conservative surgery or with bilateral mastectomies.

There are very small increases in risk reported at non-breast/ovarian sites (for example, pancreas and uterus) in female *BRCA1* mutation carriers, which do not generally warrant surveillance. *BRCA2* mutations increase the risk of developing other cancers, including pancreatic (four- to eight-fold relative risk), prostate (two- to four-fold) and male breast cancers (75-fold or absolute lifetime risk of 5%).[56,57] As the absolute risk increases are small, surveillance is not routinely recommended but is considered depending on what is found in the family history.

Patterns of inheritance

The autosomal dominant mode of genetic transmission means that both male and female children of a carrier will have a 50% chance of inheriting the *BRCA* mutation.[10] While one defective *BRCA1* or *BRCA2* allele is sufficient to predispose to cancer, the somatic loss of the wild-type allele is thought to be an obligate step driving oncogenesis. The clinical manifestation of the *BRCA* mutation is not affected by the parent of origin of the mutation; that is, imprinting is not seen. Childhood cancer risk is not increased except in rare situations where a child inherits mutated *BRCA2* genes from each parent, potentially resulting in Fanconi anaemia.[58] Individuals with one mutated *BRCA1* and one mutated *BRCA2* gene are also seen, particularly in populations with founder effects, and their clinical picture is similar to that of people with a single mutation. The main impact, however, is that their offspring have a three in four likelihood of inheriting one mutated gene (rather than the one in two risk experienced by offspring of someone with a single mutation).

Reproductive options for *BRCA* mutation carriers include prenatal testing and, more recently, pre-implantation genetic diagnosis using *in vitro* fertilisation procedures, followed by DNA analysis of early-stage embryos.[59] Such testing is rarely undertaken currently for this condition. Incomplete penetrance (the fact that the mutation does not always result in cancer) and the expectation that cancer risk will be manageable for future generations mean that many couples will elect to conceive naturally, particularly when they appreciate aspects such as conception rates being higher naturally than with *in vitro* fertilisation, if they have normal fertility.

Tissue specificity of oncogenesis

The observation that *BRCA1/2* gene mutations predispose to cancers specific to particular hormone-dependent epithelial tissues, such as breast, ovary, prostate or pancreas, has intrigued the scientific and oncology communities. Several hypotheses have now been proposed to account for this finding.

The highly proliferative nature of tissues such as the breast and ovary may result in the loss of the second *BRCA* allele at a higher frequency than in other tissues, resulting in oncogenesis. Alternatively, *BRCA* deficiency may result in an increased sensitivity of such breast and ovarian cells to the effects of local mutagens, such as estrogen metabolites. *Brca1*-deficient pre-clinical models have been reported to have alterations in mammary gland development and hormone responsiveness.[60,61] It may also be possible that *BRCA* gene products are involved in the regulation of the transcription of genes, the expression of which are limited to the breast and ovary by unknown mechanisms.

Another hypothesis is that, owing to the anti-apoptotic action of estrogens, breast and ovarian tissues are able to tolerate *BRCA1* loss of heterozygosity.[62] Since breast cancer stem cells are usually ER-negative but receive pro-survival signals from the surrounding ER-positive cells, it may be that *BRCA1*-deficient cells are able to survive as long as they are stimulated by adjacent ER-positive breast cells.[63,64]

A further theory supports the notion that the hormonal environment of susceptible tissues is the main factor responsible for the tissue specificity of *BRCA1/2*-associated cancers. For example, the progesterone receptor is aberrantly expressed in non-tumoral breast tissue of *BRCA1* mutation carriers with breast cancer.[65]

Another theory revolves around the proposed role of BRCA1 in stem cell differentiation.[10] BRCA1 depletion has been observed *in vitro* to inhibit the differentiation of stem cells, resulting in the accumulation of ER-negative early progenitors that bear some of the features of *BRCA1*-deficient breast cancer cells.[66]

Overall, it is likely that it is the combination of a number of factors, including genetic and environmental players, which contributes to the tissue-specificity of *BRCA1/2*-associated cancers.

Role of *BRCA1* and *BRCA2* gene testing

The role of *BRCA1/2* gene testing is to identify individuals with a particular genetic predisposition to developing cancer, with the goal of better estimating their risk and of increasing their survival through optimal management of their risk and of cancer, should they develop it. Testing for *BRCA1* and *BRCA2* germline mutations is mainly undertaken in the UK following referral to genetics services. The pathway of providing *BRCA* testing is undergoing change as *BRCA* status is now seen to affect some cancer treatment decisions. Genetics services are working together with oncology and surgical colleagues to develop methods of collaborating to provide fast-track genetic testing for a subset of patients, for example where a decision on bilateral mastectomies or entry to a polyadenosine diphosphate-ribose polymerase (PARP) inhibitor trial is affected by *BRCA* mutation status.

General population screening for *BRCA1/2* mutations has not been recommended owing to the low population prevalence of *BRCA1/2* mutations (estimated to be up to one in 500) and the resource implications for both laboratory and clinical services.[67]

Genetic testing in the UK

In the UK, the National Institute for Health and Clinical Excellence (NICE) guidance on familial breast cancer in 2004 designated women at high risk of breast/ovarian cancer who would be eligible for referral to cancer genetics services.[68] For example, these include those with:

- two close relatives with breast cancer diagnosed before an average age of 50 years
- three close relatives with breast cancer before an average age of 60 years
- four relatives with breast cancer at any age
- two close relatives with ovarian cancer
- one ovarian cancer and one breast cancer diagnosed before age 50 years in the woman herself, or either cancer in the woman herself and in a close relative
- male and female breast cancers in close relatives.

From this group, those assessed by a genetics service as having a 30% or greater lifetime breast cancer risk or a 20% or greater likelihood of a *BRCA* mutation in the family should be offered genetic counselling. NICE does not specify particular criteria for determining the 20% threshold of a *BRCA* mutation being present. A variety of approaches to determining this threshold has been used in practice. Different prediction models have been compared by Antoniou and colleagues.[52] The best predictor of *BRCA* status is the computer-based BOADICEA model but it is currently still being refined in research settings and is time-consuming for clinical use.

In practice, many UK genetics centres use the Manchester Scoring System.[69,70] Points are allocated for each cancer within one line of inheritance in the family according to cancer site and age at onset. If the score reaches 15, it is estimated that there is at least a 10% likelihood that an individual in the family with a relevant cancer will have a *BRCA* mutation. A close relative who is unaffected will have half the likelihood (of that of an affected sibling, parent or child) of having inherited the potential *BRCA* mutation in a dominant model. For that reason, in most situations, the individual in a family who has had a relevant cancer is the one most likely to have a *BRCA* mutation and therefore the most relevant person in whom the genetic mutation searching (the search in a family to find the particular mutation responsible by analysing the whole code of *BRCA1* and *BRCA2*) should be undertaken.

Testing is targeted in this way owing to the fact that the prior likelihood of finding a mutation may only be 10% and the resources involved in analysing the code of two large genes, for example through sequencing and multiplex ligation-dependent probe amplification (MLPA), a technique to look for large rearrangements of genes. When the mutation in a particular family has been identified, other relatives may be offered a predictive test that just looks directly at one site in the code of the relevant gene for the one specific family mutation. This predictive testing can be undertaken more quickly and cheaply than the original analysis of the whole code of the *BRCA* genes.

If a *BRCA* mutation is not seen in an affected family member, then it is likely that the family cancer picture is due to genes that are as yet unknown. In relatively few situations, it will be appropriate to undertake *BRCA* mutation searching in a second affected family member (on the grounds that one case of breast cancer could be a phenocopy; that is, a case where the cancer could be due to chance or other unidentified genes, while the remainder of the family cases are due to a *BRCA* mutation). *BRCA* testing is done in regional laboratories around the UK under the umbrella of the UK Genetic Testing Network (see www.ukgtn.nhs.uk/gtn/Search+for+a+Test for listings).

There are some situations in which the initial *BRCA* mutation searching in a family is offered to a member who has not had cancer. In general, this is appropriate when no affected relative is available to test and there is a possible founder mutation in the family, as these mutations can be tested directly rather than requiring the more expensive and time-consuming analysis of the whole of the *BRCA* codes. Founders are relevant in certain populations[42] such as Ashkenazi Jews, where up to 2.5% of the population carry one of three mutations: 185delAG or 5382insC (both in *BRCA1*) or 6174delT (in *BRCA2*).[40,41]

In some situations, a genetics service will offer an initial search of the *BRCA* codes to an unaffected person from a non-founder population when there is no affected person available to test. This is, however, generally only done when the family history is very strong and there is an increased likelihood that the unaffected person is at risk, but has just yet to manifest it.

As the cost and time needed to analyse large genes reduces with technological advances, the criteria to offer *BRCA* mutation searching will become more liberal. Ultimately, the driver for testing the germline DNA of all individuals with ovarian cancer will be whether treatment would be altered by the presence of an inherited *BRCA* mutation. Major advances in the ability to sequence large numbers of cancer genes simultaneously using 'cancer gene chips' in blood samples and in tumour specimens will change access to genetic testing in the coming decade as well as the pathways of referral between oncology and genetics services.[71]

Options for management

The main aim of identifying such high-risk *BRCA1/2* individuals has traditionally been for disease prophylactic measures, through early cancer detection with screening and prophylactic surgical measures.[72] However, it is now generally accepted that a person's *BRCA1/2* status is also a robust predictive biomarker for the optimal selection of some anti-cancer therapeutics. These treatments include platinum-based chemotherapy regimens and the newly developed PARP inhibitors.

Surveillance of *BRCA* mutation carriers

Early detection of breast and ovarian cancer is associated with improved survival and depends on the use of strategies that are both financially and medically effective. *BRCA1/2* mutation carriers or those with a positive family history of breast and/or ovarian cancer should be made aware of the issues regarding both breast and ovarian surveillance.

As *BRCA1/2* mutation carriers are at risk of breast cancer at a young age when dense breast tissue reduces the sensitivity of X-ray mammography, contrast-enhanced magnetic resonance imaging (MRI) with mammography is recommended as a strategy for screening between ages 30 and 50 years.[73] The MARIBS trial was a prospective multicentre cohort study of 649 women in the UK aged 35–49 years with a strong family history of breast cancer or a high probability of a *BRCA1*, *BRCA2* or *TP53* mutation and demonstrated that sensitivity was significantly higher for MRI (77%; 95% CI 60–90%) than for mammography (40%; 95% CI 24–58%; $P=0.01$), and was 94% (95% CI 81–99%) when both modalities were used.[73] Specificity for both procedures was acceptable. The difference between MRI and mammography sensitivities was particularly pronounced in *BRCA1* mutation carriers (13 cancers; 92% versus 23%; $P=0.004$). Annual screening, with the combination of MRI and mammography, would thus detect most tumours in this risk group. These figures are similar to those found in several international trials.[74] Women being offered breast MRI need to be aware that the increased sensitivity also results in identification of lesions that require further follow-up,[75] which occurs in about 10% of those scanned. Access to MRI surveillance remains a difficulty but is important for *BRCA* carriers owing to potential impact on survival, as recent modelling suggests similar survival advantage conferred by MRI surveillance compared to prophylactic mastectomies.[76] Breast imaging for women at high risk is becoming part of the NHS National Breast Screening Programme remit, designed to ensure that these women have a robust surveillance system.

The UK Familial Ovarian Cancer Screening Study

Ovarian screening has been offered in the UK under the national research study UKFOCSS (UK Familial Ovarian Cancer Screening Study). There is currently no conclusive evidence that monitoring the CA125 tumour marker and transvaginal ultrasound scans will result in a survival benefit. Several studies have demonstrated that annual surveillance is ineffective as the majority of tumours detected are not found at an early stage.[77,78] In the USA, annual transvaginal ultrasound and six-monthly measurements of CA125 tumour marker levels are recommended, but the efficacy of this is unknown. Women in the UKFOCSS are currently receiving annual transvaginal ultrasound scans and measurement of CA125 levels every 4 months, which are analysed with the Risk of Ovarian Cancer Algorithm (ROCA). ROCA stratifies women according to their pattern of CA125 levels over time to determine when to repeat their investigations. Women with an intermediate ROCA score have a repeat CA125 level and transvaginal ultrasound scan, while those with suspicious ultrasound scans or highly elevated ROCA scores are referred to a gynaecological oncologist for consideration of surgical investigations. Enrolment to this study is now complete and results are expected in 2013, following which clinical services will need to determine whether surveillance is to be offered as a routine service.

The mainstay of ovarian cancer risk management is currently prophylactic bilateral salpingo-oophorectomy (BSO), which is generally considered after age 40 years for *BRCA1* mutation carriers and after age 45 years for *BRCA2* mutation carriers, as the increase in ovarian cancer risk is usually later with the latter.

Prophylactic surgical options

In general, during genetic counselling, healthy female *BRCA1/2* mutation carriers are advised of their estimated increased risk of breast and ovarian cancer development, and about possible available risk-reducing procedures. Practice guidelines recommend prophylactic BSO for ovarian cancer risk reduction by age 40–45 years and support various alternatives for managing breast cancer risk: either prevention with prophylactic mastectomy (PM) or early detection with screening mammography plus MRI as discussed above.[79]

A PM with an immediate reconstruction substantially minimises future breast cancer risk[80] and appears to be acceptable surgery in *BRCA* mutation carriers if carefully prepared with a protocol including discussions with a multidisciplinary team of breast surgeons, specialist nurses and a clinical psychologist. The potential adverse effects associated with such procedures, such as psychological reactions, consequences for body image, sexuality and quality of life should be discussed and addressed.[81]

A study using a simulation modelling approach that was published in 2009 suggested that the single most effective strategy to adopt for *BRCA1/2* mutation carriers is prophylactic BSO at age 40 years, which yields a 15% absolute survival gain for *BRCA1* mutation carriers and a 7% survival gain for *BRCA2* mutation carriers.[76] The combination of PM and prophylactic BSO at age 40 years was predicted to improve survival more than any single intervention, yielding 24% survival gain for *BRCA1* mutation carriers and 11% for *BRCA2* mutation carriers. PM at age 25 years instead of age 40 years offers minimal incremental benefit (1–2%), while substituting screening for PM yields a similarly minimal decrement in survival (2–3%). These data suggest that, although PM at age 25 years and prophylactic BSO at age 40 years maximises survival probability, and provides survival approaching that of women without mutations (79% for women with *BRCA1* mutations, 83% for women with *BRCA2* mutations and 84% for the general population), substituting mammography plus MRI screening may offer comparable survival.[76] Such modelling underlines the need for these women at high risk to be offered MRI screening during the age window of 30–50 years.

Prophylactic BSO is now generally accepted as an effective prophylactic measure in women at high risk of developing ovarian cancer. Total abdominal hysterectomy is offered in conjunction in the USA but not in the UK as the small possible uterine cancer risk is not considered sufficient to warrant the increase in surgical adverse effects. Meticulous sectioning of the BSO specimen and the use of peritoneal washings are recommended to maximise the opportunity to detect occult malignancies.

In a large series of 1828 *BRCA1/2* mutation carriers from 32 centres in various countries, participants were asked to complete questionnaires at baseline and at follow-up.[82] Of the 1828 *BRCA1/2* carriers, 555 (30%) had undergone a prophylactic BSO before study entry, 490 (27%) underwent the procedure following study entry and 783 (43%) did not have the procedure. The overall (adjusted) risk reduction in cancer associated with prophylactic BSO was 80% (multivariate hazard ratio = 0.20; 95% CI 0.07–0.58; P = 0.003), but was higher in some studies that have shown risk reduction of up to 95%.[83] Prophylactic BSO performed premenopausally has also been shown to reduce breast cancer risk in *BRCA1/2* mutation carriers, even when hormone replacement therapy (HRT) is given until age 51 years (the median age of natural menopause). Thus, prophylactic BSO is associated with reduced risks of ovarian, fallopian tube and breast cancers in women at high risk, although there is a residual risk for peritoneal cancer in *BRCA1/2* mutation carriers following the procedure.

Risk-reducing BSO is, however, associated with a number of ethical and social issues, especially in the typically young women bearing *BRCA1/2* mutations, in view of the consequences of a premature menopause. There is growing awareness of the need to ensure that young women having prophylactic surgery are not unnecessarily deprived of HRT after such procedures. There is a suggestion in the literature that mortality may be increased in women having prophylactic BSO before age 45 years without HRT and that quality of life is significantly affected by menopausal symptoms, particularly if HRT is not feasible.[84] Services providing prophylactic BSO in women at high risk are developing links with menopause clinics to provide women with adequate information and access to specialist HRT management in addition to input from their GPs. HRT in a premenopausal woman who has had endogenous production largely removed by prophylactic BSO does not increase breast risk. There is evidence from the PROSE study that breast cancer risk is reduced by about half by premenopausal BSO and that breast protection is maintained even when HRT is provided to age 51 years.[83,85–87] HRT after BSO is not necessarily contraindicated for women who have had ER-negative breast cancer or those who have had ER-positive breast cancer and are on tamoxifen. For some women who have had ER-positive breast cancers, non-hormonal measures may be preferred but the decision is best made by oncology teams on an individual basis weighing up potential risks of breast cancer recurrence versus optimal symptom management and avoidance of potential long-term effects on bone and cardiovascular health.

Chemoprevention agents

Chemoprevention strategies, which could provide protection for these young women until they have completed childbearing, are also an area of interest. The oral contraceptive pill has been considered in women at high risk of developing ovarian cancer as such an approach. In one such study, a total of 207 *BRCA1/2* mutation carriers with ovarian cancer and 161 of their sisters, who acted as controls, were studied to evaluate the potential benefit of oral contraception in women at high risk of ovarian cancer.[88] The adjusted overall risk for ovarian cancer associated with any previous use of oral contraception was 0.5 (95% CI 0.3–0.8). The risk decreased with increased duration of use (P for trend <0.001), while the use for at least 6 years was associated with a 60% reduction in risk. Protection was observed in both *BRCA1* and *BRCA2* mutation carriers. The caveat to the use of oral contraception is the possible slight increased risk of breast cancer with use for over 4 years seen in women with *BRCA* mutations.[89] Given that the reduction in ovarian cancer risk is not sufficient to avoid the need for prophylactic BSO and that there may be an increase in breast cancer risk with oral contraceptive usage, the contraceptive pill is not recommended routinely as a chemopreventive option in the UK.

Other chemoprevention agents for this group of women at high risk that have been suggested include retinoids and heteroarotinoids, 1,25-dihydroxyvitamin D3, COX-2 inhibitors and peroxisome proliferator-activated receptor (PPARγ), although objective evidence of benefit is limited and these are not currently used in practice in the UK.[90]

Mitigating cancer risks in women with *BRCA* mutations remains a priority and alternative chemoprevention approaches are now urgently required. PARP inhibitors have been shown to selectively kill *BRCA2*-deficient cells *in vivo* while sparing normal tissue with heterozygous *BRCA2* loss. This may imply a chemoprophylactic potential for PARP inhibitors to kill off clones of cells with biallelic *BRCA2* loss before oncogenesis.[91] However, as with any novel developmental therapeutic, there are valid concerns about the potential of long-term adverse effects. The continuous administration of PARP inhibitors results in the chronic inhibition of key DNA repair pathways, raising the theoretical possibility of mutagenesis and development of secondary malignancies such as myelodysplasia and acute leukaemias.[92,93] As such, more chronic-exposure safety data from the use of PARP inhibitors are necessary before this strategy can be implemented. Currently, a randomised placebo-controlled trial of olaparib (AZD2281; AstraZeneca) (400 mg twice daily) as maintenance therapy in women with platinum-sensitive serous ovarian cancer at high risk of early recurrence is continuing in the UK (www.clinicaltrials.gov; NCT00753545).[94]

Medical management for *BRCA* mutation carriers

The specific oncological management of *BRCA*-mutated cancers has not differed from that of non-hereditary carriers, although differences in treatment responses do exist. There are emerging data on possible increased sensitivity to some regimens, for example very early data on complete pathological responses to neo-adjuvant platinum for breast cancer in a pilot study in *BRCA1* mutation carriers.[95] Various studies have shown that *BRCA1*-associated ovarian cancer has an improved prognosis compared with sporadic ovarian cancer.[96–98]

Tan and colleagues[99] matched 22 women with ovarian cancer with germline *BRCA1/2* mutations with 44 women with ovarian cancer in a non-hereditary control group; all patients had received primary platinum-based chemotherapies. Those with *BRCA1/2* mutations had improved overall survival compared with those in the control group (95% versus 59%; $P=0.002$), better complete response rates to first-line platinum-based chemotherapies (81.8% versus 43.2%; $P=0.004$), as well as higher response rates to second-line (91.7% versus 40.9%; $P=0.004$) and third-line treatments (100% versus 14.3%; $P=0.005$). In a separate retrospective study, *BRCA1* mRNA levels were analysed in a series of 70 sporadic ovarian cancers in women without *BRCA* germline mutations, with associated clinical outcome data.[100] Women with low to intermediate levels of *BRCA1* mRNA expression levels had a significantly increased survival compared with those with high *BRCA1* mRNA levels (57.2 versus 18.2 months; $P=0.0017$). It should be noted that the low *BRCA1* levels could be a result of mutation, methylation of the gene promoter or other associated mechanisms. These data from both studies support the notion that *BRCA1/2*-mutated carriers with ovarian cancer have increased sensitivities to platinum-based treatment and improved survival compared with those whose tumours do not have *BRCA* dysfunction. Such findings are consistent with the pre-clinical sensitivity of *BRCA1/2*-defective cells to DNA damaging agents, including platinum salts and PARP inhibitors.[101,102]

The demonstration of single-agent anti-tumour activity and the wide therapeutic index of PARP inhibitors in *BRCA1* and *BRCA2* mutation carriers with advanced ovarian and breast cancers provide strong evidence for the clinical application of this approach.[103–105] Emerging data also indicate that PARP inhibitors may be effective in sporadic cancers bearing HR defects, supporting a substantially wider role for PARP inhibitors.[106]

Conclusion

Knowledge of an individual's *BRCA* mutation status can allow them and their treating teams to manage their cancer risks.[72] The study of the function of *BRCA1* and *BRCA2* in DNA repair is leading to new approaches to anti-cancer therapy. Our improved understanding of the underlying biology of DNA damage response pathways, particular in high-grade serous ovarian cancers, has led to the development of these novel therapeutic strategies in broader groups of women with this disease. The coming years are likely to see the introduction of improved strategies for both *BRCA1/2* mutation-associated disease prophylaxis as well as individualised treatments, which will positively impact on women in the gynae-oncology clinic in the way that identification of the *BRCA1* and *BRCA2* genes has done in cancer genetics clinics over the last decade.

References

1. Easton D, Peto J. The contribution of inherited predisposition to cancer incidence. *Cancer Surv* 1990;9:395–416.
2. Claus EB, Risch N, Thompson WD. Genetic analysis of breast cancer in the cancer and steroid hormone study. *Am J Hum Genet* 1991;48:232–42.
3. Evans DG, Shenton A, Woodward E, Lalloo F, Howell A, Maher ER. Penetrance estimates for *BRCA1* and *BRCA2* based on genetic testing in a Clinical Cancer Genetics service setting: risks of breast/ovarian cancer quoted should reflect the cancer burden in the family. *BMC Cancer* 2008;8:155.
4. Vogelstein B, Kinzler KW. Cancer genes and the pathways they control. *Nat Med* 2004;10:789–99.
5. Hall JM, Lee MK, Newman B, Morrow JE, Anderson LA, Huey B, *et al.* Linkage of early-onset familial breast cancer to chromosome 17q21. *Science* 19990;250:1684–9.
6. Miki Y, Swensen J, Shattuck-Eidens D, Futreal PA, Harshman K, Tavtigian S, *et al.* A strong candidate for the breast and ovarian cancer susceptibility gene *BRCA1*. *Science* 1994;266:66–71.
7. Wooster R, Neuhausen SL, Mangion J, Quirk Y, Ford D, Collins N, *et al.* Localization of a breast cancer susceptibility gene, *BRCA2*, to chromosome 13q12–13. *Science* 1994;265:2088–90.
8. Venkitaraman AR. Cancer susceptibility and the functions of *BRCA1* and *BRCA2*. *Cell* 2002;108:171–82.
9. Bertwistle D, Ashworth A. Functions of the *BRCA1* and *BRCA2* genes. *Curr Opin Genet Dev* 1998;8:14–20.
10. Venkitaraman AR. Linking the cellular functions of *BRCA* genes to cancer pathogenesis and treatment. *Annu Rev Pathol* 2009;4:461–87.
11. Feng Z, Kachnic L, Zhang J, Powell SN, Xia F. DNA damage induces p53-dependent BRCA1 nuclear export. *J Biol Chem* 2004;279:28574–84.
12. Gudmundsdottir K, Ashworth A. The roles of BRCA1 and BRCA2 and associated proteins in the maintenance of genomic stability. *Oncogene* 2006;25:5864–74.
13. Scully R, Chen J, Plug A, Xiao Y, Weaver D, Feunteun J, *et al.* Association of BRCA1 with Rad51 in mitotic and meiotic cells. *Cell* 1997;88:265–75.
14. Paull TT, Rogakou EP, Yamazaki V, Kirchgessner CU, Gellert M, Bonner WM. A critical role for histone H2AX in recruitment of repair factors to nuclear foci after DNA damage. *Curr Biol* 2000;10:886–95.
15. Moynahan ME, Chiu JW, Koller BH, Jasin M. Brca1 controls homology-directed DNA repair. *Mol Cell* 1999;4:511–18.
16. Huen MS, Sy SM, Chen J. BRCA1 and its toolbox for the maintenance of genome integrity. *Nat Rev Mol Cell Biol* 2010;11:138–48.
17. Zhuang J, Zhang J, Willers H, Wang H, Chung JH, van Gent DC, *et al.* Checkpoint kinase 2-mediated phosphorylation of BRCA1 regulates the fidelity of nonhomologous end-joining. *Cancer Res* 2006;66:1401–8.
18. Zhuang J, Jiang G, Willers H, Xia F. Exonuclease function of human Mre11 promotes deletional nonhomologous end joining. *J Biol Chem* 2009;284:30565–73.
19. Bau DT, Fu YP, Chen ST, Cheng TC, Yu JC, Wu PE, *et al.* Breast cancer risk and the DNA double-strand break end-joining capacity of nonhomologous end-joining genes are affected by BRCA1. *Cancer Res* 2004;64:5013–19.
20. Hartman AR, Ford JM. BRCA1 induces DNA damage recognition factors and enhances nucleotide excision repair. *Nat Genet* 2002;32:180–4.
21. Chai YL, Cui J, Shao N, Shyam E, Reddy P, Rao VN. The second BRCT domain of BRCA1 proteins interacts with p53 and stimulates transcription from the $p21^{WAF1/CIP1}$ promoter. *Oncogene* 1999;18:263–8.
22. Tibbetts RS, Cortez D, Brumbaugh KM, Scully R, Livingston D, Elledge SJ, *et al.* Functional interactions between BRCA1 and the checkpoint kinase ATR during genotoxic stress. *Genes Dev* 2000;14:2989–3002.
23. Williamson EA, Dadmanesh F, Koeffler HP. BRCA1 transactivates the cyclin-dependent kinase inhibitor p27(Kip1). *Oncogene* 2002;21:3199–206.
24. Aprelikova O, Pace AJ, Fang B, Koller BH, Liu ET. BRCA1 is a selective co-activator of 14-3-3 sigma gene transcription in mouse embryonic stem cells. *J Biol Chem* 2001;276:25647–50.

25. Mullan PB, Quinn JE, Gilmore PM, McWilliams S, Andrews H, Gervin C, *et al.* BRCA1 and GADD45 mediated G2/M cell cycle arrest in response to antimicrotubule agents. *Oncogene* 2001;20:6123–31.
26. Irminger-Finger I, Siegel BD, Leung WC. The functions of breast cancer susceptibility gene 1 (*BRCA1*) product and its associated proteins. *Biol Chem* 1999;380:117–28.
27. Gorski JJ, Kennedy RD, Hosey AM, Harkin DP. The complex relationship between BRCA1 and ERalpha in hereditary breast cancer. *Clin Cancer Res* 2009;15:1514–18.
28. Fan S, Wang J, Yuan R, Ma Y, Meng Q, Erdos MR, *et al.* BRCA1 inhibition of estrogen receptor signaling in transfected cells. *Science* 1999;284:1354–6.
29. Xu J, Fan S, Rosen EM. Regulation of the estrogen-inducible gene expression profile by the breast cancer susceptibility gene *BRCA1*. *Endocrinology* 2005;146:2031–47.
30. Kawai H, Li H, Chun P, Avraham S, Avraham HK. Direct interaction between BRCA1 and the estrogen receptor regulates vascular endothelial growth factor (VEGF) transcription and secretion in breast cancer cells. *Oncogene* 2002;21:7730–9.
31. Zhang H, Somasundaram K, Peng Y, Tian H, Zhang H, Bi D, *et al.* BRCA1 physically associates with p53 and stimulates its transcriptional activity. *Oncogene* 1998;16:1713–21.
32. Parant JM, Lozano G. Disrupting TP53 in mouse models of human cancers. *Hum Mutat* 2003;21:321–6.
33. Yang H, Jeffrey PD, Miller J, , Sun Y, Thoma NH, *et al.* BRCA2 function in DNA binding and recombination from a BRCA2-DSS1-ssDNA structure. *Science* 2002;297:1837–48.
34. Davies AA, Masson JY, McIlwraith MJ, Stasiak AZ, Stasiak A, Venkitaraman AR, *et al.* Role of BRCA2 in control of the RAD51 recombination and DNA repair protein. *Mol Cell* 2001;7:273–82.
35. Tutt A, Bertwistle D, Valentine J, Gabriel A, Swift S, Ross G, *et al.* Mutation in *Brca2* stimulates error-prone homology-directed repair of DNA double-strand breaks occurring between repeated sequences. *EMBO J* 2001;20:4704–16.
36. Yuan SS, Lee SY, Chen G, *et al*: BRCA2 is required for ionizing radiation-induced assembly of Rad51 complex *in vivo*. *Cancer Res* 1999;59:3547–51.
37. Marmorstein LY, Kinev AV, Chan GK, Bochar DA, Beniya H, Epstein JA, *et al.* A human BRCA2 complex containing a structural DNA binding component influences cell cycle progression. *Cell* 2001;104:247–57.
38. Patel KJ, Yu VP, Lee H, Corcoran A, Thistlethwaite FC, Evans MJ, *et al.* Involvement of Brca2 in DNA repair. *Mol Cell* 1998;1:347–57.
39. Kraakman-van der Zwet M, Overkamp WJ, van Lange RE, Essers J, van Duijn-Goedhart A, Wiggers I, *et al.* Brca2 (XRCC11) deficiency results in radioresistant DNA synthesis and a higher frequency of spontaneous deletions. *Mol Cell Biol* 2002;22:669–79.
40. Wooster R, Weber BL. Breast and ovarian cancer. *N Engl J Med* 2003;348:2339–47.
41. Sowter HM, Ashworth A. *BRCA1* and *BRCA2* as ovarian cancer susceptibility genes. *Carcinogenesis* 2005;26:1651–6.
42. Ramus SJ, Gayther SA. The contribution of *BRCA1* and *BRCA2* to ovarian cancer. *Mol Oncol* 2009;3:138–50.
43. Malander S, Rambech E, Kristoffersson U, Halvarsson B, Ridderheim M, Borg A, *et al.* The contribution of the hereditary nonpolyposis colorectal cancer syndrome to the development of ovarian cancer. *Gynecol Oncol* 2006;101:238–43.
44. Easton DF, Pooley KA, Dunning AM, Pharoah PD, Thompson D, Ballinger DG, *et al.* Genome-wide association study identifies novel breast cancer susceptibility loci. *Nature* 2007;447:1087–93.
45. Turnbull C, Ahmed S, Morrison J, Pernet D, Renwick A, Maranian M, *et al.* Genome-wide association study identifies five new breast cancer susceptibility loci. *Nat Genet* 2010;42:504–7.
46. Antoniou A, Pharoah PD, Narod S, Risch HA, Eyfjord JE, Hopper JL, *et al.* Average risks of breast and ovarian cancer associated with *BRCA1* or *BRCA2* mutations detected in case series unselected for family history: a combined analysis of 22 studies. *Am J Hum Genet* 2003;72:1117–30.
47. Ford D, Easton DF, Bishop DT, Narod SA, Goldgar DE. Risks of cancer in *BRCA1*-mutation carriers. Breast Cancer Linkage Consortium. *Lancet* 1994;343:692–5.
48. Easton DF, Steele L, Fields P, Ormiston W, Averill D, Daly PA, *et al.* Cancer risks in two large breast cancer families linked to *BRCA2* on chromosome 13q12-13. *Am J Hum Genet* 1997;61:120–8.

49. Frank TS, Deffenbaugh AM, Reid JE, Hulick M, Ward BE, Lingenfelter B, *et al.* Clinical characteristics of individuals with germline mutations in *BRCA1* and *BRCA2*: analysis of 10,000 individuals. *J Clin Oncol* 2002;20:1480–90.
50. Antoniou AC, Sinilnikova OM, McGuffog L, Healey S, Nevanlinna H, Heikkinen T, *et al.* Common variants in LSP1, 2q35 and 8q24 and breast cancer risk for *BRCA1* and *BRCA2* mutation carriers. *Hum Mol Genet* 2009;18:4442–56.
51. Antoniou AC, Sinilnikova OM, Simard J, Léoné M, Dumont M, Neuhausen SL, *et al.* RAD51 135G-->C modifies breast cancer risk among *BRCA2* mutation carriers: results from a combined analysis of 19 studies. *Am J Hum Genet* 2007;81:1186–200.
52. Antoniou AC, Spurdle AB, Sinilnikova OM, Healey S, Pooley KA, Schmutzler RK, *et al.* Common breast cancer-predisposition alleles are associated with breast cancer risk in *BRCA1* and *BRCA2* mutation carriers. *Am J Hum Genet* 2008;82:937–48.
53. Pal T, Permuth-Wey J, Betts JA, Krischer JP, Fiorica J, Arango H, *et al.* *BRCA1* and *BRCA2* mutations account for a large proportion of ovarian carcinoma cases. *Cancer* 2005;104:2807–16.
54. Lakhani SR, Manek S, Penault-Llorca F, Flanagan A, Arnout L, Merrett S, *et al.* Pathology of ovarian cancers in *BRCA1* and *BRCA2* carriers. *Clin Cancer Res* 2004;10:2473–81.
55. Graeser MK, McCarthy A, Lord CJ, Savage K, Hills M, Salter J, *et al.* A marker of homologous recombination predicts pathologic complete response to neoadjuvant chemotherapy in primary breast cancer. *Clin Cancer Res* 2010;16:6159–68.
56. Thompson D, Easton DF. Cancer incidence in *BRCA1* mutation carriers. *J Natl Cancer Inst* 2002;94:1358–65.
57. Cancer risks in *BRCA2* mutation carriers. The Breast Cancer Linkage Consortium. *J Natl Cancer Inst* 1999;91:1310–16.
58. D'Andrea AD. Susceptibility pathways in Fanconi's anemia and breast cancer. *N Engl J Med* 2010;362:1909–19.
59. Friedman LC, Kramer RM. Reproductive issues for women with *BRCA* mutations. *J Natl Cancer Inst Monogr* 2005;(34):83–6.
60. Bennett LM, McAllister KA, Malphurs J, Ward T, Collins NK, Seely JC, *et al.* Mice heterozygous for a *Brca1* or *Brca2* mutation display distinct mammary gland and ovarian phenotypes in response to diethylstilbestrol. *Cancer Res* 2000;60:3461–9.
61. Xu X, Wagner KU, Larson D, Weaver Z, Li C, Ried T, *et al.* Conditional mutation of *Brca1* in mammary epithelial cells results in blunted ductal morphogenesis and tumour formation. *Nat Genet* 1999;22:37–43.
62. Elledge SJ, Amon A. The *BRCA1* suppressor hypothesis: an explanation for the tissue-specific tumor development in *BRCA1* patients. *Cancer Cell* 2002;1:129–32.
63. Scully R, Livingston DM. In search of the tumour-suppressor functions of *BRCA1* and *BRCA2*. *Nature* 2000;408:429–32.
64. Zeps N, Bentel JM, Papadimitriou JM, D'Antuono MF, Dawkins HJ. Estrogen receptor-negative epithelial cells in mouse mammary gland development and growth. *Differentiation* 1998;62:221–6.
65. King TA, Gemignani ML, Li W, Giri DD, Panageas KS, Bogomolniy F, *et al.* Increased progesterone receptor expression in benign epithelium of *BRCA1*-related breast cancers. *Cancer Res* 2004;64:5051–3.
66. Liu S, Ginestier C, Charafe-Jauffret E, Foco H, Kleer CG, Merajver SD, *et al.* *BRCA1* regulates human mammary stem/progenitor cell fate. *Proc Natl Acad Sci U S A* 2008;105:1680–5.
67. Levy DE, Garber JE, Shields AE. Guidelines for genetic risk assessment of hereditary breast and ovarian cancer: early disagreements and low utilisation. *J Gen Intern Med* 2009;24:822–8.
68. National Institute for Clinical Excellence. *Familial Breast Cancer: the Classification and Care of Women at Risk of Familial Breast Cancer in Primary, Secondary and Tertiary Care.* Clinical Guideline 14. London: National Institute for Clinical Excellence; 2004.
69. Evans DG, Eccles DM, Rahman N, Young K, Bulman M, Amir E, *et al.* A new scoring system for the chances of identifying a *BRCA1/2* mutation outperforms existing models including BRCAPRO. *J Med Genet* 2004;41:474–80.
70. Evans DG, Lalloo F, Wallace A, Rahman N. Update on the Manchester Scoring System for *BRCA1* and *BRCA2* testing. *J Med Genet* 2005;42:e39.

71. Summerer D, Schracke N, Wu H, Cheng Y, Bau S, Stähler CF, *et al.* Targeted high throughput sequencing of a cancer-related exome subset by specific sequence capture with a fully automated microarray platform. *Genomics* 2010;95:241–6.
72. Domchek SM, Weber BL. Clinical management of *BRCA1* and *BRCA2* mutation carriers. *Oncogene* 2006;25:5825–31.
73. Leach MO, Boggis CR, Dixon AK, Easton DF, Eeles RA, Evans DG, *et al.* Screening with magnetic resonance imaging and mammography of a UK population at high familial risk of breast cancer: a prospective multicentre cohort study (MARIBS). *Lancet* 2005;365:1769–78.
74. Sardanelli F, Boetes C, Borisch B, Decker T, Federico M, Gilbert FJ, *et al.* Magnetic resonance imaging of the breast: recommendations from the EUSOMA working group. *Eur J Cancer* 2010;46:1296–316.
75. Gilbert FJ, Warren RM, Kwan-Lim G, Thompson DJ, Eeles RA, Evans DG, *et al.* Cancers in *BRCA1* and *BRCA2* carriers and in women at high risk for breast cancer: MR imaging and mammographic features. *Radiology* 2009;252:358–68.
76. Kurian AW, Sigal BM, Plevritis SK. Survival analysis of cancer risk reduction strategies for *BRCA1/2* mutation carriers. *J Clin Oncol* 2009;28:222–31.
77. Hermsen BB, Olivier RI, Verheijen RH, van Beurden M, de Hullu JA, Massuger LF, *et al.* No efficacy of annual gynaecological screening in *BRCA1/2* mutation carriers; an observational follow-up study. *Br J Cancer* 2007;96:1335–42.
78. Evans DG, Gaarenstroom KN, Stirling D, Shenton A, Maehle L, Dørum A, *et al.* Screening for familial ovarian cancer: poor survival of *BRCA1/2* related cancers. *J Med Genet* 2009;46:593–7.
79. National Comprehensive Cancer Network. *Genetic/Familial High-Risk Assessment: Breast and Ovarian* [www.nccn.org].
80. Hartmann LC, Sellers TA, Schaid DJ, Frank TS, Soderberg CL, Sitta DL, *et al.* Efficacy of bilateral prophylactic mastectomy in *BRCA1* and *BRCA2* gene mutation carriers. *J Natl Cancer Inst* 2001;93:1633–7.
81. Brandberg Y, Sandelin K, Erikson S, Jurell G, Liljegren A, Lindblom A, *et al.* Psychological reactions, quality of life, and body image after bilateral prophylactic mastectomy in women at high risk for breast cancer: a prospective 1-year follow-up study. *J Clin Oncol 2008;*26:3943–9.
82. Finch A, Beiner M, Lubinski J, Lynch HT, Moller P, Rosen B, *et al.* Salpingo-oophorectomy and the risk of ovarian, fallopian tube, and peritoneal cancers in women with a *BRCA1* or *BRCA2* mutation. *JAMA* 2006;296:185–92.
83. Domchek SM, Friebel TM, Neuhausen SL, Wagner T, Evans G, Isaacs C, *et al.* Mortality after bilateral salpingo-oophorectomy in *BRCA1* and *BRCA2* mutation carriers: a prospective cohort study. *Lancet Oncol* 2006;7:223–9.
84. Shuster LT, Gostout BS, Grossardt BR, Rocca WA. Prophylactic oophorectomy in premenopausal women and long-term health. *Menopause Int* 2008;14:111–16.
85. Rebbeck TR, Friebel T, Lynch HT, Neuhausen SL, van 't Veer L, Garber JE, *et al.* Bilateral prophylactic mastectomy reduces breast cancer risk in *BRCA1* and *BRCA2* mutation carriers: the PROSE Study Group. *J Clin Oncol* 2004;22:1055–62.
86. Rebbeck TR, Friebel T, Wagner T, Lynch HT, Garber JE, Daly MB, *et al.* Effect of short-term hormone replacement therapy on breast cancer risk reduction after bilateral prophylactic oophorectomy in *BRCA1* and *BRCA2* mutation carriers: the PROSE Study Group. *J Clin Oncol* 2005;23:7804–10.
87. Rebbeck TR, Kauff ND, Domchek SM. Meta-analysis of risk reduction estimates associated with risk-reducing salpingo-oophorectomy in *BRCA1* or *BRCA2* mutation carriers. *J Natl Cancer Inst* 2009;101:80–7.
88. Narod SA, Risch H, Moslehi R, Dørum A, Neuhausen S, Olsson H, *et al.* Oral contraceptives and the risk of hereditary ovarian cancer. Hereditary Ovarian Cancer Clinical Study Group. *N Engl J Med* 1998;339:424–8.
89. Brohet RM, Goldgar DE, Easton DF, Antoniou AC, Andrieu N, Chang-Claude J, *et al.* Oral contraceptives and breast cancer risk in the international *BRCA1/2* carrier cohort study: a report from EMBRACE, GENEPSO, GEO-HEBON, and the IBCCS Collaborating Group. *J Clin Oncol* 2007;25:3831–6.

90. Tinelli A, Malvasi A, Leo G, Vergara D, Pisanò M, Ciccarese M, *et al.* Hereditary ovarian cancers: from *BRCA* mutations to clinical management: a modern appraisal. *Cancer Metastasis Rev* 2010;29:339–50.

91. Hay T, Jenkins H, Sansom OJ, Martin NM, Smith GC, Clarke AR. Efficient deletion of normal *Brca2*-deficient intestinal epithelium by poly(ADP-ribose) polymerase inhibition models potential prophylactic therapy. *Cancer Res* 2005;65:10145–8.

92. Tong WM, Yang YG, Cao WH, Galendo D, Frappart L, Shen Y, *et al.* Poly(ADP-ribose) polymerase-1 plays a role in suppressing mammary tumourigenesis in mice. *Oncogene* 2007;26:3857–67.

93. Nicolas L, Martinez C, Baro C, Rodríguez M, Baroja-Mazo A, Sole F, *et al.* Loss of poly(ADP-ribose) polymerase-2 leads to rapid development of spontaneous T-cell lymphomas in p53-deficient mice. *Oncogene* 2010;29:2877–83.

94. Carden CP, Yap TA, Kaye SB. PARP inhibition: targeting the Achilles' heel of DNA repair to treat germline and sporadic ovarian cancers. *Curr Opin Oncol* 2010;22:473–80.

95. Byrski T, Gronwald J, Huzarski T, Grzybowska E, Budryk M, Stawicka M, *et al.* Pathologic complete response rates in young women with *BRCA1*-positive breast cancers after neoadjuvant chemotherapy. *J Clin Oncol* 2009;28:375–9.

96. Kauff ND, Domchek SM, Friebel TM, Robson ME, Lee J, Garber JE, *et al.* Risk-reducing salpingo-oophorectomy for the prevention of *BRCA1*- and *BRCA2*-associated breast and gynecologic cancer: a multicenter, prospective study. *J Clin Oncol* 2008;26:1331–7.

97. Chetrit A, Hirsh-Yechezkel G, Ben-David Y, Lubin F, Friedman E, Sadetzki S. Effect of *BRCA1/2* mutations on long-term survival of patients with invasive ovarian cancer: the national Israeli study of ovarian cancer. *J Clin Oncol* 2008;26:20–5.

98. Ben David Y, Chetrit A, Hirsh-Yechezkel G, Friedman E, Beck BD, Beller U, *et al.* Effect of *BRCA* mutations on the length of survival in epithelial ovarian tumors. *J Clin Oncol* 2002;20:463–6.

99. Tan DS, Rothermundt C, Thomas K, Bancroft E, Eeles R, Shanley S, *et al.* "BRCAness" syndrome in ovarian cancer: a case–control study describing the clinical features and outcome of patients with epithelial ovarian cancer associated with *BRCA1* and *BRCA2* mutations. *J Clin Oncol* 2008;26:5530–6.

100. Quinn JE, James CR, Stewart GE, Mulligan JM, White P, Chang GK, *et al.* *BRCA1* mRNA expression levels predict for overall survival in ovarian cancer after chemotherapy. *Clin Cancer Res* 2007;13:7413–20.

101. Tutt AN, Lord CJ, McCabe N, Farmer H, Turner N, Martin NM, *et al.* Exploiting the DNA repair defect in *BRCA* mutant cells in the design of new therapeutic strategies for cancer. *Cold Spring Harb Symp Quant Biol* 2005;70:139–48.

102. Ashworth A. A synthetic lethal therapeutic approach: poly(ADP) ribose polymerase inhibitors for the treatment of cancers deficient in DNA double-strand break repair. *J Clin Oncol* 2008;26:3785–90.

103. Fong PC, Boss DS, Yap TA, Tutt A, Wu P, Mergui-Roelvink M, *et al.* Inhibition of poly(ADP-ribose) polymerase in tumors from *BRCA* mutation carriers. *N Engl J Med* 2009;361:123–34.

104. Tutt A, Robson M, Garber JE, Domchek SM, Audeh MW, Weitzel JN, *et al.* Oral poly(ADP-ribose) polymerase inhibitor olaparib in patients with *BRCA1* or *BRCA2* mutations and advanced breast cancer: a proof-of-concept trial. *Lancet* 2010;376:235–44.

105. Audeh MW, Carmichael J, Penson RT, Friedlander M, Powell B, Bell-McGuinn KM, *et al.* Oral poly(ADP-ribose) polymerase inhibitor olaparib in patients with *BRCA1* or *BRCA2* mutations and recurrent ovarian cancer: a proof-of-concept trial. *Lancet* 2010;376:245–51.

106. Gelmon KA, Hirte HW, Robidoux A, Tonkin KS, Tischkowitz M, Swenerton K, *et al.* Can we define tumors that will respond to PARP inhibitors? A phase II correlative study of olaparib in advanced serous ovarian cancer and triple-negative breast cancer. *J Clin Oncol* 2010;28(15s):abstr 3002.

6

Chapter 6

Implications of homologous recombination defectiveness in ovarian cancer

Richard J Edmondson, Asima Mukhopadhyay, Aiste Cerbinskaite and Nicola J Curtin

Introduction

Major advances have taken place in our understanding of the biology of cancer but it has often seemed that this has not been translated into breakthroughs in new treatments, particularly in ovarian cancer where first-line management for the disease has not changed in 20 years.

The benefits of an increasing knowledge of the biology of the disease should, however, be two-fold – identifying new targets against which drugs can be developed and being able to identify which tumours are most likely to respond to these drugs. To be able to move away from the 'one size fits all' mentality of current cytotoxic therapy towards an individualised, targeted therapy remains the holy grail of current cancer medicine.

The story of the development of polyadenosine diphosphate-ribose polymerase (PARP) inhibitors and their link with the homologous recombination (HR) DNA repair pathway is the first real example in ovarian cancer of this process being carried through from the laboratory to the clinic. This chapter outlines the DNA repair pathways involved in PARP inhibitor sensitivity, how deficiencies in these pathways are exploited by PARP inhibitors and finally how aberrations of these pathways may be identified and thus used as predictive biomarkers for treatment. The aim of this work is ultimately to allow PARP inhibitor therapy to be targeted to a group of tumours that have a very high chance of responding.

DNA damage repair pathways

The development of a cancer is defined by a pattern of genetic abnormality affecting a cell. This results in uncontrolled cell proliferation and loss of the normal cell regulatory mechanisms. Many of the genetic abnormalities identified in cancers relate to DNA repair;[1] that is, the mechanisms by which a cell recognises and repairs the frequent minor DNA defects that occur following ionising radiation or other trauma. Intracellular DNA is exposed to these damaging insults all the time. It is estimated that there are up to a million episodes of DNA damage in each cell per day.[2] Clearly, the vast majority of this damage is repaired in a fault-free manner. Repair is achieved by one of six different repair pathways. The exact mechanism used depends on the phase of the cell cycle and also whether the DNA damage affects only a single strand, in which case it is repaired using base excision repair (BER), nucleotide excision repair or DNA mismatch repair, or whether the damage affects the double strand, in which case repair is effected using HR, non-homologous end joining or microhomology-mediated end joining.[3] Evidence has suggested that there can be overlap between the various pathways under certain circumstances, for instance in repairing DNA cross-link lesions.[4]

Base excision repair

The most common form of DNA damage is the single-strand break. Mammalian cells repair this type of damage using the error-free process BER.[5] Essentially, the intact strand of DNA is used as a template to recreate the damaged strand. Base excision repair actually includes several variations, each one specific for a different base, but all the pathways have the common feature of relying on the PARP enzyme.[6] PARP-1 has the crucial role of bringing together the four elements that are required to repair the damaged site, namely XRCC1, DNA ligase III, DNA polymerase beta and a kinase.

If, for any reason, BER cannot take place then the single-strand break persists until the time of DNA replication. At this point, the replication fork becomes stalled at the damaged site and the single-strand break is converted into a double-strand break (DSB). These can then be repaired by other DNA damage repair pathways, namely HR.

Homologous recombination

HR is also an error-free mechanism for repairing DNA damage and, like BER, it uses a template to ensure that it repairs the damage accurately.[7] Unlike BER, however, where the template is the opposite strand of the DNA, HR is used when both strands of the DNA are damaged and in this situation, therefore, the sister chromatid is borrowed to be used as the template.

HR is a complex process involving the recognition of DSBs, the assembling of the relevant repair machinery and the actual repair process. The process involves the interaction of multiple protein groups (Figure 6.1) but, following recognition of the DNA damage by ATM (ataxia telangiectasia mutated protein) and ATR (ataxia telangiectasia and RAD3-related protein), the process is characterised by the initial phosphorylation of H2AX into γH2AX and a final step involving the loading of RAD51 protein onto the BRCA2 protein. These two steps are highlighted as they form the basis of the RAD51 assay described below.

Defects in HR in human cancer

Given the importance of the HR pathway, it is hardly surprising to discover that it is non-functional in a large number of cancers.[8] A defective HR pathway may be responsible for the genetic instability that is a characteristic of cancers and may be either an initiating factor or a late event within the carcinogenetic process.

Defects in HR are not limited solely to mutations of *BRCA1* and *BRCA2*. Over 40 proteins have been identified to be involved in the HR pathway, including ATM/ATR, BRCA1, BRCA2 and the Fanconi proteins. Defects in many of these have been identified in human cancers, in fact mutation or epigenetic silencing has been described in at least 33 of these genes. Genetic aberrations of almost all elements

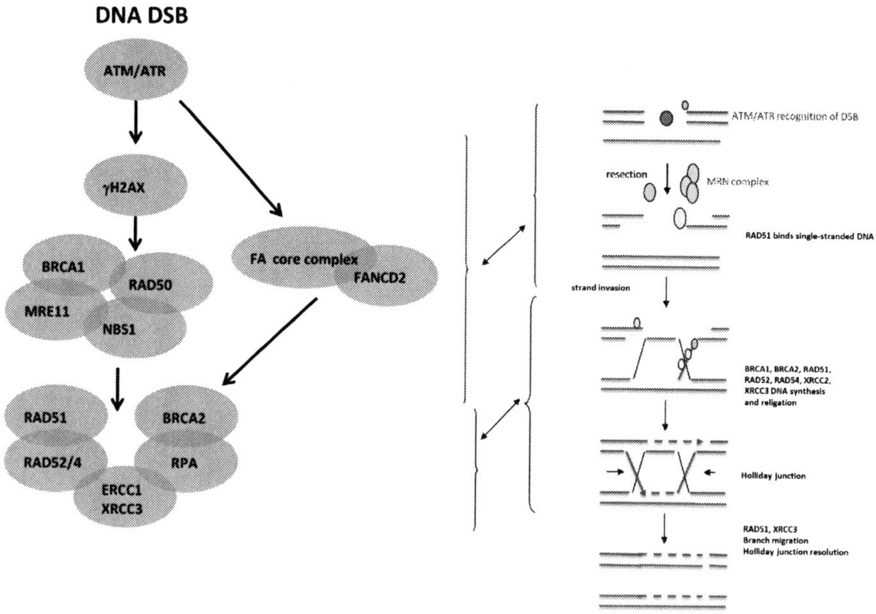

Figure 6.1 Schematic drawing of the process of homologous recombination for repair of DNA double-strand breaks (DNA DSB) demonstrating the interaction of the various protein groups (outlined on the left-hand side of the figure) with the repair process (outlined on the right-hand side of the figure). DNA DSBs are recognised by the ATM/ATR complex, resulting in phosphorylation of the H2AX protein into its gamma form. This allows assembly of the repair machinery involving several members of the Fanconi anaemia (FA) group of proteins. Repair utilises the sister chromatid to act as a template and results in a Holliday junction that is resolved by the RAD51/XRCC3 complex.

of the HR pathway have been described in human cancers. As well as germline mutations in *BRCA1* and *BRCA2*, gene silencing by methylation of *BRCA1* has also been described. Abberation of other elements that have been described include ATM, RAD50, NBS1, MRE11, EMSY, FANCA, FANCC, FANCF and XRCC3.

Furthermore, these defects are not limited to a single cancer site. In fact, disruption of the HR pathway has been described in the majority of solid tumours, including breast, ovarian, endometrial, gastric, colorectal, lung, thyroid, head and neck, testes, prostate and pancreas, as well as in some leukaemias and lymphomas.

The percentage of tumours affected by defective HR varies considerably across different cancer sites, with up to half of high-grade serous ovarian cancer having defective HR.[9] It is estimated that up to 20% of ovarian cancers have defective HR as a result of *BRCA* mutations, with roughly half of these mutations being germline and the rest being somatic.[10] This would leave approximately 30% of ovarian cancers with defective HR as a result of defects in other elements of the pathway.

Owing to the complex interactions within the HR pathway and the variable effect of gene silencing caused by methylation compared with mutation, it is essential to understand the functional significance of the genetic abberations reported. In particular, it is the effect of these mutations on the overall function of the HR pathway that needs to be understood. Further studies are thus needed to test the effects of individual and coexisting mutations on the overall HR pathway function.

BRCAness

There is substantial evidence that tumours associated with germline mutations of the *BRCA* genes are associated with a high initial sensitivity to platinum and an overall slightly improved outcome compared with other high-grade serous ovarian cancers.[11] The identification of other cancers that share this phenotype without the underlying genetic defect in *BRCA* has led to the concept of 'BRCAness'.[12]

It is now becoming clear that the tumours described as showing BRCAness are largely those tumours in which the HR pathway is defective and thus the term BRCAness is gradually being replaced by the more descriptive term homologous recombination-defective tumours.[13]

Targeting DNA damage repair pathways and the concept of synthetic lethality

DNA repair pathways would appear to be an attractive target for the development of new therapies.[13] Cancer cells are intrinsically genetically unstable and therefore susceptible to further DNA damage. Failure to repair this damage may induce apoptosis. However, it is clear that there is significant redundancy and overlap between the various DNA repair pathways. Targeting a single pathway in isolation is thus unlikely to have a significant effect, while targeting multiple pathways may well lead to unacceptable toxicity to normal cells and thus to the patient.

Synthetic lethality is a concept that exploits the vulnerability of cancer cells that have lost one mechanism of DNA repair by blocking a second/rescue pathway with a drug so that cells cannot repair DNA damage, thus leading to cell death.[14]

The advantages of a synthetically lethal system are obvious. The cancer cells have two pathways targeted, one by the drug and one as a result of an intrinsic defect, and thus cannot survive, whereas the normal cells have only one pathway affected by the drug and can rely on the rescue pathway to ensure cell survival.

Potential role of PARP inhibition

The knowledge that the BER pathway is PARP dependent led to much excitement that targeting this pathway by inhibiting PARP would increase genetic instability within a cancer cell that would promote apoptosis, making PARP inhibition a useful single-agent cytotoxic. PARP inhibitors were thus developed and the first patient underwent treatment with a PARP inhibitor in Newcastle in 2003. However, the results of a phase I study of a PARP inhibitor in conjunction with temozolomide were largely disappointing,[15] although at least there did appear to be minimal toxicity related to the PARP inhibitor.

Applying the knowledge of HR described above, and particularly the idea that tumours in women with germline mutations of *BRCA1* and *BRCA2* may be deficient in HR, suggested that PARP inhibitors may have single-agent activity in this particular group of tumours. In 2005, two simultaneously published papers from independent research groups demonstrated that this was indeed the case *in vitro*.[16,17] Both groups showed that in cell lines known to be defective in HR there was exquisite sensitivity to a PARP inhibitor with at least a 1000-fold difference between the HR-defective and HR-competent cells. This work has been expanded into cells lines of known HR status, confirming that HR-defective cells have greater sensitivity to a PARP inhibitor than cells with a functional HR pathway.[18]

The results of early-phase clinical trials in women with tumours defective in HR as a result of germline *BRCA* mutations are promising and are discussed in detail in Chapter 2.

Functional testing for homologous recombination defectiveness

The concept of personalised medicine is now well accepted.[19] Developing accurate predictive biomarkers would allow selection of patients who have a high chance of responding to treatments and would avoid subjecting those with only a low chance of responding to the inevitable adverse effects of treatment. Accurate biomarkers would also allow identification of people with tumours that are not normally recognised to respond to a particular treatment.

Predictive tests must not only have high sensitivity and specificity but should also be easy to carry out on material either normally available or easy to obtain. There is only limited use for a test carried out on a difficult-to-obtain patient sample that can be carried out only in a single laboratory. The standard material for routine pathological analysis is formalin-fixed paraffin-embedded tumour material and, while a new biomarker test would not be limited to this tissue, this remains the easiest material with which to work. In fact, most new treatments will be introduced at the time of disease relapse and therefore a new test would ideally be carried out on material collected at that time. As biopsy of small-volume disseminated disease can be difficult, the concept of identifying circulating tumour cells is attractive and worthy of further investigation.

There are several approaches possible for the development of a test for HR defectiveness. Firstly, a series of tests could be developed based on the known aberrations described in the literature. With current high-throughput techniques, this is certainly not impossible but, while we still do not understand the whole process of HR nor its interactions with other pathways, it is unlikely that such an approach will be associated with a high-enough degree of accuracy to make it useful.

Secondly, a test could be based on a functional assay that does not identify the underlying defect but merely discriminates between those cells capable of repairing DSBs with HR and those that cannot. Such an approach has many attractions but currently relies on the presence of a testable pathway, in other words a viable cell to be tested. This makes it less attractive for routine clinical use.

There are two such potential tests that have so far been described. The GFP test, first described by Pierce *et al*,[20] relies on the introduction of a vector into the cell. The vector contains a modified green flourescent protein that requires recombination of its DNA, using the host cell's HR mechanism, before it can fluoresce. A cell deficient in HR will not repair the DNA and will therefore not fluoresce.

While the test is relatively quick to perform, it requires the introduction of a vector into a viable cancer cell, a process not without its technical difficulty given the heterogeneity of ovarian cancer cells. Initial work in our laboratory suggests that transfection efficiency is widely variable in primary cultures of human ovarian cancer cells, requiring an extensive optimisation process before the test can be carried out. This would seem to rule out this test for clinical use.

A second approach is to identify markers within the cell of both DSBs and also its repair, the so-called RAD51 assay. One of the initial stages of the HR pathway is the phophorylation of H2AX to its gamma form γH2AX. Antibodies can detect this phosphorylated form using immunoflouresence. Similarly, one of the final steps in the HR pathway, the formation of RAD51 foci, can also be detected using immunoflouresence. Thus, using a two-colour technique, the number of γH2AX and RAD51 foci can be estimated in a single cell. If DSBs are created in the cell using either ionising radiation or a PARP inhibitor, the number of γH2AX foci will increase but the number of RAD51 foci will only increase in cells with intact HR. We have assessed this test in a panel of 25 primary cultures of serous ovarian cancer derived from women undergoing primary cytoreductive surgery and have found a very tight correlation between HR status as defined by the test and sensitivity to the PARP inhibitor AG014699.[9]

These results are very encouraging in suggesting that we will be able to accurately predict HR status and thus sensitivity to a PARP inhibitor but the RAD51 assay remains cumbersome, requiring the collection of viable cells and primary cell culture for approximately a week before the assay can be carried out.

To be able to assess HR status using gene expression would be attractive as mRNA can be extracted from fresh frozen tissue or even formalin-fixed paraffin-embedded tissue. Gene expression signatures have been identified that seem to correlate with BRCAness[21] and further work is now required to establish whether these signatures correlate with HR status and sensitivity to PARP inhibitors. It is not clear, however, what the effect of other epigenetic events such as methylation would have on a gene expression signature and it may be that ultimately a predictive biomarker test would require the combination of several elements, including gene expression and also methylation status of a few key genes.

Conclusion

The ultimate goal of cancer medicine must be to deliver relatively non-toxic treatments that are targeted specifically at cancer cells, individualised to patient groups with a high chance of responding. PARP inhibitor therapy in ovarian cancer seems to be promising to achieve these goals. An understanding of the biology of ovarian cancer, and specifically the role and interplay of the various DNA repair pathways, has underpinned the stratification of these drugs for use in *BRCA*-related cancers. The results of clinical trials of these drugs in this group of patients are outlined in Chapter 2. However, there also appear to be other groups of patients who may benefit from this class of drug, namely those with cancers defective in HR, including those with cancers other than breast and ovarian. The development of biomarker tests is progressing and it is hoped that these tests will soon be suitable for clinical use to allow the widest possible use of these agents.

References

1. Kastan M, Bartek J. Cell-cycle checkpoints and cancer. *Nature* 2004;432:316–23.
2. Vilenchik, MM, Knudson AG Jr. Inverse radiation dose-rate effects on somatic and germ-line mutations and DNA damage rates. *Proc Natl Acad Sci U S A* 2000;97:5381–6.
3. Warmerdam D, Kanaar R. Dealing with DNA damage: relationships between checkpoint and repair pathways. *Mutat Res* 2010;704:2–11.
4. Hinz J. Role of homologous recombination in DNA interstrand crosslink repair. *Environ Mol Mutagen* 2010;51:582–603.
5. Robertson AB, Klungland A, Rognes T, Leiros I. DNA repair in mammalian cells: base excision repair: the long and short of it. *Cell Mol Life Sci* 2009;66:981–93.

6. Almeida K, Sobol R. A unified view of base excision repair: lesion-dependent protein complexes regulated by post-translational modification. *DNA Repair (Amst)* 2007;6:695–711.
7. Li X, Heyer W. Homologous recombination in DNA repair and DNA damage tolerance. *Cell Res* 2008;18:99–113.
8. Helleday T. Homologous recombination in cancer development, treatment and development of drug resistance. *Carcinogenesis* 2010;31:955–60.
9. Mukhopadhyay A, Elattar A, Cerbinskaite A, Wilkinson SJ, Drew Y, Kyle S, *et al.* Development of a functional assay for homologous recombination status in primary cultures of epithelial ovarian tumor and correlation with sensitivity to poly(ADP-ribose) polymerase inhibitors. *Clin Cancer Res* 2010;16:2344–51.
10. Hennessy BT, Timms KM, Carey MS, Gutin A, Meyer LA, Flake DD 2nd, *et al.* Somatic mutations in *BRCA1* and *BRCA2* could expand the number of patients that benefit from poly (ADP ribose) polymerase inhibitors in ovarian cancer. *J Clin Oncol* 2010;28:3570–6.
11. Cass I, Baldwin RL, Varkey T, Moslehi R, Narod SA, Karlan BY. Improved survival in women with *BRCA*-associated ovarian carcinoma. *Cancer* 2003;97:2187–95.
12. Turner N, Tutt A, Ashworth A. Hallmarks of 'BRCAness' in sporadic cancers. *Nat Rev Cancer* 2004;4:814–19.
13. Evers B, Helleday T, Jonkers J. Targeting homologous recombination repair defects in cancer. *Trends Pharmacol Sci* 2010;31:372–80.
14. Ashworth A. A synthetic lethal therapeutic approach: poly(ADP) ribose polymerase inhibitors for the treatment of cancers deficient in DNA double-strand break repair. *J Clin Oncol* 2008;26:3785–90.
15. Plummer R, Jones C, Middleton M, Wilson R, Evans J, Olsen A, *et al.* Phase I study of the poly (ADP-ribose) polymerase inhibitor, AG014699, in combination with Temozolamide in patients with advanced solid tumours. *Clin Cancer Res* 2008;14:7917–23.
16. Bryant HE, Schultz N, Thomas HD, Parker KM, Flower D, Lopez E, *et al.* Specific killing of *BRCA2*-deficient tumours with inhibitors of poly(ADP-ribose) polymerase. *Nature* 2005;434:913–17.
17. Farmer H, McCabe N, Lord CJ, Tutt AN, Johnson DA, Richardson TB, *et al.* Targeting the DNA repair defect in *BRCA* mutant cells as a therapeutic strategy. *Nature* 2005;434:917–21.
18. Drew Y, Mulligan EA, Vong WT, Thomas HD, Kahn S, Kyle S, *et al.* Therapeutic potential of PARP inhibitor AG014699 in human cancer with mutated or methylated *BRCA1* or *BRCA2*. *J Natl Cancer Inst* 2011;103:334–46.
19. Bast R, Mills G. Personalizing therapy for ovarian cancer: BRCAness and beyond. *J Clin Oncol* 2010;28:3545–8.
20. Pierce AJ, Johnson RD, Thompson LH, Jasin M. XRCC3 promotes homology-directed repair of DNA damage in mammalian cells. *Genes Dev* 1999;13:2633–8.
21. Konstantinopoulos PA, Spentzos D, Karlan BY, Taniguchi T, Fountzilas E, Francoeur N, *et al.* Gene expression profile of BRCAness that correlates with responsiveness to chemotherapy and with outcome in patients with epithelial ovarian cancer. *J Clin Oncol* 2010;28:3555–61.

7

Chapter 7

The future of PARP inhibitors in the treatment of cancer

Yvette Drew, Timothy A Yap and Stan B Kaye

Introduction

A better understanding of the molecular biology of cancer is leading to the identification of distinct cancer sub-types, new anti-cancer targets and more individualised treatment approaches.[1] Since the discovery of the first polyadenosine diphosphate-ribose polymerase (PARP) enzyme over 40 years ago,[2] the abundant nuclear enzyme has emerged as an important novel target in cancer therapy. PARP-1 is activated by DNA damage and plays a crucial role in the repair of DNA single-strand breaks (SSBs) via the base excision repair (BER) pathway.[3] Inhibitors of PARP-1 have been shown to enhance the cytotoxic effects of ionising radiation and DNA-damaging chemotherapeutic agents.[4] In addition, pre-clinical data and early-phase clinical trial results suggest that PARP inhibitors can be used as *single* agents to selectively kill cancers defective in DNA repair pathways, specifically cancers with mutations in the tumour suppressor genes *BRCA1* and *BRCA2*.[5–9] Germline mutations in either *BRCA1* or *BRCA2* result in defective homologous recombination (HR) DNA double-strand break (DSB) repair and are associated with a high lifetime risk of breast and ovarian cancer.[10] Synthetic lethality is defined as the lethal effect of inactivating two enzymes or pathways when inactivation of either enzyme or pathway alone is non-lethal.[11] In cells with *BRCA1/2* mutations, which are defective in HR DNA repair, PARP inhibitors can induce synthetic lethality by inactivating the BER pathway. This leads to the accumulation of DNA SSBs that during replication are converted to DSBs, which are normally repaired by the HR pathway.[12] In addition, cells lacking other components of the HR repair pathway or where the *BRCA* genes have been silenced by epigenetic changes rather than mutation have been shown to be sensitive to PARP inhibitors.[13,14] Given that a substantial proportion of sporadic cancers may harbour such defects, a wider therapeutic use for PARP inhibitors is emerging. The next challenge is how to identify patients that will benefit from these agents.

This review discusses the results of recent clinical trials of PARP inhibitors, either as single agents or in combination with chemotherapy, and considers the future role of PARP inhibitors in the treatment of cancer.

PARP enzymes

The PARP super-family has 17 members. A true PARP is an enzyme that is able to transfer ADP-ribose units from nicotinamide adenine dinucleotide (NAD^+) to acceptor proteins, including itself, resulting in the formation of multiple branched and linear poly(ADP-ribose) chains, a process known as 'poly(ADP-ribosyl)ation'.[15] PARP-1 and PARP-2 are the only members known to be activated by DNA damage and PARP-1 plays the dominant role in DNA repair.[16] The *PARP1* gene, located on chromosome 1, encodes the 113 kDa PARP-1 protein, which is expressed in all nucleated human cells except neutrophils and overexpression is reported in some cancers.[17,18] PARP-1 binds with high affinity to DNA SSBs via its zinc fingers. This binding activates the enzyme to undergo 'poly(ADP-ribosyl)ation', creating a negatively charged target at the SSB facilitating recruitment of the other enzymes required for the BER pathway.[3] In addition to BER, it is now known that PARP-1 plays a role in other DNA repair processes. For example; PARP-1 has been shown to be required for MRE11-dependent restarting of stalled replication forks, which can arise following unrepaired SSBs[19] and a role in a Ku-independent non-homologous end joining DNA DSB repair pathway.[20]

PARP-1 has also been shown to regulate gene transcription, mediate p53-regulated apoptosis and initiate necrotic cell death in response to extensive DNA damage such as that occurring after myocardial infarction, stroke and septic shock, suggesting that there may be wider clinical applications for inhibitors of PARP-1.[21]

Development of PARP inhibitors

The first PARP inhibitor, 3-aminobenzamide (3-AB), was identified in 1980 following the observation that nicotinamide and 5-methylnicotinamide competed with NAD^+ as a PARP substrate.[22] In the same year, Durkacz *et al.*[23] reported that 3-AB delayed DNA repair and enhanced the cytotoxicity of DNA methylating agents in mouse leukaemic cells, the first suggestion of PARP inhibitors as chemo-potentiators. In 2003, the first PARP-1 inhibitor, AG014699 (Pfizer GRD), entered anti-cancer clinical trials in combination with the oral monofunctional alkylating agent temozolomide.[24] Subsequent PARP inhibitor development programmes have pursued two arms of investigation: PARP inhibitors as single agents selectively killing cells with genetic defects in DNA repair pathways; and PARP inhibitors as chemo-potentiators, combining them with DNA damaging agents to inhibit the repair of DNA damage. There are currently eight PARP inhibitors in anti-cancer clinical trial development (Table 7.1).[25] The most developed programmes involve the PARP inhibitors olaparib (previously known as KU-0059436; AstraZeneca/KuDOS) and BSI-201 (Sanofi-aventis/BiPar), which entered phase III clinical trials in 2010.

PARP inhibitors and the *BRCA* story

In 2005, two papers in *Nature* reported that cells deficient in *BRCA1* and *BRCA2* were 100–1000 times more sensitive to PARP inhibitors than heterozygote or wild-type cell lines.[5,6] Bryant *et al.*[5] demonstrated reduced survival in *BRCA2*-deficient cells with the PARP inhibitors NU1025 and AG14361, both forerunners to AG014699. In the sister *Nature* paper, Farmer *et al.*[6] demonstrated sensitivity of both *BRCA1*- and *BRCA2*-deficient cell lines to two small-molecule PARP-1 inhibitors, KU0058684 and KU0058948, both forerunners to olaparib. Both groups

Table 7.1 PARP inhibitors in anti-cancer clinical trial development

Agent	Company	Clinical trial phase			Therapeutic indication	References
		I	II	III		
Olaparib (AZD2281)	AstraZeneca/KuDOS	✓	✓	✓	*BRCA*-related metastatic breast and advanced ovarian cancer, high-grade serous ovarian carcinoma; combination chemotherapy studies	6–9, 41, 46
BSI-201	BiPar/Sanofi-aventis	✓	✓	✓	Triple-negative breast cancer	43
Veliparib (ABT-888)	Abbott	✓	✓		Advanced solid tumours and *BRCA* mutation breast and ovarian cancers, metastatic melanoma, brain tumours	47–49
AG014699 (PF-01367338)	Pfizer GRD	✓	✓		Metastatic melanoma in combination with temozolomide, *BRCA*-related metastatic breast and advanced ovarian cancer	24, 44
MK-4827	Merck	✓			Advanced solid tumours, *BRCA*-related metastatic breast and advanced ovarian cancer, triple-negative breast cancer	27
INO-1001	Inotek/Genentech	✓	✓		Malignant melanoma in combination with temozolomide	45
CEP-9722	Cephalon (PA)	✓			Advanced solid tumours	
GPI 21016	Guilford/MGI/Eisai				Advanced solid tumours	

concluded that *BRCA*-deficient cells were sensitive to PARP inhibition and that PARP inhibitors could selectively kill *BRCA*-deficient cancer cells by the proposed mechanism of synthetic lethality. Clinical trials investigating PARP inhibitors as single agents in *BRCA*-mutated cancers commenced in 2005.

Pivotal phase I and II olaparib trials

The first trial to report was the pivotal phase I study of the oral PARP inhibitor olaparib.[7] The phase I study was conducted in patients with advanced solid tumours ($n=60$) and enriched for *BRCA1* or *BRCA2* mutation carriers ($n=23$). Olaparib was well tolerated in all patients, including those with germline *BRCA* mutations. Dose-limiting toxicities were myelosuppression and central nervous system adverse effects with the maximum tolerated dose (MTD) of 400 mg olaparib twice daily. PARP inhibition was confirmed in surrogate and tumour tissue, and responses were seen in a number of patients with *BRCA* mutations. No responses were observed in non-mutation carriers. The study incorporated an expansion phase that focused specifically on patients with *BRCA1/2* mutations and efficacy in a total of 50 women with ovarian cancer was recently reported, with a clinical benefit rate of 46%.[26] Olaparib was subsequently taken forward in separate phase II *BRCA*-associated breast and ovarian cancer studies. Both trials investigated response and toxicity in sequential cohorts of women, who had progressed following at least one chemotherapy regimen, treated with olaparib 400 mg or 100 mg twice daily (the lowest PARP inhibitory dose with clinical activity from the phase I trial) on a 28 day cycle. The breast cancer study recruited 54 *BRCA1* or *BRCA2* mutation carriers.[8] In the 400 mg dose group ($n=27$), an objective response rate (ORR) of 41% (11 of 27 women) was seen with a progression-free survival of 5.7 months. The response rate was lower (22%) in the 100 mg group ($n=27$). The ovarian cancer study enrolled 57 *BRCA1* or *BRCA2* mutation carriers with recurrent epithelial ovarian cancer or primary peritoneal or fallopian tube carcinoma.[9] In the 400 mg dose group ($n=33$), the ORR was 33% (11 of 33 women) and again the response rate was lower (13%) in the 100 mg group ($n=24$), suggesting that the extent of PARP inhibition may be important. The toxicity profile in both studies was acceptable, with the most common toxicities being grade 1 or 2: nausea, vomiting, fatigue and anaemia (ovarian cancer study only). The breast cancer study involved women who had been heavily pretreated with chemotherapy and the overall response rate compared well with that seen with standard chemotherapy regimens in the advanced setting (20–30%). The ovarian cancer study included women who were both platinum sensitive and resistant, and the response to olaparib was seen across the groups. It is important to note that not all women with *BRCA* mutations responded to olaparib and that these are small studies with no randomised control arms and where the two dosing cohorts were not designed to be statistically compared. Thus, as with any phase II results, confirmation is required in larger phase III trials.

These are, however, proof-of-concept studies, the first to report single-agent activity of a PARP inhibitor in breast and ovarian cancer with defective HR DNA repair through *BRCA* mutation, which is an exciting breakthrough in the treatment of cancer.

In addition to olaparib, there are a number of PARP inhibitors in development for this indication (Table 7.1). Preliminary results, presented at the 2010 annual meeting of the American Society of Clinical Oncology (ASCO 2010) of a phase I study of the Merck PARP inhibitor MK-4827 reported encouraging single-agent activity in

BRCA-mutated cancers.[27] A phase II trial investigating the single-agent activity of the PARP inhibitor AG014699 (Pfizer GRD) and a phase I trial investigating the PARP inhibitor veliparib (ABT-888; Abbott) in *BRCA*-associated breast and ovarian cancers are continuing.

A role for single-agent PARP inhibitors in sporadic cancer

BRCA1/2 mutations account for the majority of hereditary breast and ovarian cancers but this represents only 5–15% of all ovarian and breast cancer cases.[28] A key question therefore is whether single-agent PARP inhibitors can be used to treat selected patients within the larger cancer population.

There is increasing evidence that inactivation of the *BRCA* genes (for example, by promoter CpG island methylation) or other components of DNA repair pathways can occur in sporadic cancers resulting in sensitivity to PARP inhibition, a characteristic now known as 'BRCAness'.[13] Somatic *BRCA1/2* mutations have been reported in sporadic cancer including ovarian cancer.[29,30] One study published in 2008 reported epigenetic loss of *BRCA1*, *BRCA1/2* germline or somatic mutations in 37% of ovarian cancer cases.[31] Dysfunction of *BRCA1* has also been reported in basal-like breast cancers (BLBC) and triple-negative breast cancers (TNBC), which are both phenotypically similar to *BRCA1* breast cancers with estrogen receptor negativity and high nuclear grade.[32] Turner *et al.*[33] reported that BLBC has reduced *BRCA1* mRNA expression and increased expression of *ID4*, a negative regulator of *BRCA1*. *BRCA2* gene methylation is rarely reported but overexpression of the BRCA2-interacting protein EMSY can result in repression of BRCA2 function which may, although this remains uncertain, include its role in HR DNA repair. *EMSY* overexpression has been observed in 13% of breast and 17% of high-grade ovarian cancers[34] suggesting another group that may benefit from PARP inhibition. Cells lacking other components of the HR pathway such as RAD51, ATR and CHK2 are sensitive to PARP inhibitors.[35] Mutations in *ATR* and *CHK2* have been reported in a number of cancers.[36,37] Cells deficient in the phosphatase and tensin homolog (*PTEN*) gene have also been shown to be sensitive to PARP inhibitors in *in vitro* and *in vivo* models.[38] *PTEN* is commonly mutated in sporadic cancers, with the highest frequencies reported in endometrial cancer.[39]

These data suggest that there is a wider role for PARP inhibitors in the treatment of cancer and clinical studies are now under way investigating the efficacy of PARP inhibitors in the non-*BRCA*-mutated cancer populations, and these are discussed below.

PARP inhibitors and high-grade serous ovarian cancers

It has been known for some years that high-grade serous ovarian carcinomas (HGSOC) frequently harbour *BRCA1/2* dysfunction, in addition to mutated *TP53*.[40] In 2008, Press *et al.*[31] reported results of a study showing *BRCA1* or *BRCA2* mutations or epigenetic loss of *BRCA1* in 60% of HGSOC cases. In light of such evidence, Gelmon *et al.*[41] embarked on a phase II study of the PARP inhibitor olaparib in HGSOC. This phase II correlative study recruited women with *BRCA*-mutated ovarian cancer and women with unknown *BRCA* status and HGSOC as well as a small cohort of women with *BRCA*-mutated and/or triple-negative breast cancers.[41] The women received continuous olaparib dosing at 400 mg twice a day. The results, presented at ASCO 2010, showed a response rate (RECIST) of 24% in the women with HGSOC, which was similar to the RECIST response rate of 28% published for *BRCA* mutation carriers.[26] Responses were seen in women who were both platinum sensitive and resistant. The study required biopsy samples to be taken pre and post olaparib to assess *BRCA* mutation status and epigenetic changes to *BRCA1*.

Importantly, this was the first study to show single-agent PARP inhibitor activity in non-*BRCA*-mutated HGSOC, indicating that sporadic ovarian cancers due to an underlying BRCA defect could be targeted with PARP inhibitors and that accurate subclassification of these cancers is essential to guide treatment.

PARP inhibitors and basal-like, triple-negative breast cancers

Gene expression profiling has clustered breast cancer into five distinct molecular subgroups, one of which is the BLBC.[42] The majority lack expression of the estrogen receptor (ER), progesterone receptor (PR) and HER2/neu receptor. Triple-negative breast cancers by definition lack ER, PR and HER2/neu expression and make up around 15% of all breast cancers. Although the terms BLBC and TNBC are often used interchangeably, it is important to note that the overlap is not complete. As there is no universal agreement on distinguishing triple-negative BLBC from TNBC, clinical trials recruiting patients are likely to be heterogeneous for both groups.

In the phase II study previously discussed, Gelmon *et al.*[41] reported no single-agent activity with the PARP inhibitor olaparib in 15 women with TNBC and there is currently no evidence of single-agent activity in TNBC using this approach. Despite this, remarkable data were presented at ASCO 2009 of a combination trial using the PARP inhibitor BSI-201.[43] This randomised phase II study, presented in abstract form only, investigated the PARP inhibitor BSI-201 in combination with carboplatin and gemcitabine in metastatic TNBC. The study randomised 120 women to receive gemcitabine ($1000\,mg/m^2$) plus carboplatin (AUC = 2) on days 1 and 8 with or without the PARP inhibitor BSI-201 given on days 1, 4, 8 and 11 of a 21 day cycle. Preliminary data analysis showed an increased ORR (48% versus 16%; $P = 0.002$), median progression-free survival of 6.9 versus 3.3 months ($P < 0.0001$) and overall survival of 9.2 versus 5.7 months ($P = 0.0005$) with the addition of BSI-201.[43] This is a significant result in a breast cancer subgroup with limited targeted treatment options. However, what is not clear from this study is the underlying mechanism of PARP inhibitor activity. The hypothesis is that the PARP inhibitor is potentiating the chemotherapy by inhibiting repair of the chemotherapy-induced DNA damage. Interestingly, in contrast to other combination studies (discussed below), no increased toxicity was seen in the BSI-201 plus chemotherapy arm. Perhaps this was due to the intermittent dosing of the inhibitor, the lower than standard dose of carboplatin used (AUC = 2) or that the PARP inhibitor is not enhancing the chemotherapy but acting via independent mechanisms. It may even be possible that the intermittent chemotherapy, by providing exogenous DNA damage, is potentiating the PARP inhibitory properties of BSI-201. Interestingly, in early 2011 Sanofi-aventis announced that the phase III study of this combination had failed to reach its primary endpoints of improvement in progression-free survival and overall survival. The study has since been discontinued and further analysis and presentation of the results are awaited.

PARP inhibitors as chemo-potentiators

PARP inhibitors were originally developed not for single-agent use but to enhance the cytotoxicity of chemotherapy.[4] The potent tricyclic indole PARP inhibitor AG014699, developed in collaboration between Newcastle University, Cancer Research UK and Agouron Pharmaceuticals (now Pfizer GRD), was the first PARP inhibitor to enter clinical trials in cancer patients.[24] At that time there were no data to support single-agent activity so AG014699 was dosed in combination with temozolomide, a combination supported by pre-clinical data. A single-agent test dose of AG014699 was given on cycle 1 to allow safety and pharmacokinetic and pharmacodynamic evaluation. This study was driven by a pharmacodynamic endpoint, establishing a PARP inhibitory dose of 12 mg/m^2, before attempting to evaluate the MTD of the combination. No AG014699 single-agent MTD was reached and the MTD of the combination was myelosuppression. Sustained PARP inhibition was demonstrated in peripheral blood lymphocytes and tumour biopsies and this combination was taken into a phase II study in metastatic melanoma. The results, reported in 2006, demonstrated enhanced temozolomide-induced myelosuppression when combined with PARP inhibitory doses of AG014699. A 25% dose reduction in the temozolomide to 150 mg/m^2 was therefore required; with this in place, the regimen was well tolerated.[44] In addition, the study reported an increase in the response rate and median time to progression compared with historical reports of temozolomide alone. These data have yet to be confirmed in a commercial trial setting.

Since these first-in-human studies, multiple phase I/II trials using various PARP inhibitors with various chemotherapy combinations have recruited patients and some results have been reported in abstract data and are discussed here.[45–49]

A phase Ib combination study of the intravenous PARP inhibitor INO-1001 (Inotek/Genentech) and temozolomide in malignant melanoma patients reported in 2009.[45] Dose-limiting toxicities were myelosuppression and elevated transaminases but, in contrast to the AG014699 phase II study, this trial established the MTD in combination with full-dose temozolomide. No pharmacodynamic data were reported so it is not clear what degree of PARP inhibition was achieved and as only 12 patients with metastatic melanoma were treated across the dose ranges it is not possible to comment of any improved efficacy. Interestingly, since these study results were published, Genentech has suspended further recruitment to the trial and returned the rights for INO-1001 to Inotek, who are currently pursuing a role for their PARP inhibitors in retinal diseases.[25] The chemo-sensitising potential of the AstraZeneca compound olaparib is being investigated in a number of combination phase I trials, for example with carboplatin, topotecan, doxorubicin, gemcitabine or irinotecan (www.clinicaltrials.gov). A National Cancer Institute-sponsored combination study of olaparib with cisplatin and gemcitabine reported dose-limiting toxicity of myelosuppression at the first dose level explored and investigators de-escalated to establish tolerable PARP inhibitory doses of olaparib with gemcitabine 400 mg/m^2 and cisplatin 40 mg/m^2 in non-heavily pretreated patients.[46] Preliminary results from three studies of the Abbott PARP inhibitor veliparib (ABT-888) in combination with topotecan, metronomic cyclophosphamide or temozolamide have been reported. In the topotecan study, dose-limiting myelosuppression was again observed at the first dose level and the MTD established with the PARP inhibitory dose was topotecan 0.6 mg/m^2 days 1–5.[47] The cyclophosphamide–veliparib combination study did not reach MTD and activity was reported in a small number of *BRCA*-mutated ovarian and triple-negative breast cancers.[48] The temozolamide–veliparib study investigated efficacy of the combination in metastatic breast cancer and again myelosuppression was seen, resulting in a dose reduction of the PARP inhibitor.[49]

A major theme emerging from these PARP inhibitor combination studies is that enhanced normal-tissue toxicity, in particular myelosuppression, is a predictable and common problem. This increased toxicity may limit the dose and choice of chemotherapy used and thus the clinical application of these PARP inhibitor combinations.

Resistance to PARP inhibitors and platinum chemotherapy

Unravelling the molecular mechanisms that result in resistance to targeted therapies not only offers insights into the biology of tumours but also provides opportunities to modify and adapt strategies for current therapies, such as the incorporation of alternative approaches to circumvent resistance. Although the response rates to novel PARP inhibitors in selected populations are encouraging thus far, not all patients respond and most responders eventually develop resistance.[7,26] Hence, dissecting the basis of resistance to PARP inhibitors is a key step to improving outcomes with such agents. While it may seem premature to determine resistance mechanisms early in the development of these novel agents, mechanism-based resistance has frequently been found to occur with targeted therapy, as it has with chemotherapy.

Studies in cancer cell lines have demonstrated that secondary mutations in *BRCA1* or *BRCA2* genes may potentially lead to resistance to PARP inhibitors.[50–52] Secondary mutations may restore *BRCA* function and HR DNA repair in the face of PARP inhibition to maintain genomic integrity. In one study, a model for drug resistance was first developed by producing cells from the *BRCA2*-deficient cell line CAPAN-1 that were insensitive to PARP inhibitors.[50] CAPAN-1 cells are derived from a pancreatic epithelial tumour arising in a carrier of a c.6174delT *BRCA2* frameshift mutation.[53] They lack a wild-type *BRCA2* gene and the c.6174delT allele encodes a truncated protein of 2002 amino acids (approximately 224 kDa), compared with the wild-type 3418 amino acid protein (approximately 390 kDa). The mutant protein lacks two whole BRC repeats, the DNA-binding/DSS1 interaction domain (DBD) and the C-terminus, which contains the TR2 RAD51-binding domain and nuclear localisation sequences.[54,55] CAPAN-1 cells are thus unable to form damage-induced RAD51 foci and are extremely sensitive to treatment with potent PARP inhibitors since they are HR deficient.[35]

PARP inhibitor-resistant (PIR) clones developed following exposure to the potent PARP inhibitor KU0058948[6] are highly resistant (more than 1000-fold).[50] PIR clones are also cross-resistant to the DNA cross-linking agent cisplatin but not to the microtubule stabilising drug docetaxel. KU0058948 and cisplatin both exert their effects on *BRCA*-deficient cells by increasing the frequency of misrepaired DSBs in the absence of effective HR, suggesting that the resistance of PIR clones to KU0058948 might be because of restored HR. This contention was supported by the acquisition in PIR cells of the ability to form RAD51 foci after KU0058948 treatment or exposure to ionising radiation. The ability of mitomycin to cause characteristic chromosome aberrations is indicative of defective HR, and such mitomycin-induced chromosomal aberrations were frequent in CAPAN-1 cells but significantly reduced in PIR cells.[50] cDNA and genomic DNA sequencing from PIR clones revealed the presence of novel *BRCA2* alleles with deletions surrounding and incorporating the c.6174delT mutation, leading to the restoration of an open reading frame and sufficient functional BRC repeats and C-terminal domains to restore HR repair functions.

Platinum chemotherapy is a well-established strategy in the treatment of women with ovarian cancer, including those with *BRCA1* or *BRCA2* mutations. Clinical observations suggest that *BRCA1/2* mutation carriers with ovarian cancer tend to respond better to platinum therapy than those with no family history of the disease, although resistance does eventually occur.[56,57] In addition, systemic chemotherapy with the platinum salts may exert their *BRCA1/2*-selective effects through similar mechanisms to PARP inhibitors.[58] In view of these findings, the *BRCA2* gene was sequenced in tumours from women with the *BRCA2* c.6174delT mutation whose ovarian carcinomas were resistant to carboplatin chemotherapy. These studies revealed deletions in the *BRCA2* gene that restored the open reading frame,[49,51] suggesting that a specific mutation (c.6174delT) in *BRCA2* and sensitivity to therapeutics in cell lines and in patients can potentially be reversed by intragenic deletion.

These findings have since been supported by data from other studies, which reported similar results in *BRCA1* tumours.[59] However, it is not yet clear whether other *BRCA1/2* mutations can be reverted in this fashion and cause resistance to PARP inhibitors and whether this will be something seen commonly in clinical practice.

Although both resistance to platinums and resistance to PARP inhibitors may be mediated by secondary mutations that restore *BRCA* function, a more complex molecular circuitry is likely to be involved as PARP inhibitor resistance does not equate to platinum resistance per se. For example, not all women with platinum-sensitive ovarian cancer were sensitive to PARP inhibition, and anti-tumour activity was seen in platinum-resistant women in the first single-agent trial of olaparib in *BRCA1/2* mutation carriers.[26] In the overall population of 50 women (11 within the dose-escalation cohort [100–400 mg olaparib twice a day] and 39 [200 mg olaparib twice a day] in the expansion cohort), the overall clinical benefit rate (GCIG CA125 and/or RECIST response or stable disease greater than 4 months) was 46%. A post-hoc analysis was conducted in these women and a significantly higher clinical benefit rate (69.2%) was seen in those who were platinum sensitive than in those who were resistant (45.8%) or refractory (23.1%) ($P<0.05$).[26]

Although clinical experience to date is limited, it appears that the use of PARP inhibitor therapy does not preclude a subsequent treatment response. Women who have progressed on PARP inhibitor therapy do respond to subsequent chemotherapy, particularly carboplatin and paclitaxel, highlighting the fact that we do not yet fully understand the mechanisms underlying clinical resistance to PARP inhibitors and platinum chemotherapy.[60]

Conclusion and future directions

PARP-1 represents an important novel target in cancer therapy. Over the past few years, potent inhibitors of PARP have entered the clinic exploring efficacy in two cancer treatment settings. Firstly, as single agents with activity in appropriately molecularly profiled patients and, secondly, as agents 'protecting' DNA SSBs caused by cytotoxic drugs potentially overcoming tumour cell resistance and resulting in enhanced anti-tumour response. The early-phase clinical trials of single-agent olaparib have confirmed the activity seen in *in vivo* models, demonstrating response rates of 33% and 41% in *BRCA*-mutated ovarian and breast cancers, respectively. The further development of a single-agent approach in both these diseases is the subject of continuing randomised trials, in the setting of recurrent disease and as maintenance therapy.

A crucial recent development has been that, in addition to *BRCA*-mutated cancers, a role for PARP inhibitors is emerging in sporadic cancers, in particular HGSOC. In order to apply the science to the wider cancer population, validated, practical and inexpensive assays are now needed to select potential patients for PARP inhibitors.

To further develop PARP inhibitors as anti-cancer agents, we need to address many unanswered questions. For example, it is not yet known to what extent PARP must be inhibited for either chemo-potentiation or to achieve optimal single-agent activity. The first trial of this class of agents demonstrated profound PARP inhibition (>95% inhibition in blood, and somewhat less in the tumour biopsies).[24] But does more PARP enzyme inhibition equal more tumour response? In the olaparib phase II studies, discussed above, there was a marked fall-off in response with reduced dose, although the duration of exposure to the inhibitor was the same. These data do suggest that degree of inhibition is important in HR-deficient patients and, with various modes of administration, scheduling, specificity and potency of PARP-1 inhibition, it may be that not all PARP-1 inhibitors are equal. It will be interesting to see whether the response seen with olaparib is repeated across the class of inhibitors.

Another question is whether there is a role for using single-agent PARP inhibitors to prevent cancer in *BRCA* mutation carriers. Although the reported studies show that these are well tolerated, there are, as yet, no data on the long-term safety of these compounds in patients. The olaparib phase I study reported significant induction of γH2AX foci, representing DNA DSB accumulation in normal tissue (eyebrow hair follicles), following treatment.[7] If this occurs continuously over time in normal tissues, could it result in secondary DNA damage? *In vivo* experiments by Tong *et al.*[61] reported that deficiency of PARP-1 resulted in mammary carcinoma formation in female mice, suggesting that PARP-1 dysfunction in humans may in fact be a risk factor for breast cancer. Intermittent scheduling or drug holidays of PARP inhibitors may be the answer to allow normal-tissue recovery but then could this result in development of drug resistance? While PARP inhibitor-induced DNA damage can be repaired when pharmacological inhibition is removed, this suggests that there may be a danger that long-term use of a PARP inhibitor could lead to secondary harmful DNA lesions. Until this risk can in some way be quantified, their use in the adjuvant or prophylactic setting must be discouraged.

In summary, a new class of drugs has entered the stage of cancer treatment. The most exciting result to come out so far is the demonstration of single-agent PARP inhibitor activity in *BRCA*-mutated ovarian and breast cancers, with a wider role being proposed in DNA-defective sporadic tumours. This selective targeting of cancer cells defective in one DNA repair pathway by inhibiting another is a major breakthrough in the treatment of cancer. Early-phase studies have shown that these agents are well tolerated in these populations. Combining PARP inhibitors with chemotherapy to overcome resistance is a valid approach but may prove more challenging, with limitations on the chemotherapy dose and drug, in view of the increased normal-tissue toxicity seen. As with the broader application of single-agent therapy, a combination approach may also require careful patient selection to identify those most likely to benefit.

To conclude, it is only a few years since the first patient received the first-ever dose of a PARP inhibitor and it is likely that, as the clinical data mature and continuing clinical trials are reported, PARP inhibitors will become key players in the targeted treatment of cancer.

References

1. Schilsky RL. Personalized medicine in oncology: the future is now. *Nat Rev Drug Discovery* 2010;9:5:363–6.
2. Okayama H, Edson CM, Fukushima M, Ueda K, Hayaishi O. Purification and properties of poly(adenosine diphosphate ribose) synthetase. *J Biol Chem* 1977;252:7000–5.
3. Rouleau M, Patel A, Hendzel MJ, Kaufmann SH, Poirier GG. PARP inhibition: PARP1 and beyond. *Nature Rev Cancer* 2010;10:293–301.

4. Calabrese CR, Almassay R, Barton S, Batey MA, Calvert AH, Canan-Koch S, *et al.* Anticancer chemosensitization and radiosensitization by the novel poly(ADP-ribose) polymerase-1 inhibitor AG14361. *J Natl Cancer Inst* 2004;96:56–67.
5. Bryant HE, Schultz N, Thomas HD, Parker KM, Flower D, Lopez E, *et al.* Specific killing of *BRCA2*-deficient tumours with inhibitors of poly(ADP-ribose) polymerase. *Nature* 2005;434:913–17.
6. Farmer H, McCabe N, Lord CJ, Tutt AN, Johnson DA, Richardson TB, *et al.* Targeting the DNA repair defect in *BRCA* mutant cells as a therapeutic strategy. *Nature* 2005;435:917–20.
7. Fong PC, Boss DS, Yap TA, Tutt A, Wu P, Mergui-Roelvink M, *et al.* Inhibition of poly(ADP-ribose) polymerase in tumors from *BRCA* mutation carriers. *N Engl J Med* 2009;361:123–34.
8. Tutt A, Robson M, Garber JE, Domchek SM, Audeh MW, Weitzel JN, *et al.* Oral poly(ADP-ribose) polymerase inhibitor olaparib in patients with *BRCA1* or *BRCA2* mutations and advanced breast cancer: a proof-of-concept trial. *Lancet* 2010;376:235–244.
9. Audeh MW, Carmichael J, Penson RT, Friedlander M, Powell B, Bell-McGuinn KM, *et al.* Oral poly(ADP-ribose) polymerase inhibitor olaparib in patients with *BRCA1* or *BRCA2* mutations and recurrent ovarian cancer: a proof-of-concept trial. *Lancet* 2010;376:245–51.
10. Gudmundsdottir K, Ashworth A. The roles of BRCA1 and BRCA2 and associated proteins in the maintenance of genomic stability. *Oncogene* 2006;25:5864–74.
11. Kaelin WG. The concept of synthetic lethality in the context of anticancer therapy. *Nat Rev Cancer* 2005;5:689–98.
12. Helleday T, Lo J, Van Gent DC, Engelward BP. DNA double-strand break repair: from mechanistic understanding to cancer treatment. *DNA Repair* 2007;6:923–35.
13. Ashworth A. A synthetic lethal therapeutic approach: poly(ADP) ribose polymerase inhibitors for the treatment of cancers deficient in DNA double-strand break repair. *J Clin Oncol* 2008;26:3785–90.
14. Drew Y, Mulligan EA, Vong WT, Thomas HD, Kahn S, Kyle S, *et al.* Therapeutic potential of poly(ADP-ribose) polymerase inhibitor AG014699 in human cancers with mutated or methylated *BRCA1* or *BRCA2*. *J Natl Cancer Inst* 2011;103:334–46.
15. Schreiber V, Dantzer F, Ame JC, de Murcia G. Poly(ADP-ribose): novel functions for an old molecule. *Nat Rev Mol Cell Biol* 2006;7:517–28.
16. Ame JC, Rolli V, Schreiber V, Niedergang C, Apiou F, Decker P, *et al.* PARP-2, a novel mammalian DNA damage-dependent poly(ADP-ribose) polymerase. *J Biol Chem* 1999;274:17860–8.
17. Oei SL, Herzog H, Hirschkauffinann M, Schneider R, Auer B, Schweiger M. Transcriptional regulation and autoregulation of the human gene for ADP-ribosyltransferase. *Mol Cell Biochem* 1994;138:99–104.
18. Alderson T. New targets for cancer chemotherapy-poly(ADP- ribosylation) processing and polyisoprene metabolism. *Biol Rev* 1990;65:623–41.
19. Bryant HE, Petermann E, Schultz N, Jemth AS, Loseva O, Issaeva N, *et al.* PARP is activated at stalled forks to mediate Mre11-dependent replication restart and recombination. *EMBO J* 2009;28:2601–15.
20. Wang M, Wu W, Wu W, Rosidi B, Zhang L, Wang H, *et al.* PARP-1 and Ku compete for repair of the DNA double strand breaks by distinct NHEJ pathways. *Nucleic Acids Res* 2006;34:6170–82.
21. Kim MY, Zhang T, Kraus WL. Poly(ADP-ribosyl)ation by PARP-1: 'PAR-laying' NAD (+) into a nuclear signal. *Genes Dev* 2005;19:1951–67.
22. Purnell MR, Whish WJ. Novel inhibitors of poly(ADP-ribose) synthetase. *Biochem J* 1980;185:775–7.
23. Durkacz B, Omidiji O, Gray D, Shall S. (ADP-ribose) participates in DNA excision repair. *Nature* 1980;283:593–6.
24. Plummer ER, Jones C, Middleton M, Wilson R, Evans J, Olsen A, *et al.* Phase 1 study of the poly(ADP-ribose) polymerase inhibitor, AG014699, in combination with temozolomide in patients with advanced solid tumours. *Clin Cancer Res* 2008;14:7917–23.
25. Ferraris D. Evolution of poly(ADP-ribose) polymerase-1 (PARP-1) inhibitors: from concept to clinic. *J Med Chem* 2010;53:4561–84.

26. Fong PC, Yap TA, Boss DS, Carden CP, Mergui-Roelvink M, Gourley C, *et al.* Poly(ADP)-ribose polymerase inhibition: frequent durable responses in *BRCA* carrier ovarian cancer correlating with platinum-free interval. *J Clin Oncol* 2010;28:2512–19.
27. Sandhu SK, Wenham RM, Wilding G, McFadden M, Sun L, Toniatti C, *et al.* First-in-human trial of a poly(ADP-ribose) polymerase (PARP) inhibitor MK-4827 in advanced cancer patients (pts) with antitumor activity in *BRCA*-deficient and sporadic ovarian cancers. *J Clin Oncol* 2010;28(15s):abstr 3001.
28. Venkitaraman AR. Cancer susceptibility and the functions of *BRCA1* and *BRCA2*. *Cell* 2002;108:171–82.
29. Turner N, Tutt A, Ashworth A. Hallmarks of 'BRCAness' in sporadic cancers. *Nat Rev Cancer* 2004;4:814–19.
30. Hennessy B, Timms K, Carey MS, Gutin A, Broaddus R, Gonzalez-Angulo A, *et al.* Somatic *BRCA* status in ovarian tumors. *J Clin Oncol* 2010;27(15s):abstr 5528.
31. Press JZ, De Luca A, Boyd N, Young S, Troussard A, Ridge Y, *et al.* Ovarian carcinomas with genetic or epigenetic *BRCA1* have distinct molecular abnormalities. *BMC Cancer* 2008;8:17.
32. Cleator S, Heller W, Coombes RC. Triple-negative breast cancer: therapeutic options. *Lancet Oncol* 2007;8:235–44.
33. Turner NC, Reis JS, Russell AM, Springall RJ, Ryder K, Steele D, *et al.* *BRCA1* dysfunction in sporadic basal-like breast cancer. *Oncogene* 2007;26:2126–32.
34. Hughes-Davies L, Huntsman D, Ruas M, Fuks F, Bye J, Chin SF, *et al.* *EMSY* links the BRCA2 pathway to sporadic breast and ovarian cancer. *Cell* 2003;115:523–35.
35. McCabe N, Turner NC, Lord CJ, Kluzek K, Bialkowska A, Swift S, *et al.* Deficiency in the repair of DNA damage by homologous recombination and sensitivity to poly(ADP-ribose) polymerase inhibition. *Cancer Res* 2006;66:8109–15.
36. Swift M, Morrell D, Massey RB, Chase CK. Incidence of cancer in 161 families affected by ataxia-telangiectasia. *N Engl J Med* 1991;325:1831–6.
37. Miller CW, Ikezoe T, Krug U, Hofmann WK, Tavor S, Vegesna V, *et al.* Mutations of the *CHK2* gene are found in some osteosarcomas, but are rare in breast, lung, and ovarian tumors. *Genes Chromosomes Cancer* 2002;33:17–21.
38. Mendes-Pereira AM, Martin SA, Brough R, McCarthy A, Taylor JR, Kim JS, *et al.* Synthetic lethal targeting of *PTEN* mutant cells with PARP inhibitors. *EMBO Mol Med* 2009;1:315–22.
39. Salmena L, Carracedo A, Pandolfi PP. Tenets of PTEN tumor suppression. *Cell* 2008;133:403–14.
40. Bell D. Origins and molecular pathology of ovarian cancer. *Mod Pathol* 2005;18 Suppl 2:S19–32.
41. Gelmon KA, Hirte HW, Robidoux KS, Tonkin KS, Tischkowitz M, Swenerton K, *et al.* Can we define tumors that will respond to PARP inhibitors? A phase II correlative study of olaparib in advanced serous ovarian cancer and triple-negative breast cancer. *J Clin Oncol* 2010;28(15s):abstr 3002.
42. Perou CM, Sorlie T, Eisen MB, van de Rijn M, Jeffrey SS, Rees CA, *et al.* Molecular portraits of human breast tumours. *Nature* 2000;406:747–52.
43. O'Shaughnessy J, Osbourne C, Pippen J, Yoffe M, Patt D, Monaghan G, *et al.* Efficacy of BSI-201, a poly(ADP-ribose) polymerase-1 (PARP-1) inhibitor, in combination with gemcitabine/carboplatin in patients with metastatic triple-negative breast cancer (TNBC): results of a randomised phase II trial. *J Clin Oncol* 2009;27(18s):abstr 3.
44. Plummer R, Lorigan P, Evans J, Steven N, Middleton M, Wilson R, *et al.* First and final report of a phase II study of the poly(ADP-ribose) polymerase (PARP) inhibitor, AG014699, in combination with temozolomide (TMZ) in patients with metastatic malignant melanoma (MM). *J Clin Oncol* 2006;24(18s):abstr 8013.
45. Bedikian AY, Papadopoulos NE, Kim KB, Hwu WJ, Homsi J, Glass MR, *et al.* A phase 1B trial of intravenous INO-1001 plus oral temozolomide in subjects with unresectable stage III or IV melanoma. *Cancer Invest* 2009;27:756–63.
46. Giaccone G, Rajan A, Kelly RJ, Gutierrez M, Kummar S, Yancey M, *et al.* A phase I combination of olaparib (AZD2281; KU-0059436) and cisplatin (C) plus gemcitabine (G) in adults with solid tumours. *J Clin Oncol* 2010;28(15s)abstr 3027.
47. Ji JJ, Kummar S, Chen AP, Zhang Y, Putvtana R, Kinders RJ, Rubinstein L, *et al.* Pharmacodynamic response in Phase I combination study of ABT-888 and topotecan in adults with refractory solid tumors and lymphomas. *J Clin Oncol* 2010;28(15s):abstr 2514.

48. Kummar S, Chen AP, Ji JJ, Allen D, Egorin MJ, Gandara DR, *et al.* A Phase I study of ABT-888 (A) in combination with metronomic cyclophosphamide (C) in adults with refractory solid tumours and lymphomas. *J Clin Oncol* 2010;28(15s):abstr 2605.
49. Isakoff SJ, Overmoyer B, Tung NM, Gelman RS, Giranda VL, Bernhard KM, *et al.* A phase II trial of the PARP inhibitor veliparib (ABT888) and temozolomide for metastatic breast cancer. *J Clin Oncol* 2010;28(15s):abstr 1019.
50. Edwards SL, Brough R, Lord CJ, Natrajan R, Vatcheva R, Levine DA *et al.* Resistance to therapy caused by intragenic deletion in *BRCA2*. *Nature* 2008;451:1111–15.
51. Sakai W, Swisher EM, Jacquemont C, Chandramohan KP, Couch FJ, Langdon SP, *et al.* Functional restoration of BRCA2 protein by secondary *BRCA2* mutations in *BRCA2*-mutated ovarian carcinoma. *Cancer Res* 2009;69:6381–6.
52. Sakai W, Swisher EM, Karlan BY, Agarwal MK, Higgins J, Friedman C, *et al.* Secondary mutations as a mechanism of cisplatin resistance in *BRCA2*-mutated cancers. *Nature* 2008;451:1116–20.
53. Goggins M, Schutte M, Lu J, Moskaluk CA, Weinstein CL, Petersen GM, *et al.* Germline *BRCA2* gene mutations in patients with apparently sporadic pancreatic carcinomas. *Cancer Res* 1996;56:5360–4.
54. Esashi F, Galkin VE, Yu X, Egelman EH, West SC. Stabilization of RAD51 nucleoprotein filaments by the C-terminal region of *BRCA2*. *Nat Struct Mol Biol* 2007;14:468–74.
55. Spain BH, Larson CJ, Shihabuddin LS, Gage FH, Verma IM. Truncated BRCA2 is cytoplasmic: implications for cancer-linked mutations. *Proc Natl Acad Sci U S A* 1999;96:13920–5.
56. Cass I, Baldwin RL, Varkey T, Moslehi R, Narod SA, Karlan BY. Improved survival in women with *BRCA*-associated ovarian carcinoma. *Cancer* 2003;97:2187–95.
57. Tan DS, Rothermundt C, Thomas K, Bancroft E, Eeles R, Shanley S, *et al.* "BRCAness" syndrome in ovarian cancer: a case–control study describing the clinical features and outcome of patients with epithelial ovarian cancer associated with *BRCA1* and *BRCA2* mutations. *J Clin Oncol* 2008;26:5530–6.
58. Tutt AN, Lord CJ, McCabe N, Farmer H, Turner N, Martin NM, *et al.* Exploiting the DNA repair defect in *BRCA* mutant cells in the design of new therapeutic strategies for cancer. *Cold Spring Harb Symp Quant Biol* 2005;70:139–48.
59. Swisher EM, Sakai W, Karlan BY, Wurz K, Urban N, Taniguchi T. Secondary *BRCA1* mutations in *BRCA1*-mutated ovarian carcinomas with platinum resistance. *Cancer Res* 2008;68:2581–6.
60. Ang JE, Yap TA, Fong PC, Carden CP, Tan DS, Hanwell J, *et al.* Preliminary experience with the use of chemotherapy (CT) following disease progression on olaparib, a poly(ADP-Ribose) polymerase inhibitor (PARP-i) in ovarian cancer patients with germline *BRCA* mutations. *J Clin Oncol* 2010;28(15s)abstr 5041.
61. Tong WM, Yang YG, Cao WH, Galendo D, Frappart L, Shen Y, *et al.* Poly(ADP-ribose) polymerase-1 plays a role in suppressing mammary tumourigenesis in mice. *Oncogene* 2007;26:3857–67.

Section 3

Imaging and therapy: state of the art

8

Chapter 8
The role of robotics and the future

Tim Mould

Introduction

Laparoscopic surgery has become an essential part of the surgical treatment for gynaecological conditions including malignancy. It has been used widely for the treatment of early cervical and endometrial cancer, and for staging in gynaecological cancers. Despite the advantages and advances of laparoscopic surgery, a number of limitations exist. These include difficulties in manipulating the camera, the two-dimensional view, the constraints of straight instruments, physical problems for the surgeon and the difficulties for trainees in learning the technique.

Robotically assisted laparoscopic surgery has the capacity to overcome the limitations of conventional laparoscopic surgery and it could enable future development of more advanced surgery with less morbidity. Initial case series show robotically assisted surgery to be as effective as conventional laparoscopic surgery, if more expensive. However, randomised studies and studies demonstrating survival data are lacking.

This chapter describes the use of conventional laparoscopic surgery in gynaecological cancer, the advantages and disadvantages of robotic surgery, and the feasibility and outcomes of the use of robotics in gynaecological cancer surgery. The final section looks at future developments.

Conventional laparoscopic surgery in gynaecological malignancy

Conventional laparoscopic surgery has been widely used for total laparoscopic hysterectomy and laparoscopically assisted vaginal hysterectomy for the treatment of endometrial cancer, and for laparoscopic radical hysterectomy for the treatment of cervical cancer.

Two large randomised controlled studies have looked at the laparoscopic treatment of endometrial cancer. The LACE trial was a two-stage randomised controlled trial that compared total laparoscopic hysterectomy with total abdominal hysterectomy for stage I endometrial cancer.[1] Quality of life was better in the laparoscopic group up to 6 months after surgery. The post-surgery adverse effects were halved in the laparoscopic group (19% versus 7.9%; $P = 0.002$). The LAP2 trial compared laparoscopy with laparotomy for comprehensive surgical staging of stage I to IIA endometrial cancer, which incorporated both pelvic and para-aortic lymphadenectomy.[2] A total of 2616 women were randomised. The conversion rate from laparoscopy to laparotomy was high at 26% but this often occurred owing to access difficuties to the para-aortic lymph nodes. Postoperative adverse effects were significantly lower in the laparoscopy group. Detection of advanced stage was the same in the two groups.

In light of these and other trials, the National Institute for Health and Clinical Excellence (NICE) has published guidance endorsing the laparoscopic treatment of endometrial cancer.[3] The meta-analysis showed that the survival and recurrence rates were similar for laparoscopic and open approaches. The postoperative complications and length of stay were lower with laparoscopic surgery.

Advantages of robotically assisted surgery

The *da Vinci*® Surgical System is the only robotic surgery device available commercially and studies reviewed in this chapter refer to this system. It has a number of features that differ from conventional laparoscopic surgery and these result in an operative platform that is inherently easier to use and on which to develop expertise. The *da Vinci* surgical robot has been developed and is marketed by Intuitive Surgical of Sunnyvale, California. The first reported procedure with the *da Vinci* system was in Belgium in 1997.[4] Since its inception, the robot has been gradually upgraded from the first three-arm system to the current four-arm, lightweight and more versatile version called the S-Type.

3-D vision

The *da Vinci* Surgical System is equipped with a three-dimensional vision system. It has a dual-lens system with two three-chip cameras spatially separated within a 12 mm casing. Hence, two complete optical systems are incorporated, representing the left and right eyes. The spatial separation of these images projected to the surgeon's eyes in the binocular viewer allows true 3-D image perception at the console.

Articulating instruments

The instruments in conventional laparoscopic surgery are rigid and provide only four degrees of motion. Furthermore, the abdominal wall adds to this a 'fulcrum effect' that reverses movements for the surgeon in laparoscopic surgery. The surgical robot provides six degrees of motion at the instrument tip and a seventh degree of freedom provided by the instrument itself (for example, grasping or cutting). Thus the robot generates a single complex movement mimicking the motion of the human wrist in open surgery.

Surgeon position and tremor

The surgeon is seated at the console in an ergonomically comfortable position with the elbows resting on a padded bar. The forehead is placed against a padded bar with eyes comfortably looking into the binocular viewer. The height and the intraocular distance can be adjusted to suit the individual surgeon. The thumb and index finger of each hand are placed in adjustable loops attached to the master controllers. Approximation of the thumb and index fingers operate the jawed instruments. The multi-joint master controller permits movement freely in all dimensions. The movement is translated from the surgeon's fingers to the tip of the surgical instruments, allowing intuitive control of the instruments and the camera. Position sensing occurs approximately 1500 times per second. During this process, any physiological tremor is eliminated by the robotic system. This allows the surgeon to conduct more precise surgical manoeuvres during surgery.

These advantages offer significant technical ease in performing complicated surgical procedures, including suturing and tying of knots by the surgeon. It provides a familiar environment similar to that of the open approach. The use of a robotic system in preset laboratory drills has been associated with faster performance times, increased accuracy, enhanced dexterity, faster suturing and reduced number of errors when compared with conventional laparoscopic instrumentation.[5]

A shorter learning curve, training and virtual reality training

The technical difficulty of conventional laparoscopic surgery is an obstacle to more widespread use of minimally invasive approaches in gynaecological oncology. However, the features of the robotic system discussed above result in a shorter learning curve in laparoscopic surgery with robotic assistance as opposed to traditional straight-stick laparoscopy. Suturing and dexterity skills can be acquired more quickly in robotic surgery than in conventional laparoscopy.[6,7] Seamon *et al.*[8] demonstrated that the learning curve for endometrial cancer staging with the robot platform required only 20 cases to reach an efficient standard, which was shorter than that with conventional laparoscopic surgery. Although there was a lack of data for the learning curve of robotic surgery in radical hysterectomy, all investigators who assessed the feasibility of robotic radical hysterectomy compared with laparotomy reported acceptable surgical outcomes in their initial experiences with the robotic system.

Robotic surgery is well suited to virtual reality training as the operation is computer guided. 3-D virtual reality images can be projected into the console of the robot. A number of virtual reality training simulators have been created.

Disadvantages of robotic surgery

Cost

Robotically assisted surgery is more expensive than conventional laparoscopy, which is the main reason preventing its more widespread use. However, because of the reduced length of stay achieved by the minimal access approach, it is not more expensive than open surgery. The cost to install the *da Vinci* robotic platform in an institution ranges from $1,000,000 to $1,500,000 and there is a 10% annual maintenance fee. The articulating robotic instruments cost $250 each and they can only be used ten times. Other costs include increased length of time of surgery during the learning curve, and the additional time involved in setting up the robot.

Sarlos *et al.*[9] conducted a prospective matched case–control study of 40 robotic and 40 laparoscopic hysterectomies for benign indications. The average cost of the robotic cases was €4,067 compared with €2,151 for the conventional laparoscopic cases. A retrospective study of endometrial cancer treatment in 33 women used operating room time, instrument use, disposable item use and length of hospital stay to calculate costs. Total hospital costs were higher for robotic surgery, at $5,084 versus $3,615 ($P$=0.002).[10]

A study examining all published articles since 2005 relating to cost in robot-assisted surgery across 20 different procedures including hysterectomy estimated that the increase in cost was 6% with robotically assisted surgery compared with conventional laparoscopy.[11] According to a report by Bell *et al*,[12] total average cost, including hospital charges, for endometrial cancer staging surgery with laparotomy, conventional laparoscopy and robot-assisted laparoscopy were approximately $13,000, $7,600 and $8,200, respectively.

The cost for surgical treatment differs according to whether a hospital uses the laparoscopic or laparotomy approach, the medical insurance system, the volume of cases and the culture of the country. Many cost analyses do not include indirect costs such as the cost of the hospital bed. If use of the robot reduces the length of hospital stay, then the cost may be competitive. Thus hospitals that use the open laparotomy approach, and that may be able to train more easily to a laparoscopic approach with robotic assistance, are the most likely to have competitive costing with a robot.

Tactile feel and size of ports

The robotic system removes any tactile feedback from the instruments. This is a change from conventional laparoscopy and should be viewed as a disadvantage. However, it has not been demonstrated to reduce the safety or effectiveness of robotically assisted surgery.

Robotic surgery requires 8 mm ports for the instruments compared with 5 mm ports in conventional laparoscopic staging surgery. Trocar site herniation develops more frequently when 10 mm ports or larger are used and is rare with ports smaller than 10 mm, ranging from 0 to 0.09%.[13] Seamon *et al.*[14] reported a case of small bowel evisceration through an 8 mm robotic port site after endometrial cancer staging surgery.

While no published evidence could be found, it would be expected that larger sized ports would cause aggravated postoperative pain and produce poorer cosmetic results. In principle, port sizes should be kept as small as possible to reduce complication rates. As robotically assisted surgery requires an increase in port size, this should be viewed as a potential disadvantage.

Feasibility and outcomes in gynaecological oncology surgery

The feasibility of robotically assisted surgery has been demonstrated by numerous case series. Unlike the case with conventional laparoscopy, randomised trials are lacking in assessing the outcomes of robotically assisted surgery.

Sert and Eraker[15] reported on 125 gynaecological oncology procedures performed robotically in 53 women. The operations included radical hysterectomy, pelvic and para-aortic node dissection, and omentectomy. There were no conversions to laparoscopy or laparotomy and no complications.

Cervical cancer

Geisler *et al.*[16] compared the first 30 cases of robotic radical hysterectomy in their institution to the previous 30 cases of open radical hysterectomy. The cases were similar in terms of patient characteristics. There were no significant differences in complications, length of operation, or nodal yield and margins. Blood loss was less in the robotic cases. Interestingly, hospital stay was similar in both groups, with the mean length of stay being 2.8 days for the open cases.

Boggess *et al.*[17] conducted a case–control study of robotically assisted laparoscopic radical hysterectomy compared with the open laparotomy approach. This study found that robotically assisted laparoscopic radical hysterectomy was superior to open radical hysterectomy with regard to blood loss, operative time, hospital stay and lymph node retrieval. In another study, Lowe *et al.*[18] reported the experience of a multi-institution consortium that consisted of five gynaecological oncologists in distinct geographical regions of the USA for radical hysterectomy using the *da Vinci* robotic platform. The study comprised 42 women who underwent a type II or III robotic radical hysterectomy. Robotically assisted laparoscopic type II/III radical hysterectomy was associated with a shortened hospital stay, few operative complications, acceptable lymph node yields, and acceptable operative times.

A phase III randomised clinical trial comparing laparoscopic or robotically assisted radical hysterectomy with abdominal radical hysterectomy in women with early-stage cervical cancer is currently being conducted under the auspices of the American Association of Gynecologic Laparoscopists (AAGL).[19]

Endometrial cancer

Several authors have reported that robotically assisted staging surgery in endometrial cancer is comparable to conventional laparoscopic and open laparotomy approaches in terms of surgical outcomes.[20–26] However, there are no randomised studies and no reports concerning survival.

Obese women and endometrial cancer

Gehrig *et al.*[27] conducted a comparative study to examine which is the optimal minimally invasive surgical approach between conventional laparoscopy and robotically assisted surgery for obese women with endometrial cancer. The authors reported that robotically assisted surgery was associated with shorter operative time, less blood loss, increased number of resected lymph nodes and shorter hospital stay compared with traditional laparoscopy.

Seamon *et al.*[28] performed a comparative study to compare outcomes between robotic and laparoscopic staging for endometrial cancer in obese women. The authors reported that robotic staging surgery for endometrial carcinoma in heavier women resulted in shorter operation times, shorter hospital stays, lower transfusion rates and less frequent conversion to laparotomy when compared with conventional laparoscopic staging.

Staging procedures

In a prospective study of 109 women requiring surgical staging for endometrial cancer, Jung *et al.*[29] compared laparotomy, laparoscopy and robotic operative outcomes. The number of pelvic lymph nodes removed was equal for open and robotic surgery but lower for laparoscopy. The number of resected para-aortic nodes and the operative time was the same for all three groups. Hospital stay, operative complications and transfusions were worse in the laparotomy group.

A retrospective series by Cardenas-Goicoechea *et al.*[30] reviewed 102 robotic cases and 173 laparoscopic cases of women undergoing surgical staging for endometrial cancers. There was no significant difference in major complications, and the operative time was longer but blood loss was less in the robotic group. Time to discharge and reoperation rates were not significantly different.

Feasibility trials have been published for retroperitoneal para-aortic nodal staging in cervical cancer and transperitoneal para-aortic nodal staging in ovarian cancer but no survival outcomes have been reported.[31,32]

Exenterative surgery

Pruthi *et al.*[33] described the technique of robotically assisted laparoscopic anterior pelvic exenteration performed in 12 women for clinically localised bladder cancer. Nine women underwent ileal conduit diversion and three underwent an orthotopic neobladder construction. In all cases, the urinary diversion was performed extracorporeally. The mean operating room time was 4.6 hours, the mean surgical blood loss was 221 ml and the mean time to discharge was 4.8 days. There were two postoperative complications (17%) in two women. Davis *et al.*[34] presented a further two cases of robotically assisted laparoscopic anterior pelvic exenteration with acceptable operative, pathological and short-term clinical outcomes.

Survival data were not presented in these papers and thus they should be viewed as feasibility studies only. More experience is required to adequately evaluate and validate these procedures as appropriate surgical and oncological options.

Survival

Studies concerning long-term survival in women with gynaecological cancers who have undergone robotically assisted laparoscopic surgery are limited. The effectiveness of robotic surgery compared with other approaches needs to be supported by prospectively designed multicentre studies, as have been performed in conventional laparoscopy.

Some retrospective evidence concerning survival exists. Cantrell *et al.*[35] conducted a retrospective analysis to demonstrate progression-free survival (PFS) and overall survival (OS) for women with cervical cancer undergoing robotic radical hysterectomy. Survival data for 71 women were compared with a group of historical open radical hysterectomies. Analysis at 3 years showed no statistical difference in PFS or OS between the robotic and historical groups. A phase III randomised clinical trial comparing laparoscopic or robotically assisted surgery in women with early-stage cervical cancer is under way.[19]

The future

Decreasing costs

It is arguable that the advantages of robotically assisted surgery outweigh the disadvantages, if cost is removed from the equation. The capital outlay for the system, plus its operating cost, prevents increased numbers of systems being used across the world. Despite this, more than 1000 systems have now been set up, with the majority of them being in the USA. The number of robotically assisted operations increased from 80 000 in 2007 to 205 000 in 2009.[11]

It is expected that the number of systems and operations will continue to increase. It is hoped that the cost will decrease as the number of users increase. However, with only one company producing a robotic system, there is no competition to drive down prices. If costs decrease, it would be expected that the numbers of systems will increase dramatically. This would allow systems to be integrated into minimally invasive operating theatres, rather than be standalone systems as at present.

Prospective randomised trials

There are many case series looking at surgical outcomes with robotic surgery. They confirm the feasibility of the technique and show that surgical outcomes are as good as or better than the laparotomy or conventional laparoscopic approaches. However, the most important outcome in oncology is survival and this has not been studied in anything other than a limited number of case–control studies.

Prospective randomised studies are required to demonstrated survival at least as good as open or conventional laparoscopy approaches before robotically assisted gynaecological oncology surgery can be widely adopted. In view of the potential increase in costs with robotic surgery, improved survival figures may be required. However, the survival rates in early endometrial and cervical cancers are high in any case, and it is likely that studies will show comparable survival figures rather than improvements.

Single-port laparoscopic surgery

Single-port laparoscopic surgery (SPLS) uses a 3 cm umbilical port with a number of channels through which the necessary instruments are passed. As the instruments all pass through a central port, articulated instruments are more effective for this technique than traditional straight instruments. Thus, robotically assisted surgery is ideal for use in SPLS. There are possible advantages of SPLS in gynaecology. Firstly, operative complications related to trocar insertion such as epigastric vessel injury, visceral organ herniation, wound infection and visceral organ damage might be reduced by eliminating the need for ancillary ports. Secondly, postoperative pain, which results from skin incision and from penetrating muscle and fascia with the trocar, might be reduced. Thirdly, a better cosmetic result may be obtained. Fourthly, resected specimens can be more easily extracted through the larger umbilical incision of the SPLS than that of conventional ports.

However, there is no literature which examines the potential benefits of SPLS in gynaecology compared with the conventional laparoscopic approach. Therefore, the advantages of a single-port approach compared with conventional laparoscopic ports should be evaluated in a randomised prospective study.

Fusion of imaging

The latest S-Type system is able to show magnetic resonance imaging (MRI) and computed tomography (CT) images on the console. This is likely to be expanded to include any relevant information that may be needed during surgery.

Telerobotic surgery

The capacity for remote surgery using robotic assistance is exciting, although there are as yet no substantial reports concerning this. The speed and reliability of the connection between the console and the robot is critical. Communication with the surgical assistant beside the patient is a potential problem. When these issues are overcome, telerobotic surgery could be used in many remote or hostile arenas.

Summary

Laparoscopic treatment for early cervical and endometrial cancers plus staging is common. In the case of endometrial cancer, randomised trials show significant advantages for laparoscopic surgery. The difficulties associated with conventional laparoscopic surgery can be overcome with robotic assistance, which may enable increased use of minimal access surgical approaches in gynaecological oncology operations. The cost of the operating platform remains a significant disadvantage that impedes its wider use. Cost increases are less where a hospital could change an open laparotomy approach to a laparoscopic approach using robotic assistance. The effectiveness in terms of surgical outcomes has been demonstrated in gynaecological oncology by numerous case series. However, there are no studies looking at survival outcomes and no prospective randomised studies to demonstrate survival. As survival in early-stage cancers will in any case be high, studies will need to be multicentre to achieve the required numbers. A phase III randomised clinical trial comparing laparoscopic with robotically assisted surgery in women with early-stage cervical cancer is under way.

References

1. Janda M, Gebski V, Brand A, Hogg R, Jobling TW, Land R, *et al.* Quality of life after total laparoscopic hysterectomy versus total abdominal hysterectomy for stage I endometrial cancer (LACE): a randomised trial. *Lancet Oncol* 2010;11:772–80.
2. Walker JL, Piedmonte MR, Spirtos NM, Eisenkop SM, Schlaerth JB, Mannel RS, *et al.* Laparoscopy compared with laparotomy for comprehensive surgical staging of uterine cancer: Gynecologic Oncology Group Study LAP2. *J Clin Oncol* 2009;27:5331–6.
3. National Institute for Health and Clinical Excellence. *Laparoscopic Hysterectomy (including Laparoscopic Total Hysterectomy and Laparoscopically Assisted Vaginal Hysterectomy) for Endometrial Cancer.* London: NICE; 2010 [guidance.nice.org.uk/IPG356].
4. Himpens J, Lemans G, Cadiere GB. Telesurgical laparoscopic cholecystectomy. *Surg Endosc* 1998;12:1091.
5. Magrina JF. Robotic surgery in gynecology. *Eur J Gynaecol Oncol* 2007;28:77–82.
6. Yohannes P, Rotariu P, Pinto P, Smith AD, Lee BR. Comparison of robotic versus laparoscopic skills: is there a difference in the learning curve? *Urology* 2002;60:39–45.
7. Hernandez JD, Bann SD, Munz Y, Moorthy K, Datta V, Martin S, *et al.* Qualitative and quantitative analysis of the learning curve of a simulated surgical task on the da Vinci system. *Surg Endosc* 2004;18372–8.
8. Seamon LG, Fowler JM, Richardson DL, Carlson MJ, Valmadre S, Phillips GS, *et al.* A detailed analysis of the learning curve: robotic hysterectomy and pelvic-aortic lymphadenectomy for endometrial cancer. *Gynecol Oncol.* 2009;114:162–7.
9. Sarlos D, Kots L, Stevanovic N, Schaer G. Robotic hysterectomy versus conventional laparoscopic hysterectomy: outcome and cost analyses of a matched case–control study. *Eur J Obstet Gynecol Reprod Biol* 2010;150:92–6.
10. Holtz DO, Miroshnichenko G, Finnegan MO, Chernick M, Dunton CJ. Endometrial cancer surgery costs: robot vs laparoscopy. *J Minim Invasive Gynecol* 2010;17:500–3.
11. Barbash G, Glied S. New technology and health care costs: the case of robot-assisted surgery. *N Engl J Med* 2010;363:701–3.
12. Bell MC, Torgerson J, Seshadri-Kreaden U, Suttle AW, Hunt S. Comparison of outcomes and cost for endometrial cancer staging via traditional laparotomy, standard laparoscopy and robotic techniques. *Gynecol Oncol* 2008;111:407–11.
13. Tonouchi H, Ohmori Y, Kobayashi M, Kusunoki M. Trocar site hernia. *Arch Surg* 2004;139:1248–56.
14. Seamon LG, Backes F, Resnick K, Cohn DE. Robotic trocar site small bowel evisceration after gynecologic cancer surgery. *Obstet Gynecol* 2008;112:462–4.
15. Sert MB, Eraker R. Robot-assisted laparoscopic surgery in gynaecological oncology; initial experience at Oslo Radium Hospital and 16 months follow-up. *Int J Med Robot* 2009;5:410–14.
16. Geisler JP, Orr CJ, Khurshid N, Phibbs G, Manahan KJ. Robotically assisted laparoscopic radical hysterectomy compared with open radical hysterectomy. *Int J Gynecol Cancer* 2010;20:438–42.
17. Boggess JF, Gehrig PA, Cantrell L, Shafer A, Ridgway M, Skinner EN, *et al.* A case–control study of robot-assisted type III radical hysterectomy with pelvic lymph node dissection compared with open radical hysterectomy. *Am J Obstet Gynecol* 2008;199:357.e1–7.
18. Lowe MP, Chamberlain DH, Kamelle SA, Johnson PR, Tillmanns TD. A multi-institutional experience with robotic-assisted radical hysterectomy for early stage cervical cancer. *Gynecol Oncol* 2009;113:191–4.

19. Obermair A, Gebski V, Frumovitz M, Soliman PT, Schmeler KM, Levenback C, *et al.* A phase III randomized clinical trial comparing laparoscopic or robotic radical hysterectomy with abdominal radical hysterectomy in patients with early stage cervical cancer. *J Minim Invasive Gynecol* 2008;15:584–8.
20. Boggess JF, Gehrig PA, Cantrell L, Shafer A, Ridgway M, Skinner EN, *et al.* A comparative study of 3 surgical methods for hysterectomy with staging for endometrial cancer: robotic assistance, laparoscopy, laparotomy. *Am J Obstet Gynecol* 2008;199:360–9.
21. DeNardis SA, Holloway RW, Bigsby GE, Pikaart DP, Ahmad S, Finkler NJ. Robotically assisted laparoscopic hysterectomy versus total abdominal hysterectomy and lymphadenectomy for endometrial cancer. *Gynecol Oncol* 2008;111:412–17.
22. Lowe MP, Johnson PR, Kamelle SA, Kumar S, Chamberlain DH, Tillmanns TD. A multi-institutional experience with robotic-assisted hysterectomy with staging for endometrial cancer. *Obstet Gynecol* 2009;114:236–43.
23. Peiretti M, Zanagnolo V, Bocciolone L, Landoni F, Colombo N, Minig L, *et al.* Robotic surgery: changing the surgical approach for endometrial cancer in a referral cancer center. *J Minim Invasive Gynecol* 2009;16:427–31.
24. Seamon LG, Cohn DE, Henretta MS, Kim KH, Carlson MJ, Phillips GS, *et al.* Minimally invasive comprehensive surgical staging for endometrial cancer: robotics or laparoscopy? *Gynecol Oncol* 2009;113:36–41.
25. Seamon LG, Cohn DE, Richardson DL, Valmadre S, Carlson MJ, Phillips GS, *et al.* Robotic hysterectomy and pelvic-aortic lymphadenectomy for endometrial cancer. *Obstet Gynecol* 2008;112:1207–13.
26. Veljovich DS, Paley PJ, Drescher CW, Everett EN, Shah C, Peters WA. Robotic surgery in gynecologic oncology: program initiation and outcomes after the first year with comparison with laparotomy for endometrial cancer staging. *Am J Obstet Gynecol* 2008;198:679.e1–9; discussion 679.e9-1.
27. Gehrig PA, Cantrell LA, Shafer A, Abaid LN, Mendivil A, Boggess JF. What is the optimal minimally invasive surgical procedure for endometrial cancer staging in the obese and morbidly obese woman? *Gynecol Oncol* 2008;111:41–5.
28. Seamon LG, Bryant SA, Rheaume PS, Kimball KJ, Huh WK, Fowler JM, *et al.* Comprehensive surgical staging for endometrial cancer in obese patients: comparing robotics and laparotomy. *Obstet Gynecol* 2009;114:16–21.
29. Jung YW, Lee DW, Kim SW, Nam EJ, Kim JH, Kim JW, *et al.* Robot-assisted staging using three robotic arms for endometrial cancer: comparison to laparoscopy and laparotomy at a single institution. *J Surg Oncol* 2010;101:116–21.
30. Cardenas-Goicoechea J, Adams S, Bhat SB, Randall TC. Surgical outcomes of robotic-assisted surgical staging for endometrial cancer are equivalent to traditional laparoscopic staging at a minimally invasive surgical center. *Gynecol Oncol* 2010;117:224–8.
31. Querleu D, Dargent D, Ansquer Y, Leblanc E, Narducci F. Extraperitoneal endosurgical aortic and common iliac dissection in the staging of bulky or advanced cervical carcinomas. *Cancer* 2000;88:1883–91.
32. Magrina JF, Long JB, Kho RM, Giles DL, Montero RP, Magtibay PM. Robotic transperitoneal infrarenal aortic lymphadenectomy: technique and results. *Int J Gynecol Cancer* 2010;20:184–7.
33. Pruthi RS, Stefaniak H, Hubbard JS, Wallen EM. Robotic-assisted laparoscopic anterior pelvic exenteration for bladder cancer in the female patient. *J Endourol* 2008;22:2397–402; discussion 2402.
34. Davis MA, Adams S, Eun D, Lee D, Randall TC. Robotic-assisted laparoscopic exenteration in recurrent cervical cancer. Robotics improved the surgical experience for 2 women with recurrent cervical cancer. *Am J Obstet Gynecol* 2010;202:663.e1.
35. Cantrell LA, Mendivil A, Gehrig PA, Boggess JF. Survival outcomes for women undergoing type III robotic radical hysterectomy for cervical cancer: a 3-year experience. *Gynecol Oncol* 2010;117:260–5.

Chapter 9
'Ultra-radical' surgery in advanced ovarian cancer

Oliver Zivanovic and Dennis S Chi

Introduction

Over the past four decades, increased understanding of the pathophysiology and behaviour of gynaecological peritoneal surface malignancies has led to significant advances in effective treatment modalities. Numerous studies have shown that surgical cytoreduction of all visible tumour in the peritoneal cavity plays a crucial role in optimising survival from these diseases. Consequently, the surgical management of advanced ovarian, primary peritoneal and fallopian tube cancers has evolved from basic gynaecological oncology procedures (hysterectomy, salpingo-oophorectomy, omentectomy, and pelvic and para-aortic lymph node dissection) to the incorporation of more comprehensive surgical cytoreductive procedures as part of a maximal surgical effort. These extensive procedures often target peritoneal surfaces that involve multiple 'non-gynaecological' organs and sites such as the small intestine, colon, diaphragm, liver, porta hepatis, gall bladder, spleen, pancreas, stomach, coeliac axis, mediastinal lymph nodes and pleural cavity.

Individually, each of the procedures used in a maximal cytoreductive effort are performed by surgeons throughout the world. However, the performance of many if not all of the various upper abdominal and pelvic procedures in women with gynaecological malignancies is not necessarily done nor accepted internationally, and hence some refer to the combination of these procedures in individual women for cytoreductive purposes as 'ultra-radical'. Unquestionably, these procedures require detailed knowledge of upper abdominal anatomy not generally taught in gynaecological oncology training programmes. Consequently, there is a potential for 'non-gynaecological' perioperative complications in addition to those that may be encountered in more standard gynaecological oncology surgery. Anticipating, avoiding and adequately managing the perioperative complications allows for timely initiation of combination platinum-based chemotherapy, which is a critical component of standard initial therapy. The advanced operative approach to women with gynaecological peritoneal surface malignancies and the understanding, anticipation and management of perioperative complications represent cornerstones of surgical management. This chapter provides an outline for the rationale and implementation of a comprehensive cytoreductive surgical approach in advanced ovarian cancer.

Surgical resection of advanced ovarian cancer

The clinical course of women with advanced stage epithelial ovarian cancer can be characterised by clinical remission after primary cytoreductive surgery and postoperative chemotherapy, followed by disease recurrence in the majority. Surgical cytoreduction and platinum-based chemotherapy have improved the median overall survival from 1 year in 1975 (stages II and III) to approximately 5 years in 2005 (optimally debulked stage III).[1,2] The long-term cure rates, however, languish between 20% and 30%.[2,3] The most important prognostic factors are primary surgical outcome and the response to postoperative chemotherapy. Surgical cytoreduction (also called tumour debulking) of advanced stage ovarian cancer is defined as an attempt to maximally resect all visible and palpable disease. As tumour debulking is also used in patients with advanced fallopian tube and peritoneal carcinomas with similar results, references to advanced ovarian cancer in this chapter include these other two primary disease sites as well. Although the approach of cytoreduction of the primary site as well as of metastatic implants is a rare surgical strategy in the field of surgical oncology (and is not applicable for the majority of other solid tumours), there is a large body of evidence demonstrating a survival benefit for women with ovarian cancer who are left with minimal ('optimal') disease after the surgical procedure. It has been known for more than 30 years that women with advanced ovarian cancer who initiate systemic chemotherapy with an apparent smaller volume of residual disease after primary surgery experience a superior outcome compared with those who have larger disease volume after initial surgery.[1]

Multiple retrospective studies, pooled exploratory analyses and meta-analyses have demonstrated that the amount of residual disease after cytoreductive surgery inversely correlates with progression-free survival (PFS) and overall survival (OS).[4–14] Although the benefit of surgical cytoreduction has not yet been prospectively established through a prospective phase III trial (surgery plus chemotherapy versus chemotherapy alone), cytoreductive surgery with the goal of achieving minimal residual disease in combination with platinum- and taxane-based chemotherapy is currently the accepted standard management. The removal of large malignant masses substantially increases the likelihood that effective concentrations of active cytotoxic agents will be delivered to residual cancer populations. Furthermore, intraperitoneal cytotoxic agents directly penetrate to a depth of only a few millimetres beneath the tumour surface. Consequently, those whose tumours are cytoreduced to small-volume disease (≤ 1 cm) can be expected to benefit most from this approach, while those left with bulkier tumour masses may not. A further rationale for surgical cytoreduction is that it allows for the removal of cancer deposits from specific locations such as those causing partial bowel obstruction, which will lead to an improvement in the woman's nutritional and immunological status, and consequently have a positive effect on the overall tolerability to subsequent cytotoxic therapy.[15]

Residual disease

Residual disease is defined as the maximum diameter of the largest tumour mass measured in centimetres remaining after cytoreductive surgery. For ovarian cancer, the term 'optimal' residual disease refers to a threshold below which patients are thought to have a survival benefit. This threshold has decreased over the past three decades, with variably defined cut-off values of 3 cm down to 0 cm being advocated as the 'optimal' goal of primary cytoreduction.[5,12–14]

Advances in operative technology have allowed surgeons to maximise cytoreductive effort in women with bulky advanced stage (IIIC and IV) ovarian cancer, enabling them to remove all visible disease in a growing subset of patients. In light of these advances, many investigators propose defining optimal cytoreduction as cytoreduction to no gross residual disease.[5,12–14] However, there is controversy as to how much surgical effort should be undertaken to achieve optimal residual disease status before reaching the point of subjecting the woman to the potential excessive additional morbidity associated with a surgical procedure that will not clearly result in a significant survival benefit.[15,16]

Published data have demonstrated that if cytoreductive surgery is performed by physicians with training in gynaecological oncology then a survival advantage can be achieved when compared with surgery performed by general surgeons or generalist gynecologists. However, despite that knowledge, the actual reported percentage of women with advanced ovarian cancer whose tumours are optimally cytoreduced varies widely, from 15% to more than 85%.[17] While this wide variation can partially be explained by the variable cut-off values used by the authors for 'optimal' cytoreduction as well as the inconsistent inclusion or exclusion criteria for patients with advanced disease offered primary cytoreduction, it is also due to variable surgical philosophy, practice, training and effort. Reports of optimal cytoreduction rates above 50% generally include a substantial number of women who have undergone intestinal tract surgery and extensive upper abdominal procedures to attain optimal residual status.[18–20]

While the best exact cut-off point for 'optimal' versus 'suboptimal' cytoreduction still remains somewhat controversial, a consistent point demonstrated by studies by the Gynecologic Oncology Group (GOG) and others is that women left with residual disease of 1–2 cm do not derive a survival benefit from primary cytoreductive surgery.[5,9,11–14] Thus, those who undergo suboptimal cytoreduction sustain the morbidity of a cytoreductive attempt without the associated survival benefit.

In an attempt to avoid the potential morbidity of primary cytoreduction, some advocate the use of neoadjuvant chemotherapy before attempted cytoreduction.[21] A phase III trial led by the European Organisation for Research and Treatment of Cancer (EORTC) and published in 2010 randomised women with stage IIIC or IV ovarian cancer to primary debulking surgery followed by platinum-based chemotherapy or to neoadjuvant platinum-based chemotherapy followed by debulking surgery (so-called interval debulking surgery). The median OS was 29 months in the primary-surgery arm and 30 months in the neoadjuvant chemotherapy group, with a median PFS of 12 months in both arms. Postoperative rates of adverse effects and mortality tended to be higher after primary debulking than after interval cytoreduction. The authors concluded that the neoadjuvant chemotherapy and interval cytoreduction approach was not inferior to primary debulking surgery followed by chemotherapy and therefore represents a treatment option for women with bulky stage IIIC or IV ovarian carcinoma.[21] However, many have criticised the low PFS and OS rates in the primary debulking arm of this study in that the survival rates were similar to those reported in prospective and retrospective studies of only suboptimally cytoreduced patients and the OS rate was substantially less than those reported in subsets of optimally cytoreduced patients.[5,9,11–14] Possible explanations for the poor survival rates in the primary cytoreduction arm are that almost 60% of the women who underwent primary debulking were suboptimally cytoreduced and therefore would not be expected to have had improved survival due to the surgery, and almost a quarter of the women in each arm had stage IV disease, which could potentially blunt the beneficial effects of primary cytoreduction. The results also demonstrated that complete resection of all macroscopic disease, whether performed as primary treatment or after neoadjuvant chemotherapy, was the strongest independent variable predicting OS, and therefore remains the objective whenever cytoreduction is performed.

Therefore, while the neoadjuvant chemotherapy and interval cytoreduction approach may potentially be associated with lower morbidity and mortality than a primary debulking approach, the data in the literature consistently demonstrate that those women who have optimal primary surgical outcomes have the best survival. Thus, predicting which patients can and cannot undergo primary optimal cytoreduction in order to not deprive those who can the survival benefits associated with primary optimal debulking, while sparing those destined to be suboptimally debulked a non-beneficial and potentially harmful procedure, represents a critical decision-making point in the treatment of these women.

However, to date, no preoperative predictor of cytoreductive outcome has been demonstrated to accurately predict surgical outcome. Variable surgical practice and surgical effort among different institutions and individual surgeons makes it difficult to generalise and broadly apply preoperative risk factors of surgical outcome. Furthermore, the evolution of the surgical cytoreductive approach has been able to overcome many of the factors previously associated with suboptimal surgical outcomes.[22,23] While there is a need to identify and investigate new prognostic models that will be able to predict with accuracy and consistency whether a patient will undergo optimal surgical debulking, currently it is incumbent on the surgeon making the decision to be knowledgable about all the surgical options and procedures available, their potential benefits and limitations, and the appropriate circumstances in which they can be used, so that patients are not denied the survival benefits of a primary cytoreductive approach.

Improving cytoreductive outcome

Advanced ovarian cancer is heterogeneous, ranging from focal intra-abdominal disease to diffuse carcinomatosis involving the majority of parietal and visceral peritoneal surfaces (Figure 9.1). Disease involving the upper abdomen cephalad to the greater omentum (UAD) is frequently seen in women with ovarian cancer. Historically, the rate of optimal primary cytoreduction for women with advanced disease has been 40% or less. The use of intestinal resections and extensive upper abdominal resections were not routinely part of the surgical armamentarium of advanced disease management in many centres. Consequently, large-volume intestinal and upper abdominal tumour involving the diaphragm, liver and/or spleen was deemed 'unresectable' and the woman was left with a suboptimal surgical result. A step-wise increase over time in optimal cytoreduction rates parallels the learning curve of cytoreductive surgery. As an example of this, in Figure 9.2, the thin grey line demonstrates the success rate of optimal cytoreduction of advanced FIGO (International Federation of Gynecology and Obstetrics) stage IIIC epithelial ovarian cancer patients at Memorial Sloan-Kettering Cancer Center (MSKCC) over a 15 year time period starting with an optimal cytoreduction rate of 30% in 1989 and improving to 78% in 2002/2003. This line demonstrates the learning curve and the challenges of a gynaecological oncology service in the surgical management of advanced ovarian cancer patients. The introduction of more radical pelvic cytoreduction including intestinal resections and upper abdominal procedures has played an important role in the positive step-wise development of advanced cytoreductive surgery.

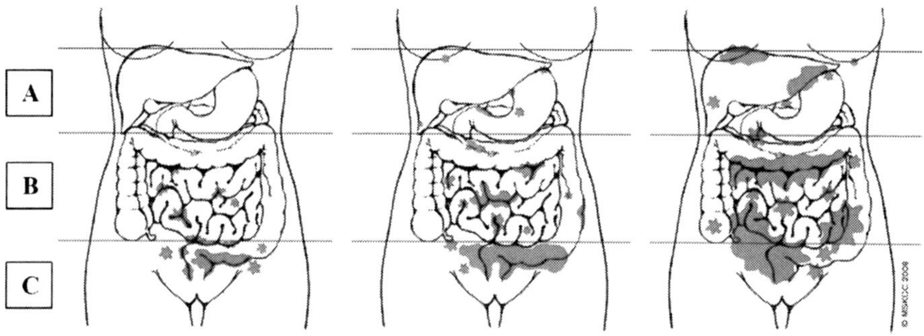

Figure 9.1 Three different groups of patients presenting with FIGO stage IIIC ovarian carcinoma (uterus, fallopian tubes/ovaries, and omentum removed) and their peritoneal disease distribution at the beginning of the operative procedure. (A) upper abdomen cephalad to the greater omentum; (B) mid-abdomen; (C) pelvis. UAD is upper abdominal disease cephalad to the greater omentum and is defined as metastatic implants involving the diaphragm, liver, porta hepatis, spleen, pancreas, stomach, coeliac axis and lesser sac. Group 1 (left) includes women without visible or palpable UAD (region A) at the time of exploration, group 2 (middle) consists of women with minimal UAD (1 cm or less) and group 3 (right) consists of women with bulky UAD (larger than 1 cm). Figure reproduced by courtesy of Memorial Sloan-Kettering Cancer Center.

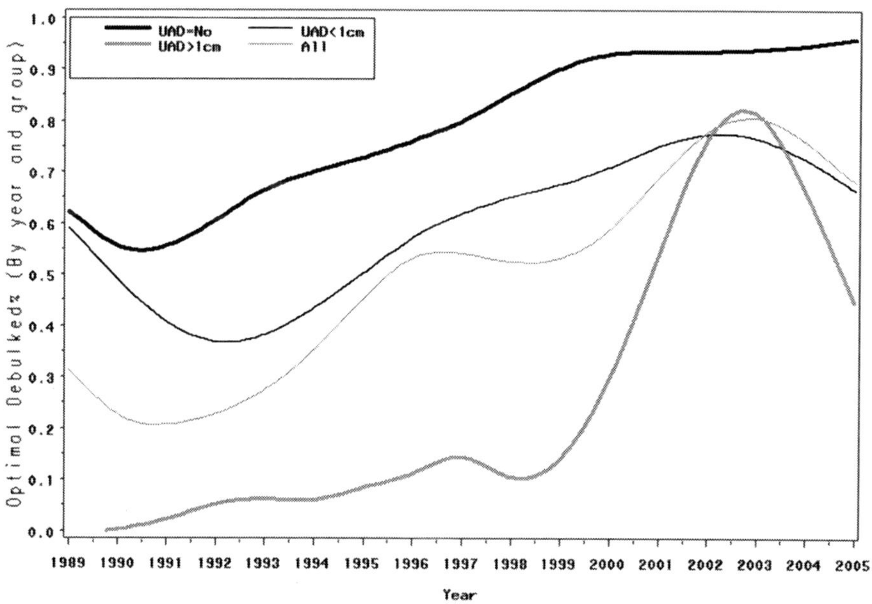

Figure 9.2 Rates of optimal cytoreduction by year and group, showing improved surgical outcomes in 474 women with FIGO stage IIIC ovarian cancer over the course of time. A significant increase in optimal cytoreduction was observed beginning in 2000. This effect was most pronounced in women with bulky upper abdominal disease (UAD >1 cm).

'Clearing' the pelvis

Among women requiring intestinal resection to achieve optimal cytoreduction, low anterior resection and rectosigmoid colectomy in the context of a modified posterior exenteration with or without a pelvic peritonectomy (stripping) are the most commonly required procedures to completely remove (or 'clear') all visible tumour in the pelvis.[18–20,24] This procedure almost always allows for a complete cytoreduction of pelvic disease even in cases of tumour encasing multiple organs and obliterating the cul-de-sac. Enhanced familiarity, training and use of these procedures has resulted in an increase in optimal cytoreduction rates at MSKCC for patients with FIGO stage IIIC ovarian cancer from 30% to 50% between 1989 and 1996 (Figure 9.2). Bowel-related morbidity and complications, including anastomotic leak, have been reported to range from 2% to 30.5%.[25,26] However, with the preferred use of stapled (double-stapling technique) rather than hand-sewn techniques and by performing tension-free and adequately perfused anastomoses, low anastomotic leak rates of less than 2% are achievable in women with advanced ovarian cancer undergoing multiple complex primary cytoreductive procedures.[27]

Targeting upper abdominal disease

Although advances have been reported in the successful and safe resection of pelvic disease and disease involving the intestinal tract, bulky tumour (> 1 cm) involving the upper abdomen cephalad to the greater omentum has been cited as the principal obstacle to achieving an optimal cytoreductive outcome. A survey of Society of Gynecologic Oncologists (SGO) members showed that tumour involving the diaphragm, bowel mesentery, coeliac axis and portal triad consistently precluded optimal cytoreduction.[28]

In general, over 50% of women with stage IIIC disease present with UAD.[29] Historically, at MSKCC and at other centres, disease involving the upper abdomen was associated with suboptimal surgical outcomes. In this setting, the physician is faced with one of two options:

- rely on postoperative chemotherapy for those found to have bulky UAD at primary cytoreduction or do not even take these women to the operating room but rather give them neoadjuvant chemotherapy, or
- attempt to expand the surgical approach to match the advanced disease involvement and thereby increase the percentage of patients who have optimal primary cytoreduction.

At MSKCC, we followed the latter approach and incorporated into our surgical armamentarium procedures such as diaphragm peritonectomy and/or resection, splenectomy, distal pancreatectomy, partial liver resection and cholecystectomy, and resection of tumour from the porta hepatis, coeliac axis or the thoracic cavity in cases where the primary surgeon deemed them necessary to achieve optimal cytoreduction. A significant increase in optimal cytoreduction rates was achieved after incorporation of these comprehensive surgical efforts targeting the upper abdomen. Following this programmatic change in surgical approach at MSKCC, the rate of optimal cytoreduction for women with stage IIIC ovarian cancer increased from 50% in the mid-1990s to greater than 75% starting in 2001 (Figure 9.2).

Moreover, the incorporation of extensive upper abdominal surgical procedures had a significant impact on survival outcomes. Eisenhauer *et al.*[30] reported that women who required extensive upper abdominal surgery to achieve optimal surgical outcome had a similar initial response to chemotherapy and similar PFS and OS compared with those who had optimal cytoreduction by standard surgical techniques, and a significantly improved outcome when compared with those left with residual disease greater than 1 cm in greatest diameter.

We have analysed the effect of surgical outcome on PFS and OS in women with advanced ovarian carcinoma stratified by the initial presence and volume of UAD found at the time of exploration.[31] Women with bulky UAD who underwent optimal cytoreduction through the incorporation of 'ultra-radical' procedures had a 28% decreased risk of relapse (hazard ratio 0.72; 95% CI 0.53–0.99; $P=0.04$) and a 33% decreased risk of death (hazard ratio 0.67; 95% CI 0.47–0.96; $P=0.03$) compared with those who underwent suboptimal cytoreduction.

When comparing all women with stage IIIC and IV ovarian cancer who underwent primary cytoreduction at MSKCC before and after the incorporation of extensive upper abdominal procedures, we found not only increased optimal cytoreduction rates but also significantly improved PFS and OS with the more comprehensive surgical approach.[32] Overall, these results suggest that the presence of large-volume disease (even diffuse peritoneal carcinomatosis) found during surgical exploration does not preclude the benefits of optimal cytoreduction. The findings support the management strategy of maximising surgical efforts with increasing tumour burden in women with stage IIIC and IV ovarian cancer.

New sources of perioperative morbidity

As a consequence of targeting the upper abdomen, there is a potential for 'non-gynaecological' complications that add to the usually encountered perioperative morbidity. Given that the most commonly identified site of disease precluding optimal cytoreduction by gynaecological oncologists is the upper abdomen, knowledge of the types and frequencies of complications associated with the addition of surgical procedures in this area to those already performed in the pelvis and mid-abdomen is crucial for gynaecological oncologists contemplating this comprehensive approach. Only a few studies in the gynaecological oncology literature have evaluated the complications associated with extensive upper abdominal surgery in the primary cytoreductive setting.

Eisenhauer *et al.*[33] reported on the incidence and management of pleural effusions after diaphragm peritonectomy or full-thickness resection in 59 women with advanced ovarian cancer. More than half of the women developed ipsilateral pleural effusions. Most were managed conservatively without requiring a thoracentesis or chest tube for relief of pulmonary symptoms. The overall rate of postoperative thoracentesis or chest tube placement was 15%. In 75% of the women requiring intervention, thoracentesis or chest tubes were placed within 5 days of the surgery. The incidence of symptomatic pleural effusions was not high enough to recommend routine intraoperative chest tube placement. However, in cases of extensive liver mobilisation with large diaphragm peritonectomies and/or resections, we often place chest tubes intraoperatively to prevent potential postoperative pulmonary compromise.

Complications involving the debulking of the left upper quadrant during cytoreduction have also been evaluated. Magtibay *et al.*[34] analysed the complications in 112 women who underwent splenectomy as part of cytoreductive surgery. Reported complications included thromboembolic events (8%), wound infections (6%), postoperative pneumonia (4%) and sepsis (4%). Eisenkop *et al.*[35] also examined a cohort of 49 women requiring splenectomy during cytoreduction. The rate of complications was not substantially different from that in a similar cohort of patients who underwent optimal cytoreduction but did not require splenectomy. Kehoe *et al.*[36] reported on the incidence and management of pancreatic leaks after distal pancreatectomy performed during primary cytoreductive surgery for advanced ovarian cancer. Of the 17 women in the study, four developed a pancreatic leak. The leak usually occurred within 2 weeks of surgery but also was seen in the late postoperative period in one woman. Conservative management with percutaneous drainage was effective, and no patient required reoperation or prolonged restriction of oral intake. Although the length of hospital stay for those with a pancreatic leak or fistula was increased, postoperative treatment with chemotherapy was not delayed for any of these women compared with those who did not have a leak.

In addition to the complications specific to upper abdominal procedures, the introduction of these procedures increases operative time and blood loss. Increased operative time and blood loss are both associated with an increased risk of general surgical complications not directly related to the upper abdominal procedures. Abu-Rustum *et al.*[37] showed that women with advanced ovarian cancer who require blood transfusion after primary cytoreduction have an increased risk of developing venous thrombosis and/or pulmonary emboli compared with those who do not. Rather than the transfusion of packed red blood cells, the liberal use of fresh frozen plasma (FFP) was hypothesised to be the main cause of thromboembolism and subsequently we have used more strict criteria for transfusing FFP. In a follow-up study by Black *et al*,[38] blood transfusions did not have an adverse effect on overall survival in this patient population.

In a continuing attempt to monitor the morbidity and mortality of this comprehensive surgical approach, the incidence of major surgical complications during primary cytoreduction of stage IIIC–IV ovarian cancer was analysed and reported in 2010 (Table 9.1).[27] During the study period, 141 women underwent one or more extensive upper abdominal surgical procedure as part of their primary cytoreduction. The extensive upper abdominal surgical procedures included 101 diaphragm peritonectomies, 45 splenectomies, 19 full-thickness diaphragm resections, 18 partial hepatectomies, 16 distal pancreatectomies, 15 cholecystectomies and 14 resections of porta hepatis tumour. The cytoreductive outcomes were 42 women (30%) with no gross residual, 85 women (60%) with residual up to 1 cm and 14 women (10%) with residual greater than 1 cm.

Major complications occurred in 31 women (21%), including two (1.4%) postoperative mortalities. However, 21 (68%) of the 31 women with major complications had their complication successfully managed by interventional radiological placement of percutaneous drains for infected or non-infected collections. The 1.4% postoperative mortality rate after extensive surgical cytoreduction compares favourably to other single-centre and population-based studies that report an average perioperative mortality rate of 2.5–3.7%.[39] Given the relatively low postoperative mortality rate, the ability to manage approximately two-thirds of the major complications by percutaneous drainage of infected and non-infected collections, and an overall median survival of 57 months in a cohort of patients with a large tumour burden, this rate of morbidity and mortality appears very acceptable.

In 'expert' centres, which patients should be considered for neoadjuvant chemotherapy?

In an analysis of a cohort of 576 women with stage IIIC and IV ovarian cancer who underwent primary cytoreductive surgery at four 'expert' centres, Aletti *et al.*[40] found age, tumour extent and residual disease after surgery to be independent prognostic

Table 9.1 Characteristics of women undergoing extensive upper abdominal procedures for advanced ovarian cancer at Memorial Sloan-Ketting Cancer Center from January 2001 to December 2006 (*n* = 141)

Variable	Number of patients (%)[a]
Age (median and range)	60 years (38–82 years)
Body mass index (median and range)	24 kg/m² (16–39 kg/m²)
Preoperative serum albumin (median and range)	4.0 g/dl (2.0–5.0 g/dl)
American Society of Anesthesiologists class	
I	12 (8%)
II	87 (62%)
III	37 (26%)
Unknown	5 (4%)
Primary site of disease	
Ovary	108 (77%)
Fallopian tube	19 (13%)
Peritoneum	14 (10%)
FIGO stage	
IIIC	103 (73%)
IV	38 (27%)
Tumour grade	
1	5 (4%)
2	10 (7%)
3	122 (86%)
Unknown	4(3%)
Histology	
Serous	131 (93%)
Other	10 (7%)
Preoperative serum CA125 (median and range)	942 Units/ml (18–20 888 Units/ml)
Ascites (median and range)	1625 ml (0–12 000 ml)
Estimated blood loss (median and range)	1000 ml (100–7500 ml)
Surgical time (median and range)	327 min (120–750 min)
Residual disease	
No gross residual	42 (30%)
0.1–1.0 cm	85 (60%)
>1 cm	14 (10%)
Surgical procedures	
Extensive upper abdominal procedures	
Diaphragm peritonectomy	101 (72%)
Splenectomy	45 (32%)
Full-thickness diaphragm resection	19 (14%)
Partial hepatectomy	18 (13%)
Distal pancreatectomy	16 (11%)
Cholecystectomy	15 (11%)
Other procedures	
Unilateral/bilateral salpingo-oophorectomy	128 (91%)
Hysterectomy	127 (90%)
Omentectomy	126 (89%)
Large bowel resection	79 (56%)
Pelvic lymph node dissection	51 (36%)
Para-aortic lymph node dissection	47 (33%)
Appendectomy	35 (25%)
Thoracoscopy	10 (7%)
Small bowel resection	9 (6%)
Ileostomy	9 (6%)
Colostomy	5 (4%)
Inguinal lymph node dissection	2 (1%)

[a] unless specified otherwise

Most of the 141 patients had multiple procedures

factors. They identified a high-risk group of patients ($n = 38$; 6.6% of the overall cohort) who had all three of the following characteristics:

- age 75 years or older
- American Society of Anesthesiologist score greater than 3 or preoperative serum albumin less than 3 g/dl
- stage IV disease or large initial tumour extent.

This high-risk group had a high rate of perioperative morbidity (64%) with limited survival benefit to optimal cytoreduction and appears to comprise patients who may best be served with a neoadjuvant chemotherapy approach.

Summary

The primary management of patients with advanced ovarian cancer is exceptionally challenging. Effective chemotherapy allows for the performance of surgical cytoreduction with improved outcomes when the outcome of the surgery is optimal. However, not all surgical patients achieve optimal cytoreduction and not all women who have been left with optimal residual disease have prolonged disease-free and overall survival. While there is a need to identify and investigate new prognostic models that will be able to predict with accuracy and consistency whether a specific woman will undergo optimal surgical debulking and whether that cytoreductive effort will be associated with improved survival, currently it is critical for the physicians taking care of these women to be knowledgable about the various surgical options available, their potential benefits and limitations, and the appropriate circumstances where they can be used, so that patients are not denied the survival benefits of a primary cytoreductive approach. In centres where a comprehensive primary surgical approach can be offered, it should be the standard of care except for the high-risk group of women who meet all three of the following criteria:

- age 75 years or older
- American Society of Anesthesiologist score greater than 3 or preoperative serum albumin less than 3 g/dl
- stage IV disease or large initial tumour extent.

References

1. Griffiths CT. Surgical resection of tumor bulk in the primary treatment of ovarian carcinoma. *Natl Cancer Inst Monogr* 1975;42:101–4.
2. Armstrong DK, Bundy B, Wenzel L, Huang HQ, Baergen R, Lele S, *et al.* Intraperitoneal cisplatin and paclitaxel in ovarian cancer. *N Engl J Med* 2006;354:34–43.
3. Ozols RF, Bundy BN, Greer BE, Fowler JM, Clarke-Pearson D, Burger RA, *et al.* Phase III trial of carboplatin and paclitaxel compared with cisplatin and paclitaxel in patients with optimally resected stage III ovarian cancer: a Gynecologic Oncology Group study. *J Clin Oncol* 2003;21:3194–200.
4. Hacker NF, Berek JS, Lagasse LD, Nieberg RK, Elashoff RM. Primary cytoreductive surgery for epithelial ovarian cancer. *Obstet Gynecol* 1983;61:413–20.
5. Chi DS, Eisenhauer EL, Lang J, Huh J, Haddad L, Abu-Rustum NR, *et al.* What is the optimal goal of primary cytoreductive surgery for bulky stage IIIC epithelial ovarian carcinoma (EOC)? *Gynecol Oncol* 2006;103:559–64.
6. Eisenkop SM, Spirtos NM, Montag TW, Nalick RH, Wang HJ. The impact of subspecialty training on the management of advanced ovarian cancer. *Gynecol Oncol* 1992;47:203–9.

7. Piver MS, Baker T. The potential for optimal (less than or equal to 2 cm) cytoreductive surgery in advanced ovarian carcinoma at a tertiary medical center: a prospective study. *Gynecol Oncol* 1986;24:1–8.
8. Omura GA, Bundy BN, Berek JS, Curry S, Delgado G, Mortel R. Randomized trial of cyclophosphamide plus cisplatin with or without doxorubicin in ovarian carcinoma: a Gynecologic Oncology Group Study. *J Clin Oncol* 1989;7:457–65.
9. Hoskins WJ, McGuire WP, Brady MF, Homesley HD, Creasman WT, Berman M, *et al.* The effect of diameter of largest residual disease on survival after primary cytoreductive surgery in patients with suboptimal residual epithelial ovarian carcinoma. *Am J Obstet Gynecol* 1994;170:974–9; discussion 979–80.
10. Bristow RE, Montz FJ, Lagasse LD, Leuchter RS, Karlan BY. Survival impact of surgical cytoreduction in stage IV epithelial ovarian cancer. *Gynecol Oncol* 1999;72:278–87.
11. Piver MS, Lele SB, Marchetti DL, Baker TR, Tsukada Y, Emrich LJ. The impact of aggressive debulking surgery and cisplatin-based chemotherapy on progression-free survival in stage III and IV ovarian carcinoma. *J Clin Oncol* 1988;6:983–9.
12. du Bois A, Reuss A, Pujade-Lauraine E, Harter P, Ray-Coquard I, Pfisterer J. Role of surgical outcome as prognostic factor in advanced epithelial ovarian cancer: A combined exploratory analysis of 3 prospectively randomized phase 3 multicenter trials: by the Arbeitsgemeinschaft Gynaekologische Onkologie Studiengruppe Ovarialkarzinom (AGO-OVAR) and the Groupe d'Investigateurs Nationaux Pour les Etudes des Cancers de l'Ovaire (GINECO). *Cancer* 2009;115:1234–44.
13. Winter WE 3rd, Maxwell GL, Tian C, Carlson JW, Ozols RF, Rose PG, *et al.* Prognostic factors for stage III epithelial ovarian cancer: a Gynecologic Oncology Group Study. *J Clin Oncol* 2007;25:3621–7.
14. Winter WE 3rd, Maxwell GL, Tian C, Sundborg MJ, Rose GS, Rose PG, *et al.* Tumor residual after surgical cytoreduction in prediction of clinical outcome in stage IV epithelial ovarian cancer: a Gynecologic Oncology Group Study. *J Clin Oncol* 2008;26:83–9.
15. Markman M. Concept of optimal surgical cytoreduction in advanced ovarian cancer: a brief critique and a call for action. *J Clin Oncol* 2007;25:4168–70.
16. Crawford SC, Vasey PA, Paul J, Hay A, Davis JA, Kaye SB. Does aggressive surgery only benefit patients with less advanced ovarian cancer? Results from an international comparison within the SCOTROC-1 Trial. *J Clin Oncol* 2005;23:8802–11.
17. Earle CC, Schrag D, Neville BA, Yabroff KR, Topor M, Fahey A, *et al.* Effect of surgeon specialty on processes of care and outcomes for ovarian cancer patients. *J Natl Cancer Inst* 2006;98:172–80.
18. Berek JS, Hacker NF, Lagasse LD. Rectosigmoid colectomy and reanastomosis to facilitate resection of primary and recurrent gynecologic cancer. *Obstet Gynecol* 1984;64:715–20.
19. Clayton RD, Obermair A, Hammond IG, Leung YC, McCartney AJ. The Western Australian experience of the use of en bloc resection of ovarian cancer with concomitant rectosigmoid colectomy. *Gynecol Oncol* 2002;84:53–7.
20. Sonnendecker EW, Beale PG. Rectosigmoid resection without colostomy during primary cytoreductive surgery for ovarian carcinoma. *Int Surg* 1989;74:10–12.
21. Vergote I, Trope CG, Amant F, Kristensen GB, Ehlen T, Johnson N, *et al.* Neoadjuvant chemotherapy of primary surgery in stage IIIC or IV ovarian cancer. *N Engl J Med* 2010;363:943–53.
22. Chi DS, Zivanovic O, Palayekar MJ, Eisenhauer EL, Abu-Rustum NR, Sonoda Y, *et al.* A contemporary analysis of the ability of preoperative serum CA-125 to predict primary cytoreductive outcome in patients with advanced ovarian, tubal and peritoneal carcinoma. *Gynecol Oncol* 2009;112:6–10.
23. Axtell A, Lee M, Bristow R, Dowdy SC, Cliby WA, Raman S, *et al.* Computed tomography predictors of primary suboptimal cytoreduction in patients with advanced ovarian cancer: a multi-institutional reciprocal validation study. *J Clin Oncol* 2007;25:384–9.
24. Mourton SM, Temple LK, Abu-Rustum NR, Gemignani ML, Sonoda Y, Bochner BH, *et al.* Morbidity of rectosigmoid resection and primary anastomosis in patients undergoing primary cytoreductive surgery for advanced epithelial ovarian cancer. *Gynecol Oncol* 2005;99:608–14.
25. Tebes SJ, Cardosi R, Hoffman MS. Colorectal resection in patients with ovarian and primary peritoneal carcinoma. *Am J Obstet Gynecol* 2006;195:585–9; discussion 589–90.

26. Estes JM, Leath CA 3rd, Straughn JM Jr, Rocconi RP, Kirby TO, Huh WK, *et al.* Bowel resection at the time of primary debulking for epithelial ovarian carcinoma: outcomes in patients treated with platinum and taxane-based chemotherapy. *J Am Coll Surg* 2006;203:527–32.
27. Chi DS, Zivanovic O, Levinson KL, Kolev V, Huh J, Dottino J, *et al.* The incidence of major complications after the performance of extensive upper abdominal surgical procedures during primary cytoreduction of advanced ovarian, tubal, and peritoneal carcinomas. *Gynecol Oncol* 2010;119:38–42.
28. Eisenkop SM, Spirtos NM. What are the current surgical objectives, strategies, and technical capabilities of gynecologic oncologists treating advanced epithelial ovarian cancer? *Gynecol Oncol* 2001;82:489–97.
29. Zivanovic O, Eisenhauer EL, Zhou Q, Iasonos A, Sabbatini P, Sonoda Y, *et al.* The impact of bulky upper abdominal disease cephalad to the greater omentum on surgical outcome for stage IIIC epithelial ovarian, fallopian tube, and primary peritoneal cancer. *Gynecol Oncol* 2008;108:287–92.
30. Eisenhauer EL, Abu-Rustum NR, Sonoda Y, Levine DA, Poynor EA, Aghajanian C, *et al.* The addition of extensive upper abdominal surgery to achieve optimal cytoreduction improves survival in patients with stages IIIC–IV epithelial ovarian cancer. *Gynecol Oncol* 2006;103:1083–90.
31. Zivanovic O, Sima CS, Iasonos A, Hoskins WJ, Pingle PR, Leitao MM Jr, *et al.* The effect of primary cytoreduction on outcomes of patients with FIGO stage IIIC ovarian cancer stratified by the initial tumor burden in the upper abdomen cephalad to the greater omentum. *Gynecol Oncol* 2010;116:351–7.
32. Chi DS, Eisenhauer EL, Zivanovic O, Sonoda Y, Abu-Rustum NR, Levine DA, *et al.* Improved progression-free and overall survival in advanced ovarian cancer as a result of a change in surgical paradigm. *Gynecol Oncol* 2009;114:26–31.
33. Eisenhauer EL, D'Angelica MI, Abu-Rustum NR, Sonoda Y, Jarnagin WR, Barakat RR, *et al.* Incidence and management of pleural effusions after diaphragm peritonectomy or resection for advanced mullerian cancer. *Gynecol Oncol* 2006;103:871–7.
34. Magtibay PM, Adams PB, Silverman BM, Cha SS, Podratz KC. Splenectomy as part of cytoreductive surgery in ovarian cancer. *Gynecol Oncol* 2006;102:369–74.
35. Eisenkop SM, Spirtos NM, Lin WM. Splenectomy in the context of primary cytoreductive operations for advanced epithelial ovarian cancer. *Gynecol Oncol* 2006;100:344–8.
36. Kehoe SM, Abu-Rustum NR, Sonoda Y. Incidence and management of pancreatic leaks after splenectomy with distal pancreatectomy performed during primary cytoreductive surgery for advanced ovarian cancer. 38th Annual Meeting on Women's Cancer of the Society of Gynecologic Oncologists, March 2007, San Diego, CA, USA.
37. Abu-Rustum NR, Richard S, Wilton A, Lev G, Sonoda Y, Hensley ML, *et al.* Tranfusion utilization during adnexal or peritoneal cancer surgery: effects on symptomatic venous thromboembolism and survival. *Gynecol Oncol* 2005;99:320–6.
38. Black D, Iasonos A, Ahmed H, Chi DS, Barakat RR, Abu-Rustum NR. Effect of perioperative venous thromboembolism on survival in ovarian, primary peritoneal, and fallopian tube cancer. *Gynecol Oncol* 2007;107:66–70.
39. Gerestein CG, Damhuis RA, Burger CW, Kooi GS. Postoperative mortality after surgery for ovarian cancer: a systematic review. *Gynecol Oncol* 2009;114:523–7.
40. Aletti GD, Eisenhauer EL, Santillan A, Axtell A, Aletti G, Holschneider C, *et al.* Identification of patient groups at highest risk from traditional approach to ovarian cancer treatment. *Gynecol Oncol* 2011;120:23–8.

10

Chapter 10
Antivascular therapy in gynaecological cancers

Leena Mukherjee and Gordon Rustin

The great majority of women with advanced ovarian cancer will relapse and die from their disease. There is therefore a great need for new agents that can extend remission and prolong survival. One approach is to introduce agents that target the vasculature that maintains a tumour's ability to survive and grow. These can be divided into agents that act against established blood vessels (vascular disrupting agents or VDAs) or inhibit the formation of new blood vessels (anti-angiogenic drugs). Angiogenesis inhibitors are considered to be cytostatic in nature, in contrast to VDAs, which are thought to be cytotoxic, but there is considerable overlap between the two groups, with agents classified according to their primary site of action (Box 10.1).[1,2]

Angiogenesis is under dynamic regulation by stimulatory pro-angiogenic factors released by tumour and host cells, such as vascular endothelial growth factor (VEGF), platelet-derived growth factor (PDGF), basic fibroblast growth factor (bFGF), interleukin 8 (IL-8), matrix metalloproteinases (MMPs) and inhibitory anti-angiogenic factors (tumour necrosis factor [TNF], 5-HT, angiostatin, endostatin). Diffusion of nutrients and oxygen from nearby capillaries beyond a tumour size of 2 mm is insufficient to sustain cell function. An imbalance of pro- and anti-angiogenic factors[3] stimulates an angiogenic switch so that the tumour develops an angiogenic phenotype to grow and metastasise.[4–6] Several process are thereafter involved, such as endothelial cell proliferation, proteolytic degradation of the extracellular matrix and migration of endothelial cells, leading to the formation of a functioning vessel with a lumen.[7]

Tumour hypoxia is an important stimulus for angiogenesis.[8] The release of hypoxia-inducable factor 1 (HIF-1), controlled by the Von Hippel–Lindau tumour

Box 10.1 Differences between angiogenesis inhibitors and vascular disrupting agents; CEPs = circulating endothelial progenitor cells

Angiogenesis inhibitors	Vascular disrupting agents
• effects within days	• effects within minutes
• chronic dosing	• acute dosing
• oral and intravenous	• mostly intravenous
• decrease CEPs	• increase CEPs
• decreased permeability	• increased permeability
• cytostatic	• cytotoxic

suppressor gene, is crucial, and upregulates VEGF transcription. Other pathways are also upregulated as a result of the hypoxic tumour microenvironment, such as nitric oxide synthase (NOS), PDGF, angiopoeitin 2 and acidic and basic fibroblast growth factors. The hypoxic tumour microenvironment can also lead to enhanced survival, by selecting for tumour cells that will evade apoptosis.

The VEGF pathway was initially identified in the 1980s.[9] VEGF-A was identified as a vascular permeability factor in 1983 and later characterised as an endothelial-specific mitogen in the late 1980s.[10] Seven glycoproteins, VEGF-A to E and placental growth factors 1 and 2, signal through three tyrosine kinase receptors, VEGFR-1 to 3. The resultant receptor dimerisation causes activation of downstream cascades leading to angiogenesis (Figure 10.1). This is done by increasing vessel permeability, leading to the induction of endothelial cell migration and proliferation and the formation of endothelial sprouts that anastomose to form a vascular network.

VEGF also recruits circulating endothelial progenitor cells (CEPs) from bone marrow to the site of angiogenesis; these differentiate *in situ* to form mature endothelial cells in a process called vasculogenesis.[7,11,12] VEGFR-1 and VEGFR-2 promote angiogenesis and mediate the effects of VEGF-A. VEGF-A is also thought to have a direct effect on tumour cell proliferation via the mTOR pathway and it affects the expression of MMPs, thereby regulating the invasiveness of tumour cells.[13–15] Although VEGFR-1 has a more than ten-fold higher affinity for VEGF-A, its activation has a lesser impact on the downstream intracellular intermediates than

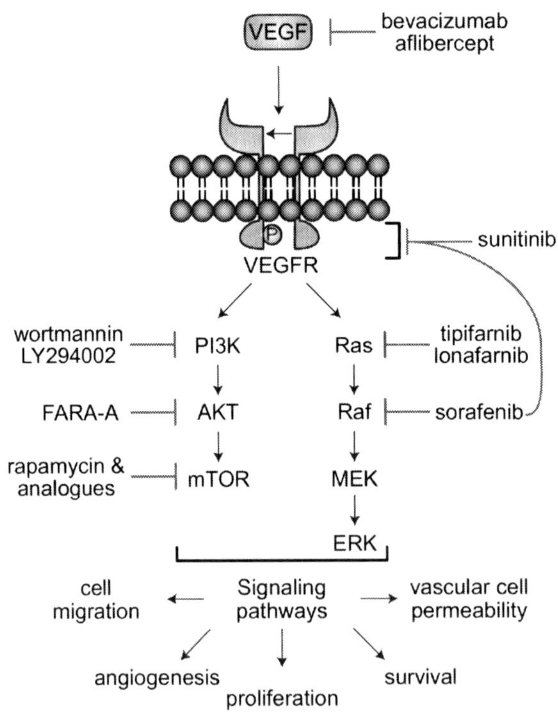

Figure 10.1 Angiogenesis pathway and pre-clinical/clinical compounds that inhibit the pathway; reproduced from Cook and Figg[79] with permission of John Wiley & Sons, Inc.

VEGFR-2. VEGFR-2 has therefore been the target for research into anti-angiogenic therapies. VEGFR-3 mediates lymphangiogenesis.

Aberrant angiogenesis produces abnormal vessels, which results in heterogeneous blood flow, increased permeability causing interstitial extravasation of plasma, perpetuation of the hypoxic microenvironment and further angiogenesis. There are important differences between normal and tumour blood vessels, as listed in Box 10.2.

Hypoxia renders tumour cells resistant to chemotherapy and radiation, and pretreatment oxygenation levels correlate with response to radiotherapy and the likelihood of tumour progression and metastatic disease.[16–19] Normalisation of the vasculature may enhance drug delivery and radiosensitivity by improving oxygenation. Therefore antivascular therapies that normalise vasculature may aid delivery of traditional cytotoxic chemotherapy or radiotherapy.[20]

Box 10.2 Characteristics of tumour blood vessels compared with normal blood vessels[2]

- increased vessel tortuosity and varied diameter
- thin walled and fragile
- constant remodelling
- vessel immaturity with lack of smooth muscle and pericytes
- poor connections between pericytes and endothelial cells
- irregular basement membrane and endothelial cell shape
- increased vessel permeability
- increased interstitial pressure within tumour
- variable flowrates, leading to regional hypoxia
- huge variability in vascular density
- lack of lymphatic drainage effects

Ovarian cancer and angiogenesis

Angiogenesis is particularly relevant in ovarian cancer.[21] VEGF is important in both ovarian physiology and pathology. VEGF-A levels change cyclically with the menstrual cycle and blockage of the pathway can suppress ovulation.[22] In ovarian cancer, intratumoral VEGF and VEGFR-2 expression and the carriage of VEGF gene polymorphisms associated with increased VEGF excretion are independent poor prognostic factors.[23–25] Increased levels of VEGF have been shown in multivariate analysis to be an independent prognostic indicator of poor survival in early and advanced ovarian disease. Tumour VEGF overexpression is associated with tumour angiogenesis, malignant progression and metastasis, ascites formation and early recurrence and death from disease. In animal models, blockage of VEGF slows tumour growth and inhibits ascites formation.[26–28]

Angiogenesis inhibitors

Bevacizumab

Bevacizumab is a humanised monoclonal antibody that binds to VEGF-A, preventing it from binding to receptors (Figure 10.1). It is approved by the US Food and Drug Administration (FDA) in combination with interferon for metastatic renal cell carcinoma, as a single agent for second-line treatment of glioblastoma, in combination with paclitaxel for metastatic breast cancer, in combination with carboplatin and paclitaxel for non-small cell lung cancer, and as combination therapy for first- or second-line treatment of metastatic colorectal cancer. Approval was based on improved survival in colorectal and lung cancer trials, improved progression-free survival (PFS) in breast and renal cell cancer trials, and on response in the glioblastoma trial.[29]

Single-agent activity in ovarian carcinoma

Several phase II studies have shown single-agent activity in recurrent ovarian cancer. Burger *et al.*[30] showed using 15 mg/kg every 21 days that, in 62 women with persistent or recurrent ovarian carcinoma, of whom 40% were platinum resistant, 13 patients (21%) had clinical response (3% complete and 18% partial) and 25 (40%) were alive and progression-free at 6 months. The median overall survival (OS) of 16.9 months was longer than all other Gynecologic Oncology Group (GOG) trials performed in this patient group. There was no evidence that number of prior regimens or performance status altered response, and no gastrointestinal (GI) perforations occurred. In addition to the predictable anti-angiogenic effects, there was a reduction in tumour burden seen, suggesting that endothelial and tumour cells expressed VEGF.

Cannistra *et al.*[31] used 3-weekly 15 mg/kg single-agent bevacizumab in 44 women with platinum-resistant ovarian cancer progressing within 3 months of second-line doxorubicin or topotecan. In this study, seven of the women (16%) had a partial response, which was comparable with the Burger *et al.* study.[30] The median PFS was 4.4 months and median OS was 10.7 months. However, in this study, GI perforation occurred in five women (11%) and the study was terminated early. This trial also had a higher than expected rate of arterial thromboembolic events, at 7%, and three treatment-related deaths.

In combination with cytotoxic agents

Bevacizumab 10 mg/kg 2-weekly was investigated in combination with 50 mg oral cyclophosphamide in 15 women with heavily pretreated recurrent ovarian cancer in a retrospective analysis.[32] There was a response rate of 53%, with two women (13%) showing a complete response and six (40%) a partial response. The median duration of response was 3.8 months, and three women (20%) had stable disease for 4.0, 5.2 and 5.5 months. There were no GI perforations.

Garcia *et al.*[33] carried out a prospective analysis of 50 mg cyclophosphamide once daily with 10 mg/kg bevacizumab 2-weekly in 70 women with recurrent ovarian carcinoma. A partial response was seen in 17 women (24%) in this less heavily pretreated cohort. There was no difference in response between platinum-resistant and platinum-sensitive disease. This study had GI perforations or fistulae in four women (6%) and there were three treatment-related deaths. The probability of being alive and progression-free at 6 months was 56%, with a median time to progression of 7.2 months and OS of 16.9 months.

A retrospective analysis[34] of 23 heavily pretreated recurrent, platinum-refractory patients observed a 35% partial response rate of bevacizumab combined with various regimens including doxorubicin, gemcitabine, docetaxol, 5-fluorouracil and cyclophosphamide. The women achieving a response could expect a median PFS of 5.6 months.

Randomised trials

Two phase III trials of first-line bevacizumab with carboplatin (AUC = 6) and paclitaxel (175 mg/m^2) in advanced epithelial ovarian carcinoma were reported in 2010,[35,36] with important differences between the two trials (Table 10.1; Box 10.3). The GOG-218 trial randomised patients between a control arm of paclitaxel and carboplatin for six cycles versus the same with bevacizumab 15 mg/kg, and a third arm where bevacizumab maintenance continued for a further 16 cycles. It showed a significant increase in PFS (14.1 versus 10.3 months; HR 0.701) in the maintenance bevacizumab arm, but no significant improvement in the arm where bevacizumab was given just during cytotoxic chemotherapy.

In the two-arm ICON7 trial, the bevacizumab arm received 7.5 mg/kg for six cycles followed by 12 cycles as maintenance therapy. The median PFS was 17.3 months in the control arm and 19.0 months in the bevacizumab arm (HR 0.81; P=0.0041). Analysis of the benefit from bevacizumab in these two trials is confusing as the curves actually cross over in the more mature ICON7 trial, thus making a PFS analysis unreliable. Furthermore, as the patients in GOG-218 had a worse prognosis, the PFS graphs showed the maximum separation at the median survival. However, in ICON7, where the patients had a better prognosis, the maximum separation of the curves was some months prior to when the curve had fallen to the median, and by the time the curve had fallen to the median the curves had come closer together. A more

Table 10.1 Phase III trials of targeted agents in ovarian carcinoma

Agent	Group or sponsor	Line of therapy	Primary efficacy endpoint(s)	Status
Bevacizumab	GOG-218	First	PFS	ASCO 2010
	ICON7 (GCIG study)	First	PFS and OS	ESMO 2010
	OCEANS	Recurrent	PFS	Closed
	GOG-213	Recurrent	OS	Active
	AURELIA	Recurrent	PFS	Closed
BIBF 1120	AGO-OVAR12 (Boehringer Ingelheim)	First	PFS	Active
Cediranib	ICON6 (GCIG study)	Recurrent	PFS and OS	Active
Pazopanib	GlaxoSmithKline	First (maintenance only)	PFS	Active

AGO = Arbeitsgemeinschaft Gynäkologische Onkologie; ASCO 2010 = data presented at the 2010 annual meeting of the American Society for Clinical Oncology; ESMO 2010 = data presented at the 2010 congress of the European Society for Medical Oncology; GCIG = Gynecologic Cancer Intergroup; GOG = Gynecologic Oncology Group; OS = overall survival; PFS = progression-free survival

Box 10.3 Differences between the GOG-218 and ICON7 phase III trials of bevacizumab

GOG-218

- three arms
- bevacizumab 15 mg/kg for six cycles followed by 16 cycles as maintenance therapy
- placebo controlled
- more advanced disease

ICON7

- two arms
- bevacizumab 7.5 mg/kg for six cycles followed by 12 cycles as maintenance therapy
- open label

reliable method of ascertaining benefit is to measure the area between the curves of the treatment arms. If this so-called restricted-mean analysis is calculated in the more advanced patients in ICON7, a similar group to those in GOG-218, the hazard ratio becomes 0.68 in favour of bevacizumab with a 3.2 month improvement in PFS. Thus both trials appear to delay progression by a similar amount. These trials demonstrate the dangers of relying on median PFS and also demonstrate that if the curves cross even hazard ratios are unreliable.

Hypertension was the only toxicity significantly increased in the bevacizumab arm in both trials. There is considerable debate as to whether bevacizumab should be a standard of care for first-line ovarian cancer management. It is too early to show whether there is any survival benefit from adding bevacizumab but it is clear that, as the PFS curves come together at about 24 months, there will not be an increase in the proportion of long-term survivors (i.e. cures). It is still possible that there could be a modest prolongation of survival.

Other randomised trials

The OCEANS trial is a randomised phase III trial investigating carboplatin, gemcitabine and bevacizumab versus carboplatin and gemcitabine alone in women with relapsed ovarian cancer and should report results in 2011.

GOG-213 is a randomised trial in recurrent ovarian cancer. Patients are stratified as to whether they are surgical candidates. If they are surgical candidates, they are randomised to surgery or no surgery followed by randomisation thereafter to chemotherapy or no chemotherapy. If patients are randomised to no surgery, they are subsequently randomised to receive carboplatin/paclitaxel or carboplatin/paclitaxel plus bevacizumab.

AURELIA is a randomised open-label two-arm study of bevacizumab added to chemotherapy in women with platinum-resistant ovarian cancer, and should also report in 2011. It evaluates the efficacy and safety of bevacizumab added to chemotherapy versus chemotherapy alone in platinum-resistant patients with epithelial ovarian, fallopian tube or primary peritoneal cancer. All patients received standard chemotherapy with either paclitaxel or topotecan or liposomal doxorubicin. Patients randomised to the test arm of the study received concomitant 10 mg/kg intravenous 2-weekly or 15 mg/kg intravenous 3-weekly bevacizumab. Anticipated time on study treatment is until disease progression.

Other pathways

The mTOR pathway has been shown to regulate VEGF expression in cancer cells and, in pre-clinical studies, in combination with bevacizumab, everolimus has been shown to reduce tumour growth by 94% and prolong survival.[37] A phase II trial is therefore under way.

Tyrosine kinase inhibitors

EGFR tyrosine kinase inhibitor

Epidermal growth factor receptor (EGFR) is expressed in 35–70% of advanced epithelial ovarian carcinoma, and expression correlates with advanced stage and poor survival. EGFR activation has been suggested to promote VEGF secretion, and VEGF upregulation independent of EGFR signalling appears to contribute to resistance to EGFR inhibition.[38]

In combination with bevacizumab Nimieri *et al.*[39] studied a combination of erlotinib, an orally available EGFR tyrosine kinase inhibitor, with bevacizumab in recurrent or refractory ovarian cancer. The response rate in ovarian cancer was comparable to that with single-agent bevacizumab, and there was a 15% perforation rate – although both of these women had documented evidence of prior bowel wall involvement. The trial was therefore terminated.

VEGFR tyrosine kinase inhibitors

There are many VEGFR tyrosine kinase inhibitors being tested in patients with ovarian cancer (Table 10.2).

Cediranib Cediranib is an orally available tyrosine kinase inhibitor of VEGFR-1, VEGFR-2, VEGFR-3, platelet-derived growth factor receptor (PDGFR) and c-Kit. Matulonis *et al.*[40] studied cediranib therapy in 46 patients with up to two prior lines of therapy, 65% of whom were platinum resistant. The study reported that 17% of patients had a partial response and 13% had stable disease of more than 16 weeks. Toxicities included hypertension in 46% and hypothyroidism in 56%, and there was significant diarrhoea and fatigue. Median PFS was 5.2 months. There were no GI perforations or fistulae, but 23% of patients were removed from the study due to treatment adverse effects.

Hirte *et al.*[41] showed response or disease stabilisation in 41% of platinum-sensitive and 29% of platinum-resistant patients out of a total of 46 patients receiving cediranib with one line of prior therapy. Adverse effects were hypertension (33%) and fatigue (20%).

A phase III trial is under way evaluating standard carboplatin and paclitaxel chemotherapy with or without concurrent cediranib and also the effect of maintenance cediranib in relapsing platinum-sensitive ovarian cancer (ICON6) (Table 10.1).

Vargatef Vargatef™, also known as BIBF 1120, is a combined inhibitor of VEGFR, fibroblast growth factor receptor (FGFR) and PDGFR, and there is magnetic resonance imaging (MRI) evidence of effects on vascular perfusion. A randomised phase II trial examined its effects as maintenance therapy in 83 women who had responded to chemotherapy for relapse.[42] The 36 week PFS rate was 14% and 5% in the BIBF 1120

Table 10.2 Tyrosine kinase inhibitors that target VEGFR

Inhibitor	Other names	Inhibits
Axitinib	AG013736	VEGFR, PDGFR, c-Kit
Cediranib	Recentin®, AZD2171	VEGFR-1 to 3, PDGFR-B, c-Kit
Motesanib	AMG 706	VEGFR, PDGFR, c-Kit
Pazopanib	Armala™, GW786034	VEGFR, PDGFR-B, c-Kit
Regorafenib	BAY 73-4506	VEGFR-2 and Tie-2
Semaxinib	SU5416	VEGFR
Sorafenib	Nexavar®, BAY439006	Raf, VEGFR-2,VEGFR-3 PDGFR, c-Kit
Sunitinib	Sutent®, SU11248	VEGFR, PDGFR, Flt-3, c-Kit, RET, CSF-1R
Vandetanib	Zactima™, ZD6474	VEGFR-2, PDGFR-B, EGFR, RET
Vargatef™	BIBF 1120	VEGFR, PDGFR, FGFR

and placebo groups, respectively (HR 0.68; 95% CI 0.44–1.07; $P=0.09$). Adverse effects included gastrointestinal toxicities (in fewer than 10%), asymptomatic elevation of liver enzymes (51%) and grade 3 or 4 hypertension (4.6%). A randomised trial in women receiving first-line chemotherapy plus Vargatef or placebo is under way (Table 10.1).

Pazopanib Pazopanib inhibits VEGFR, PDGFR and c-Kit. In a phase II trial, a CA125 response (a fall of 50% or more from baseline) was seen in 11 (31%) of the 36 women in the study.[43] The most common toxicities were fatigue, diarrhoea, vomiting and disturbance in liver function tests. Hypertension was relatively uncommon. Pazopanib is now being compared with placebo as maintenance following first-line therapy with carboplatin and paclitaxel (AGO-OVAR16/GSK [NCT00866697]) (Table 10.1).

Other tyrosine kinase inhibitors Biagi *et al.*[44] have shown one partial response and three CA125 responses in 30 patients, with up to two prior lines of therapy, with sunitinib maleate, an oral, multitargeted tyrosine kinase inhibitor that inhibits VEGFR, c-Kit and PDGFR. Adverse effects seen were hand-foot syndrome, neutropenia and thrombocytopenia. Matei *et al.*[45] demonstrated stable disease in 12 (20%) and a partial response in two (3%) of 59 patients, with up to two prior lines of therapy, treated with sorafenib, an oral, small-molecule, multitargeted tyrosine kinase inhibitor that inhibits the MAP kinase pathway. Adverse effects were rash (17%), metabolic (15%) and gastrointestinal (4%).

VEGF-Trap

Aflibercept (VEGF-Trap) is a fusion protein of the human extracellular domains of VEGFR-1 and VEGFR-2 and the Fc portion of human immunoglobulin IgG which binds VEGF and prevents it binding to its receptor. Trials in pre-clinical ovarian cancer models have shown a reduction in tumour burden and ascites,[28,46] and phase I data from solid tumours has shown a partial response in a woman with ovarian cancer.[47] Several phase II studies are currently under way in recurrent, platinum-resistant ovarian cancer, with one reporting an overall response rate of 13.8%.[48] Interim reporting of a study examining patients resistant to platinum, topotecan and doxorubicin treated with aflibercept showed a partial response in 11% (ARD 6122, ARD 6772). A phase II trial combining VEGF-Trap with docetaxol in women with persistent or recurrent ovarian cancer is currently continuing (NCT00436501).

Other anti-angiogenic agents

Metronomic cytotoxic chemotherapy

Metronomic chemotherapy – the delivery of frequent low doses of cytotoxic chemotherapy – suppresses tumour growth in experimental models, potentially via inhibiting angiogenesis through stimulation of thrombospondin release. Previous clinical trials have shown encouraging activity with minimal toxicity, and animal studies of combination with anti-angiogenic agents have shown marked inhibition of tumour growth.[33,49]

Chemotherapy and VDAs can cause mobilisation of bone marrow progenitor cells, including CEPs, which could theoretically increase angiogenesis. Indeed, CEPs have been shown to increase after delivery of maximum tolerated dose (MTD) chemotherapy in keeping with the repair process that occurs in both healthy and cancerous cells.[50,51]

Evaluation of microvascular density during 3-weekly chemotherapy with carboplatin and paclitaxel using antibodies shows a significant increase in CD31 and CD105, endothelial surface and proliferation markers, respectively. This would appear to show that MTD chemotherapy promotes tumour vascularisation, possibly due to secondary recovery. Metronomic chemotherapy allows lower total exposure but constant administration, thereby preventing vascular repair and regrowth. Cyclophosphamide has been shown to have antivascular effects, possibly through release of thrombospondin.[33] After delivery of metronomic chemotherapy, CEPs decreased, showing a sustained anti-angiogenic effect. Maintenance therapy with anti-angiogenic agents would capitalise on the gains from cytotoxic treatments.[51]

Thalidomide

Thalidomide inhibits expression of VEGF and bFGF via mechanisms involving TNF-α and transcriptional activation of the VEGF promoter. A randomised phase III trial of daily low-dose tamoxifen versus thalidomide in 138 women with biochemically recurrent but asymptomatic epithelial ovarian, primary peritoneal or fallopian tube cancer found that those randomised to the thalidomide arm did not have a longer remission. They had a statistically significant similar PFS, but 9 month shorter median survival, worse OS (24.0 versus 33.2 months) and a higher risk of death (HR 1.76; 95% CI 1.16–2.68). There was a higher incidence of grade 3 and 4 toxicities (55% versus 3%) in the thalidomide arm and a higher rate of treatment discontinuation due to adverse effects (16% versus 1%). This suggests that there is no role for using thalidomide in ovarian cancer.[52]

AMG 386

Angiopoietin 1 and 2 bind to the vascular receptor tyrosine kinase Tie-2 and are key cytokines regulating pro-angiogenic pathways. Angiopoietin 1 promotes recruitment of pericytes to vascular tubes, promoting vessel stabilisation and maturation. Angiopoietin 2 is expressed primarily at sites of vascular remodelling, and its actions can be pro-angiogenic or anti-angiogenic depending on the signalling environment. Angiopoietin 2 expression is upregulated at sites of tumour angiogenesis and overexpression leads to increased angiogenesis and tumour growth in experimental cancer models. AMG 386 is a recombinant peptide-Fc fusion protein containing a peptide sequence that binds angiopoietin 1 and 2. By selectively neutralising these cytokines, their interaction with Tie-2 is blocked, which has been shown to inhibit tumour growth and even cause disappearance of tumour in animal models. A randomised phase II study in relapsed ovarian cancer showed that weekly administration at a dose of 3 or 10 mg/kg with paclitaxel led to improved PFS and CA125 response rate compared with the paclitaxel plus placebo arm.[53] Further randomised trials in ovarian cancer are due to start soon.

Enzastaurin

Enzastaurin, an acyclic bisindolylmaleimide, was initially developed for anti-angiogenic cancer therapy as a specific inhibitor of protein kinase C-beta (PKCB). It inhibits PKCB- and VEGF-mediated angiogenesis.[54] In addition to this major target, enzastaurin also inhibits other PKC isoforms. Recent pre-clinical studies have shown that enzastaurin exerts pro-apoptotic, growth-inhibitory and anti-angiogenic properties in a variety of human cancers. Enzastaurin was shown to target the PI3K/AKT pathway, to inhibit

GSK3b and ribosomal protein S6 phosphorylation, to decrease the expression of VEGF and also to show a synergism with SUI174 and pemetrexed.

In clinical studies, enzastaurin was well tolerated but early results of randomised clinical trials have been disappointing.[55]

Integrins as targets

Integrins are a super-family of widely expressed transmembrane glycoprotein receptors for extracellular matrix ligands and act in concert with VEGF to regulate, orchestrate and amplify angiogenesis and tumour metastasis. Endothelial cell expression of the $\alpha_5\beta_1$ integrin and the ligand fibronectin are both upregulated during tumour angiogenesis. In pre-clinical models, selective antagonists targeted to $\alpha_5\beta_1$ integrin inhibit tumour growth. This is therefore an attractive target for antivascular research. Clinical trials of volociximab and cilengitide, two agents that target integrins, are under way.[56,57]

Use of CA125 measurements in patients receiving VEGF inhibitors

There are concerns from laboratory studies that molecular targeting agents such as enzastaurin might increase shedding of CA125 and thus make it an unreliable marker for monitoring therapy.[58] Two trials of combination therapy that included bevacizumab have suggested discrepancies between CA125 and RECIST response evaluation.[32,59] However, on closer inspection of the data, it is probable that the discrepancies are due to rising CA125 levels being an earlier and more sensitive indicator of progression than RECIST, or being a more sensitive indicator of response that is not durable or long enough to be accepted by RECIST. It is important to realise that novel agents might be slowing the rate of tumour growth so, even if CA125 levels might be slowly rising, they might be rising more slowly than if the patient were not on therapy. Therefore therapy should not be automatically stopped just because of a rise in CA125 levels. High CA125 response rates have been seen in trials of pazopanib.[43] To validate the use of CA125 in this situation requires that the hazard ratio for PFS be similar whether RECIST or CA125 criteria are used.[60]

Other gynaecological cancers

Cervical cancer is caused by human papillomavirus (HPV). Continuing HPV infection, usually associated with genomic HPV integration, leads to dysregulation of p53. The dysregulation of p53 is mediated by the oncogenic protein HPV E6 via two mechanisms. The first involves blockage of induction of p53 following DNA damage, which normally causes the damaged cell to enter cell cycle arrest and undergo DNA repair, or, if irreparable, triggers apoptosis. The second involves E6-induced ubiquitination of p53 and subsequent protein degradation. The downregulation of the tumour suppressor gene p53 increases angiogenic potential through subsequent upregulation of VEGF. HPV E6 also independently enhances induction of HIF-1α in experimental models, increasing VEGF through a second mechanism. There is a strong association with VEGF expression and poor prognosis in cervical carcinoma, and levels correlate with stage of disease and prognosis.

Higher intratumoral microvessel density (MVD) has been shown on multivariate analysis to be a significant independent prognostic factor with poorer OS and locoregional control. Tumours with high levels of CD31-MVD (a non-specific endothelial marker) and low levels of CA-1X (a marker for tumour hypoxia) have been shown to have the poorest survival and both factors have been shown on Cox regression analysis to be independent factors influencing PFS and OS. This implies that better tumour vascularisation and oxygenation allows improved treatment delivery.

Advanced or recurrent cervical cancer has a median OS of 9 months with conventional platinum-containing cytotoxic regimens. There is therefore a rationale for treating cervical cancer lesions with antivascular therapies.

A phase II trial looked at the effect of 15 mg/kg bevacizumab every 21 days in 46 women with recurrent and/or advanced cervical cancer. The endpoint was PFS, which was comparable to other treatment modalities at 3.4 months, with a median OS of 7.3 months. The response rate was 11%, with a 24% probability of being progression-free at 6 months. On closer analysis, there were no definitive predictors of response, but factors indicating a poor outcome were being young, of African-American origin, and poor performance status. The acceptable and predictable adverse effect profile suggests that bevacizumab is active in advanced/recurrent cervical cancer, and phase III trials are warranted.[61]

A randomised phase II trial compared EGF-based therapy (lapatinib, an oral EGFR tyrosine kinase inhibitor with HER2 activity) with anti-angiogenesis therapy (pazopanib, an oral tyrosine kinase inhibitor targeting VEGFR, PDGFR and c-Kit) in 130 women with advanced or recurrent cervical cancer. This study convincingly suggested the superiority of anti-angiogenesis therapy. Pazopanib improved PFS (HR 0.66; 90% CI 0.48–0.91; P=0.013) and OS (HR 0.67; 90% CI 0.46–0.99; P=0.045). The only grade 3 adverse event that occurred in more than 10% of patients was diarrhoea (11% with pazopanib and 13% with lapatinib).[62]

Vascular disrupting agents

VDAs selectively target pre-existing tumour vasculature, leading to rapid tumour cell ischaemia and death. Pre-clinical studies have shown that they induce vascular shutdown within 30 minutes of administration.[63–65]

In animal models, VDAs are able to induce extensive vascular shutdown and haemorrhagic necrosis at the tumour core, but tend to leave a periphery of active cells that easily repopulate. VDAs have therefore been trialled alongside conventional therapies to maximise tumour necrosis. There are two types of VDA – biological or ligand-directed, which have not been tested in gynaecological cancers and are not discussed further, and small-molecule VDAs.

Small-molecule vascular disrupting agents

Flavonoids

Flavonoids damage the actin cytoskeleton, leading to DNA strand breaks and induction of endothelial cell apoptosis. Cytokines such as TNF are also released from activated macrophages, and activated platelets and serotonin augment the antivascular effect. Flavone-8-acetic acid (FAA), a flavonoid developed initially as a nonsteroidal anti-inflammatory drug, was the first agent shown to cause haemorrhagic necrosis in animal tumours and opened the field of vascular disruptive therapy. Although active in pre-clinical studies, no activity was seen in humans. This led to the development of 5,6-dimethylxanthenone-4-acetic acid (DMXAA), a more potent analogue.

DMXAA causes vascular shutdown in murine tumours within 30 minutes.[66] It damages the tumour vascular endothelium, causing DNA strand breaks and the induction of apoptosis.[67] The exact target remains elusive, but the nuclear transcription factor NF-κB is upregulated, producing TNF and other cytokines. Tumour and plasma TNF synthesis is induced by DMXAA and 5H1AA levels – a marker for vascular damage – increase in a dose-dependent fashion. Tumour blood flow decreases, and levels of 5-HT, probably released from platelets, together with nitric oxide and TNF in plasma and tumour tissue increase.[67,68] This cascade is probably required for the vascular effects of DMXAA, and induces production of TNF, which mediates its anti-tumour effects and toxicity.

Phase II data in previously untreated non-small cell lung cancer patients with 1800 mg/m^2 DMXAA in combination with carboplatin and paclitaxel showed that it was well tolerated, with a response rate of 38% and stable disease in 43%, with a median survival of 14.9 months. It has an acceptable adverse effect profile and no adverse pharmacokinetic interactions, but so far no proven survival benefit when added to systemic chemotherapy.[69]

Gabra *et al.*[70] conducted a randomised phase II study of DMXAA (1200 mg/m^2) in addition to standard carboplatin (AUC = 6) and paclitaxel (175 mg/m^2) chemotherapy in recurrent platinum-sensitive ovarian carcinoma. There was no increase in toxicity with the addition of DMXAA, but unfortunately also no improvement in PFS. A planned interim analysis of data from the ATTRACT-1 phase III trial of DMXAA (also known as ASA404) in previously untreated non-small cell lung cancer showed that continuation of the trial would be futile, as there was little or no prospect of demonstrating a survival benefit with ASA404 in this setting. The ATTRACT-1 trial was therefore halted and there is unlikely to be further development of this agent.

Tubulin-binding agents

Tubulin-binding agents such as combretastatin A-4 phosphate (CA4P) work by attaching to an alternative binding site on the tubulin molecule from that which colchicine binds to, leading to tubulin depolymerisation and disruption of the actin and tubulin. The consequent change in endothelial shape leads to vascular blockage, reduction in blood flow, exposure of the basement membrane and, ultimately, increased vessel permeability. Increased interstitial pressure leads to further congestion and decreased blood flow. Exposure of the basement membrane activates the coagulation cascade.[63,71]

CA4P is selectively toxic to tumour vasculature but within hours of administration viable tumour cells at the periphery regrow, supplied by nutrients from the surrounding vasulature, as seen on dynamic contrast-enhanced (DCE) MRI and histological slides.[72]

Single-agent activity *in vitro*, therefore, has been minimal in four phase I studies, but has confirmed vascular disruption on functional imaging.[73]

Enhanced tumour control is achieved *in vivo* when combined with cytotoxic agents, radiotherapy and angiogenesis inhibitors. Enhanced activity is seen when CA4P is combined *in vivo* with cisplatin and irinotecan, suggesting the need for human combination studies.[73]

In a phase Ib study combining carboplatin (AUC = 5) with an infusion of CA4P (27–36 mg/m^2) after 1 hour, nine of 16 patients (56%) experienced grade 3 or 4 neutropenia.[74] This increased myelotoxicity was postulated to be due to decreased renal perfusion after infusion of CA4P leading to accumulation of carboplatin. Subsequently, it has been shown in breast xenograft models that administration after 24 hours is as effective as before chemotherapy. It has also been shown that regrowth at the periphery, perhaps stimulated by CEPs, can be seen 24 hours after administration of CA4P, therefore perhaps this would be the ideal time to administer cytotoxic therapy.[75]

A phase 1b dose-escalation trial with administration of CA4P 20 hours before carboplatin and paclitaxel chemotherapy for treatment of heavily pretreated advanced cancer was therefore undertaken. This demonstrated a response rate of 39% in 18 women with ovarian carcinoma. Toxicity was improved with this method of delivery – grade 3 or 4 neutropenia in 17%, pain in 65% and hypertension in 26% of 46 patients – and was dose dependent.[76]

A phase II trial of 44 patients given 63 mg/m^2 CA4P 18–20 hours before carboplatin (AUC = 5) and paclitaxel (175 mg/m^2) has since been completed in platinum-resistant ovarian cancer. Grade 3 or 4 neutropenia was seen in 25% and hypertension was the most common drug-related toxicity. Other adverse effects were similar to those expected from traditional cytotoxic chemotherapy. Hypertension was easily controlled by glyceryl trinitrate (GTN) and prophylactic amlodipine. Responses were seen in 14 of the patients (32%), with one additional unconfirmed partial response. The addition of CA4P to paclitaxel/carboplatin chemotherapy seems to increase response rate with a favourable adverse effect profile and phase III trials are planned.[77]

OXi4503

OXi4503 (combretastatin A-1 phosphate) is a prodrug of OXi4500 (combretastatin A-1). In pre-clinical studies it is at least ten times more toxic in terms of vascular shutdown, with similar MTD, and thus potentially offers a wider therapeutic window. It also has quinolone metabolites, which may confer additional cytotoxic effects.[73]

OXi4503 (0.06–15.4 mg/m^2 dose escalation) was given to 42 patients with advanced solid tumours. Common adverse events were hypertension, tumour pain, fatigue, myelosuppression and nausea. Drug-related dose-limiting toxicities were seen in both of the patients at 15.4 mg/m^2 (atrial fibrillation and bowel fistula with septic shock secondary to tumour lysis) and two of the patients at 11 mg/m^2 (CTCAE grade 3 hypertension). Seven of 16 evaluable patients (44%) showed DCE-MRI changes consistent with VDA activity. Responses were reported in two women with epithelial ovarian cancer (one at 11 mg/m^2 and one at 14 mg/m^2) and a further patient benefited from control of ascites.[78]

Methods of predicting response and measuring activity

In view of the modest activity and great expense of the currently licensed anti-angiogenic therapies, there is a great need to determine which patients are most likely to benefit from these agents and also to obtain an early signal of activity. So far, there has been no clear predictor of response or resistance to angiogenesis inhibitors. VEGF, E-selectin, thrombospondin and EGFR levels have not been shown to correlate with response.[33] Evaluation of response based on RECIST criteria can contradict that dependent on CA125, suggesting that both methods should be used in conjunction with clinical status. The decrease in vascular tumour perfusion seen using dynamic contrast imaging suggests dynamic methods such as DCE-MRI, positron emission tomography-computed tomography (PET/CT) and MR spectroscopy in phase I and II trials may give an early indication of antivascular effect. We await trials that demonstrate whether these early signals of activity correlate with improvement in response or in PFS.

References

1. Siemann DW, Bibby MC, Dark GG, Dicker AP, Eskens FA, Horsman MR, *et al.* Differentiation and definition of vascular-targeted therapies. *Clin Cancer Res* 2005;11:416–20.
2. Patterson DM, Rustin GJ. Vascular damaging agents. *Clin Oncol (R Coll Radiol)* 2007;19:443–56.
3. Bergers G, Benjamin LE. Tumorigenesis and the angiogenic switch. *Nat Rev Cancer* 2003;3:401–10.
4. Hanahan D, Folkman J. Patterns and emerging mechanisms of the angiogenic switch during tumorigenesis. *Cell* 1996;86:353–64.
5. Folkman J, Watson K, Ingber D, Hanahan D. Induction of angiogenesis during the transition from hyperplasia to neoplasia. *Nature* 1989;339:58–61.
6. Carmeliet P. VEGF gene therapy: stimulating angiogenesis or angioma-genesis? *Nat Med* 2000;6:1102–3.
7. Risau W Mechanisms of angiogenesis. *Nature* 1997;386:671–4.
8. Carmeliet P. Mechanisms of angiogenesis and arteriogenesis. *Nat Med* 2000;6:389–95.
9. Senger DR, Galli SJ, Dvorak AM, Perruzzi CA, Harvey VS, Dvorak HF. Tumour cells secrete a vascular permeability factor that promotes accumulation of ascites fluid. *Science* 1983;219:983–5.
10. Ferrara N, Henzel WJ. Pituitary follicular cells secrete a novel heparin-binding growth factor specific for vascular endothelial cells. *Biochem Biophys Res Commun* 1989;161:851–8.
11. Jain RK, Duda DG. Role of bone marrow-derived cells in tumor angiogenesis and treatment. *Cancer Cell* 2003;3:515–16.
12. Li B, Sharpe EE, Maupin AB, Teleron AA, Pyle AL, Carmeliet P *et al.* VEGF and PIGF promote adult vasculogenesis by enhancing EPC recruitment and vessel formation at the site of tumor neovascularization. *FASEB J* 2006;20:1495–7.
13. Ferrara N, Frantz G, LeCouter J, Dillard-Telm L, Pham T, Draksharapu A, *et al.* Differential expression of the angiogenic factor genes vascular endothelial growth factor (VEGF) and endocrine gland-derived VEGF in normal and polycystic human ovaries. *Am J Pathol* 2003;162:1881–93.
14. Trinh XB, Tjalma WA, Vermeulen PB, Van den Eynden G, Van der Auwera I, Van Laere SJ, *et al.* The VEGF pathway and the AKT/mTOR/p70S6K1 signalling pathway in human epithelial ovarian cancer. *Br J Cancer* 2009;100:971–8.
15. Zhang A, Meng L, Wang Q, Xi L, Chen G, Wang S, *et al.* Enhanced *in vitro* invasiveness of ovarian cancer cells through up-regulation of VEGF and induction of MMP-2. *Oncol Rep* 2006;15:831–6.
16. Okunieff P, Hoeckel M, Dunphy EP, Schlenger K, Knoop C, Vaupel P. Oxygen tension distributions are sufficient to explain the local response of human breast tumors treated with radiation alone. *Int J Radiat Oncol Biol Phys* 1993;26:631–6.
17. Nordsmark M, Overgaard M, Overgaard J. Pretreatment oxygenation predicts radiation response in advanced squamous cell carcinoma of the head and neck. *Radiother Oncol* 1996;41:31–9.
18. Knocke TH, Weitmann HD, Feldmann HJ, Selzer E, Pötter R. Intratumoral pO_2-measurements as predictive assay in the treatment of the uterine cervix. *Radiother Oncol* 1999;53:99–104.
19. Young SD, Marshall RS, Hill RP. Hypoxia induces DNA over-replication and enhances metastatic potential of murine tumor cells. *Proc Natl Acad Sci U S A* 1988;85:9533–7.
20. Jain RK. Normalization of tumor vasculature: an emerging concept in antiangiogenic therapy. *Science* 2005;307:58–62.
21. Campos SM, Ghosh S. A current review of targeted therapeutics for ovarian cancer. *J Oncol* 2010;2010:149362.
22. Fraser HM, Duncan WC. SRB Reproduction, Fertility and Development Award Lecture 2008. Regulation and manipulation of angiogenesis in the ovary and endometrium. *Reprod Fertil Dev* 2009;21:377–92.
23. Shen GH, Ghazizadeh M, Kawanami O, Shimizu H, Jin E, Araki T, *et al.* Prognostic significance of vascular endothelial growth factor expression in human ovarian carcinoma. *Br J Cancer* 2000;83:196–203.
24. Goodheart MJ, Ritchie JM, Rose SL, Fruehauf JP, De Young BR, Buller RE. The relationship of molecular markers of p53 function and angiogenesis to prognosis of stage I epithelial ovarian cancer. *Clin Cancer Res* 2005;11:3733–42.

25. Hefler LA, Mustea A, Könsgen D, Concin N, Tanner B, Strick R, *et al.* Vascular endothelial growth factor gene polymorphisms are associated with prognosis in ovarian cancer. *Clin Cancer Res* 2007;13:898–901.
26. Dvorak HF. Vascular permeability factor/vascular endothelial growth factor: a critical cytokine in tumor angiogenesis and a potential target for diagnosis and therapy. *J Clin Oncol* 2002;20:4368–80.
27. Ferrara N, Kerbel RS. Angiogenesis as a therapeutic target. *Nature* 2005;438:967–74.
28. Byrne AT, Ross L, Holash J, Nakanishi M, Hu L, Hofmann JI, *et al.* Vascular endothelial growth factor-trap decreases tumor burden, inhibits ascites, and causes dramatic vascular remodeling in an ovarian cancer model. *Clin Cancer Res* 2003;9:5721–8.
29. Van Meter ME, Kim ES. Bevacizumab: current updates in treatment. *Curr Opin Oncol* 2010;22:586–91.
30. Burger RA, Sill MW, Monk BJ, Greer BE, Sorosky JI. Phase II trial of bevacizumab in persistent or recurrent epithelial ovarian cancer or primary peritoneal cancer: A Gynaecologic Oncology Group study. *J Clin Oncol* 2007;25:5165–71.
31. Cannistra SA, Matulonis UA, Penson RT, Hambleton J, Dupont J, Mackey H, *et al.* Phase II study of bevacizumab in patients with platinum-resistant ovarian cancer or peritoneal serous cancer. *J Clin Oncol* 2007;25:5180–6. Erratum in: *J Clin Oncol* 2008;26:1773.
32. Chura JC, Van Iseghem K, Downs LS Jr, Carson LF, Judson PL. Bevacizumab plus cyclophosphamide in heavily pretreated patients with recurrent ovarian cancer. *Gynaecol Oncol* 2007;107:326–30.
33. Garcia A, Hirte H, Fleming G, Yang D, Tsao-Wei DD, Roman L, *et al.* Phase II trial of bevacizumab and low-dose metronomic oral cyclophosphamide in recurrent ovarian cancer: A trial of the California, Chicago, and Princess Margaret Hospital Phase II consortia. *J Clin Oncol* 2008;26:76–82.
34. Wright JD, Hagemann A, Rader JS, Viviano D, Gibb RK, Norris L, *et al.* Bevacizumab combination therapy in recurrent, platinum-refractory epithelial ovarian cancer: a retrospective analysis. *Cancer* 2006;107:83–9.
35. Burger R, Brady M, Bookman M, Walker JL, Homesley HD, Fowler J, *et al.* Phase III trial of bevacizumab (BEV) in the primary treatment of advanced epithelial ovarian cancer (EOC), primary peritoneal cancer (PPC), or fallopian tube cancer (FTC): A Gynecologic Oncology Study Group. 2010 ASCO Meeting Proceedings. *J Clin Oncol* 2010;28(18s):abstr LBA1.
36. Perren T, Swart A.M, Pfisterer J, Ledermann J, Lortholary A, Kristensen G, *et al.* Icon7: A phase III randomised Gynaecologic Cancer Intergroup trial of concurrent bevacizumab and chemotherapy followed by maintenance bevacizumab, versus chemotherapy alone in women with newly diagnosed epithelial ovarian (EOC), primary peritoneal (PPC) or fallopian tube cancer (FTC). *Ann Oncol* 2010;21:VIII2.
37. Huynh H, Teo CCM, Khee CS. Bevacizumab and rapamycin inhibit tumor growth in peritoneal model of human ovarian cancer. *Mol Cancer Ther* 2007;11:2959–66.
38. Tabernero J. The role of VEGF and EGFR inhibition: implications for combining anti-VEGF and anti-EGFR agents. *Mol Cancer Res* 2007;5:203–20.
39. Nimieri HS, Oza AM, Morgan RJ, Friberg G, Kasza K, Faoro L, *et al.* Efficacy and safety of bevacizumab plus erlotinib for patients with recurrent ovarian, primary peritoneal, and fallopian tube cancer: A trial of the Chicago, PMH and California Phase II consortia. *Gynaecol Oncol* 2008;110:49–55.
40. Matulonis UA, Berlin S, Ivy P, Tyburski K, Krasner C, Zarwan C, *et al.* Cediranib, an oral inhibitor of vascular endothelial growth factor receptor kinases, is an active drug in recurrent epithelial ovarian, fallopian tube, and peritoneal cancer. *J Clin Oncol* 2009;27:5601–6.
41. Hirte H, Vidal L, Fleming GF, Sugimoto AK, Morgan RJ, Biagi JJ, *et al.* A phase II study of cediranib (AZD 2171) in recurrent or persistent ovarian, peritoneal or fallopian tube cancer: final results of a PMH, Chicago and California consortia trial. *J Clin Oncol* 2008;26(15s):5521.
42. Ledermann J A, Rustin G J, Hackshaw A, Kaye SB, Jayson G, Gabra H, *et al.* A randomized phase II placebo-controlled trial using maintenance therapy to evaluate the vascular targeting agent BIBF 1120 following treatment of relapsed ovarian cancer (OC). *J Clin Oncol* 2009;27(15s):abstr 5501.
43. Friedlander M, Hancock KC, Rischin D, Messing MJ, Stringer CA, Matthys GM, *et al.* A phase II, open-label study evaluating pazopanib in patients with recurrent ovarian cancer. *Gynecol Oncol* 2010;119:32–7.

44. Biagi JJ, Oza AM, Chalchal HI, Grimshaw R, Ellard SL, Lee U, *et al.* A phase II study of sunitinib in patients with recurrent epithelial ovarian and primary peritoneal carcinoma: an NCIC Clinical Trials Group study. *Ann Oncol* 2011;22:335–40.
45. Matei D, Sill MW, DeGreest K, Bristow RE. Phase II trial of sorafenib in persistent or recurrent epithelial ovarian cancer (PPC): a Gynaecologic Oncology Group (GOG) study. *J Clin Oncol* 2008;26(suppl):abstr 5537.
46. Hu L, Hoffman J, Holash J, Yancopoulos GD, Sood AK, Jaffe RB. Vascular endothelial growth factor trap combined with paclitaxel strikingly inhibits tumour and ascites, prolonging survival in a human ovarian cancer model. *Clin Cancer Res* 2005;11:6966–71.
47. Dupont J, Rothenberg ML, Spriggs DR, Cedarbaum JM, Furfine ES, Cohen DP, *et al.* Safety and pharmacokinetics of intravenous VEGF trap in a phase I clinical trial of patients with advanced solid tumours. *J Clin Oncol* 2005;23(16s):abstr 3029.
48. Tew WP, Colombo N, Ray-Coquard I, Oza A, del Campo J, Scambia G, *et al.* VEGF-Trap for patients with recurrent platinum-resistant epithelial ovarian cancer (EOC): preliminary results of a randomized, multicenter phase II study. *J Clin Oncol* 2007;25(18s):abstr 5508.
49. Colleoni M, Rocca A, Sandri MT, Zorzino L, Masci G, Nolè F, *et al.* Low-dose oral methotrexate and cyclophosphamide in metastatic breast cancer: antitumor activity and correlation with vascular endothelial growth factor levels. *Ann Oncol* 2002;13:73–80.
50. Browder T, Folkman J, Hahnfeldt P, Heymach J, Hlatky L, Kieran M, *et al.* Antiangiogenic therapy and p53. *Science* 2002;297:471; discussion 471.
51. Bertolini F, Paul S, Mancuso P, Monestiroli S, Gobbi A, Shaked Y, *et al.* Maximum tolerable dose and low-dose metronomic chemotherapy have opposite effects on the mobilization and viability of circulating endothelial progenitor cells. *Cancer Res* 2003;63:4342–6.
52. Hurteau JA, Brady MF, Darcy KM, McGuire WP, Edmonds P, Pearl ML, *et al.* Randomized phase III trial of tamoxifen versus thalidomide in women with biochemical-recurrent-only epithelial ovarian, fallopian tube or primary peritoneal carcinoma after a complete response to first-line platinum/taxane chemotherapy with an evaluation of serum vascular endothelial growth factor (VEGF): A Gynecologic Oncology Group study. *Gynecol Oncol* 2010;119:444–50.
53. Karlan B, Oza A, Hansen V, Richardson GE, Provencher DM, Ghatage P, *et al.* Randomized, double-blind, placebo-controlled phase 2 study of AMG 386 combined with weekly paclitaxel in patients (pts) with recurrent ovarian carcinoma. *J Clin Oncol* 2010;28(15s):abstr 5000.
54. Chen YB, LaCasce AS. Enzastaurin. *Expert Opin Investig Drugs* 2008;17:939–44.
55. Casey EM, Harb W, Bradford D, Bufill J, Nattam S, Patel J, *et al.* Randomized, double-blinded, multicenter, phase II study of pemetrexed, carboplatin, and bevacizumab with enzastaurin or placebo in chemonaïve patients with stage IIIB/IV non-small cell lung cancer: Hoosier Oncology Group LUN06-116. *J Thorac Oncol* 2010;5:1815–20.
56. Carter A. Integrins as target: first phase III trial launches, but questions remain. *J Natl Cancer Inst* 2010;102:675–7.
57. Ricart AD, Tolcher AW, Liu G, Holen K, Schwartz G, Albertini M, *et al.* Volociximab, a chimeric monoclonal antibody that specifically binds alpha5 beta1 integrin: a phase I, pharmacokinetic, and biological correlative study. *Clin Cancer Res* 2008;14:7924–9.
58. Cadron I, Van Gorp T, Mihalyi A, Luyten C, Drijkoningen K, Amant F, *et al.* The impact of enzastaurin (LY317615.HCl) on CA125 biosynthesis and shedding in ovarian cancer cells. *Gynecol Oncol* 2010;118:64–8.
59. Azad NS, Annunziata CM, Steinberg SM, Minasian L, Premkumar A, Chow C, *et al.* Lack of reliability of CA125 response criteria with anti-VEGF molecularly targeted therapy. *Cancer* 2008;112:1726–32.
60. Rustin GJ, Timmers P, Nelstrop A, Shreeves G, Bentzen SM, Baron B, *et al.* Comparison of CA-125 and standard definitions of progression of ovarian cancer in the intergroup trial of cisplatin and paclitaxel versus cisplatin and cyclophosphamide. *J Clin Oncol* 2006;24:45–51.
61. Monk BJ, Sill MW, Burger RA, Gray HJ, Buekers TE, Roman LD. Phase II trial of bevacizumab in the treatment of persistent or recurrent squamous cell carcinoma of the cervix: a gynecologic oncology group study. *J Clin Oncol* 2009;27:1069–74.
62. Monk BJ, Willmott LJ, Sumner DA. Anti-angiogenesis agents in metastatic or recurrent cervical cancer. *Gynecol Oncol* 2010;116:181–6.

63. Tozer GM, Prise VE, Wilson J, Cemazar M, Shan S, Dewhirst MW, *et al.* Mechanisms associated with tumor vascular shut-down induced by combretastatin A-4 phosphate: intravital microscopy and measurement of vascular permeability. *Cancer Res* 2001;61:6413–22.
64. Zwi LJ, Baguley BC, Gavin JB, Wilson WR. Correlation between immune and vascular activities of xanthenone acetic acid antitumor agents. *Oncol Res* 1994;6:79–85.
65. Denekamp J. Review article: angiogenesis, neovascular proliferation and vascular pathophysiology as targets for cancer therapy. *Br J Radiol* 1993;66:181–96.
66. Lash CJ, Li AE, Rutland M, Baguley BC, Zwi LJ, Wilson WR. Enhancement of the anti-tumour effects of the antivascular agent 5,6-dimethylxanthenone-4-acetic acid (DMXAA) by combination with 5-hydroxytryptamine and bioreductive drugs. *Br J Cancer* 1998;78:439–45.
67. Ching LM, Cao Z, Kieda C, Zwain S, Jameson MB, Baguley BC. Induction of endothelial cell apoptosis by the antivascular agent 5,6-dimethylxanthenone-4-acetic acid. *Br J Cancer* 2002;86:1937–42.
68. Baguley BC, Zhuang L, Kestell P. Increased plasma serotonin following treatment with flavone-8-acetic acid, 5,6-dimethylxanthenone-4-acetic acid, vinblastine, and colchicine: relation to vascular effects. *Oncol Res* 1997;9:55–60.
69. McKeage MJ, Reck M, Jameson MB, Rosenthal MA, Gibbs D, Mainwaring PN, *et al.* Phase II study of ASA404 (vadimezan, 5,6-dimethylxanthenone-4-acetic acid/DMXAA) 1800mg/m(2) combined with carboplatin and paclitaxel in previously untreated advanced non-small cell lung cancer. *Lung Cancer* 2009;65:192–7.
70. Gabra H, AS1404-202 Study Group Investigators. Phase II study of DMXAA combined with carboplatin and paclitaxel in recurrent ovarian cancer. *J Clin Oncol* 2006;24(18s):abstr 5032.
71. Galbraith SM, Chaplin DJ, Lee F, Stratford MR, Locke RJ, Vojnovic B, *et al.* Effects of combretastatin A4 phosphate on endothelial cell morphology *in vitro* and relationship to tumour vascular targeting activity *in vivo*. *Anticancer Res* 2001;21:93–102.
72. Beauregard DA, Thelwall PE, Chaplin DJ, Hill SA, Adams GE, Brindle KM. Magnetic resonance imaging and spectroscopy of combretastatin A4 prodrug-induced disruption of tumour perfusion and energetic status. *Br J Cancer* 1998;77:1761–7.
73. Zweifel M, Rustin G. The clinical development of tubulin binding agents. In: Meyer T, editor. *Vascular Disruptive Agents for the Treatment of Cancer*. New York: Springer; 2010. p. 183–216.
74. Bilenker JH, Flaherty KT, Rosen M, Davis L, Gallagher M, Stevenson JP, *et al.* Phase I trial of combretastatin A-4 phosphate with carboplatin. *Clin Cancer Res* 2005;11:1527–33.
75. Shaked Y, Tang T, Woloszynek J, Daenen LG, Man S, Xu P, *et al.* Contribution of granulocyte colony-stimulating factor to the acute mobilization of endothelial precursor cells by vascular disrupting agents. *Cancer Res* 2009;69:7524–8.
76. Rustin GJ, Shreeves G, Nathan PD, Gaya A, Ganesan TS, Wang D, *et al.* A phase Ib trial of CA4 P (combretastatin A-4 phosphate), carboplatin, and paclitaxel in patients with advanced cancer. *Br J Cancer* 2010;102:1355–60.
77. Zweifel M, Jayson GC, Reed NS, Osborn R, Hassan B, Lederman J, *et al.* Phase II trial of combretastatin A4 phosphate, carboplatin and paclitaxel in patients with platinum-resistant ovarian cancer. *Ann Oncol* 2011 Jan 27 [Epub ahead of print].
78. Zweifel M, Patterson DM, Taylor NJ, Padhani AR, Middleton MR, Price P. Phase I pharmacokinetic and pharmacodynamic evaluation of the vascular disrupting agent OXi4503 in patients with advanced solid tumors. *J Clin Oncol* 2010;28(15s): abstr 2594.
79. Cook KM, Figg WD. Angiogenesis inhibitors: current strategies and future prospects. *CA Cancer J Clin* 2010;60:222–43.

11

Chapter 11

Oncolytic viral gene therapy in ovarian cancer

Iain A McNeish

Introduction

Oncolytic viruses are a novel treatment for cancer. These agents infect cancer cells and replicate selectively within them, causing death with release of mature virions that can subsequently infect neighbouring cells. A series of viruses have been developed and are being taken towards clinical trials in women with relapsed ovarian cancer. However, the majority of data derive from research on adenoviruses. In this chapter, I review the biology of adenoviruses, clinical trials of oncolytic viral gene therapy in ovarian cancer and recent developments that may give cause for cautious optimism.

DNA viruses and cancer

Successful completion of any DNA virus life cycle requires the virus to overcome many cellular pathways and checkpoints in order to permit replication of the viral DNA and generation of new virions. Many of the pathways targeted by DNA viruses are the same as those deregulated in cancer and it is this overlap between virus and cancer biology that makes replicating viruses potential treatments for human malignancy.

The first description of viruses as anti-cancer agents came over 100 years ago and, in 1953, a clinical trial to investigate the therapeutic potential of adenoviruses was conducted in women with cervical cancer and some short-lived responses were seen.[1] More recently, there have been anecdotal descriptions of lymphoma regressing following measles infection.[2]

Adenoviruses are attractive candidates for cancer gene therapy – their biology is very well understood, they can be produced in sufficiently large quantities for clinical studies, they are able to infect a wide range of cells and the wild-type infection is generally mild and self-limiting. Their natural mode of transmission as a respiratory infection does, however, pose problems for systemic delivery, as will be discussed.

Adenovirus life cycle

There are 49 serotypes of human adenoviruses, divided into six groups (Table 11.1). However, the structure and overall life cycle differ little among the serotypes and groups. The adenovirus genome is contained within a capsid comprising 12 penton

Table 11.1 Classification of adenoviruses

Group	Serotype
A	12, 18, 31
B	3, 7, 11, 14, 16, 21, 34, 35
C	1, 2, 5, 6
D	8, 9, 10, 13, 15, 17, 19, 20, 22–30, 32, 33, 36–39, 42–49
E	4
F	40, 41

and 240 hexon subunits, plus minor structural proteins. Adenoviral DNA is linear, approximately 36 kb in length and is tightly wrapped around viral proteins V and VII in the core. It contains five early transcription units named E1A, E1B, E2, E3 and E4, two delayed early units IX and IVa2, and the major late transcription unit, which produces five species of late mRNA designated L1–L5. Transcription occurs from both the leftward and rightward strands of the adenoviral chromosome. With the exception of the E4 region, each transcription unit encodes proteins with similar functions.

The life cycle commences with binding of the adenovirus to its primary receptor, with attachment utlilising the knob domain of the fibre protein projecting from each apex of the virus. For groups A, C, D, E and F, this receptor is CAR, the coxsackie and adenovirus receptor,[3] a component of tight junctions[4] whose knockout in mice leads to cardiac conduction defects.[5] For group B adenoviruses, the two primary receptors are CD46 and desmoglein 2.[6,7] Following attachment to the primary receptor, there is interaction between Arg-Gly-Asp (RGD) motifs in penton proteins, located at the base of the fibre, with the secondary receptors, $\alpha v\beta 3$ and $\alpha v\beta 5$ integrins, whereupon the virus is internalised into an endosome. Following internalisation, the virus capsid escapes the endosome and attaches to microtubules via hexon/cytoplasmic dynein interactions,[8] prompting predominantly minus end-directed microtubule transport.[9] The capsid then binds nuclear protein import pathway components to allow viral DNA to enter the nucleus,[10] where transcription of viral genes commences.

The first viral gene to be transcribed, and the only one whose expression is entirely dependent on host cell factors, is E1A. Because the host cell is the entire determinant of E1A expression and E1A is the sine qua non of productive virus infection, host cell factors have a significant influence on the initiation of viral replication. We have shown that the rate and extent of E1A expression within malignant cells correlates directly with eventual cytotoxicity and that expression of $p21^{Waf1}$ within ovarian cancer cells before infection is a potential marker of a host environment conducive to E1A expression.[11] The E1A product contains three conserved regions, CR1, CR2 and CR3, and it is through these domains that E1A exerts its control over the cell cycle to drive the infected cell into S phase (Figure 11.1),[12] the phase most conducive to replication of the viral genome. E1A CR1 and CR2 both bind to pRb; CR2 binds with high affinity to the B-domain of the pRb pocket while E1A CR1 subsequently binds to pRb directly at the E2F binding site with lower affinity, displacing E2F from the E1A CR2/pRb complex. Free E2F can then transactivate genes necessary for DNA replication and S phase entry. E2F also transactivates the E2 region of the adenovirus, which is how E2F was first described. Thus, normal control of the cell cycle is bypassed by the adenoviral early coding regions in order to facilitate preferential replication of the viral genome.

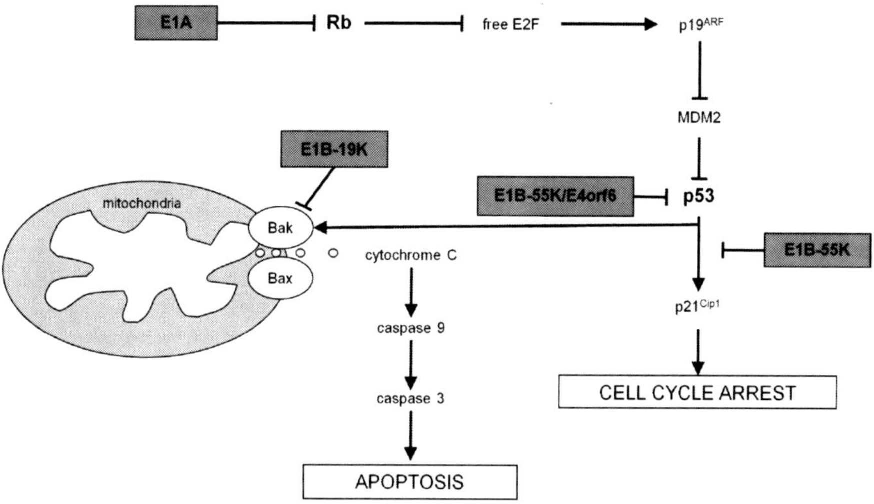

Figure 11.1 Control of cell cycle progression and the intrinsic apoptotic pathway after adenoviral infection; E1 adenoviral early gene products are shown in dark grey

Such deregulation of the host cell cycle will activate pro-apoptotic responses – indeed, E1A has been used as a therapeutic gene in its own right in ovarian cancer gene therapy trials.[13] The two other E1 gene products, E1B-55K and E1B-19K, act to combat premature apoptotic cell death via inhibition of p53 and by functioning as a Bcl-2 homologue, respectively. E1B-55K has been the subject of considerable interest following the development of a first-generation oncolytic vector, dl1520, that was deleted in this gene. E1B-55K functions in two ways to inhibit the activity of p53: it forms a complex with E4orf6 that binds to p53 and targets it for proteasomal destruction, and it binds to the MDM2-binding site of p53, forming a complex that acts as a transcriptional repressor for p53 target genes thus blocking both apoptosis and cell cycle arrest.[14] Finally, E1B-55K also promotes the export of late viral mRNA from the nucleus to the cytoplasm.

The remaining early adenovirus genes have a wide variety of functions. E2 promotes viral DNA replication, E3 encodes for proteins that subvert the host immune response and allow persistence of the infected cell,[15] while the multiple open reading frames from the E4 region have functions that are incompletely understood but that include targeting cellular proteins for proteasomal destruction,[16–18] inhibition of the mTOR pathway to promote translation of viral mRNA species[19] and potentially inducing cell death at the end of the life cycle.[20,21]

The late adenovirus genes (L1–L5) encode all the viral structural proteins required to generate new virions. All five genes are transcribed as a single giant mRNA species from a single promoter, the major late promoter (MLP), which is activated approximately 16 hours post-infection. Final assembly of the viral capsid and insertion of the replicated viral DNA both remain poorly understood, as is the mode of virus-induced cell death. The E3 11.6kDa protein, adenovirus death protein (ADP), has been reported to be essential for cell lysis.[22,23] However, we have shown that in cancer cells its deletion has no effect on virus replication, virion production or cell death.[24] We and others have also shown that adenovirus infected cells do not die by classical apoptosis,[24,25] but it is unclear what role non-apoptotic modes of death such as autophagy[26] and necrosis[24] play in the final demise of the infected cell.

Clinical trials of adenovirus gene therapy in ovarian cancer

There have only been a small number of clinical trials of gene therapy in ovarian cancer. Given that mutations in p53 are almost universal in high-grade serous ovarian cancer,[27] there were early attempts to re-introduce wild-type p53 gene expression using a non-replicating adenovirus. Phase I/II trials indicated that intraperitoneal (IP) delivery of the virus SCH58500, in which wild-type p53 expression lay under transcriptional control of the cytomegalovirus immediate-early promoter/enhancer, was safe up to doses of 7.5×10^{13} particles/day for 5 days when given either alone or in combination with carboplatin and paclitaxel chemotherapy to women with recurrent ovarian cancer.[28] There was no dose-limiting toxicity, although abdominal pain and nausea were common. Vector-specific p53 expression was detected in both ascites and tumour in 17 of 20 samples taken. There were reductions in CA125 of 50% or greater in eight of 16 women who completed three cycles of combination treatment, but no objective responses on computed tomography (CT) scanning. To assess whether the virus-encoded p53 was functional, tumour biopsies from five women were assessed for expression of p53 target genes, such as p21, *BAX* and *MDM2*. Four of the five samples showed increases in these target genes,[29] although there was large inter-patient variability in the degree of induction.

Armed with these largely positive data, a randomised phase II/III trial was conducted in women with advanced ovarian cancer at first presentation. Following primary debulking surgery, women whose tumours had demonstrable p53 mutations were randomised to conventional platinum and paclitaxel chemotherapy with or without IP SCH58500. Sadly, the study has never been published, but it was terminated early after an interim analysis showed no clinical benefit. There was also increased toxicity in the SCH58500 arm.[30] This disappointing outcome led to a reassessment of gene therapy in ovarian cancer and a questioning of the role of gene replacement as a strategy.

The next generation of gene therapy trials involved an oncolytic vector, dl1520, also known as Onyx-015 and H101. This adenovirus type 2/5 vector is deleted in the E1B-55K region as well as in the E3B region. Given the role of E1B-55K in blocking the function of p53 in infected cells, it was hypothesised the dl1520 would replicate only in cells that lacked wild-type p53 function (i.e. many malignant cells). In non-malignant cells, with normal p53 function, the absence of E1B-55K would lead to premature failure of virus replication and prevent lytic infection. Early results appeared to support this hypothesis,[31] including in models of ovarian cancer,[32] although there were siren voices suggesting that dl1520 activity was more complex than the p53 hypothesis suggested.[33,34] Following successful early-phase trials in head and neck squamous cell cancer (in which p53 mutations are common),[35] pancreas cancer[36] and colorectal cancer,[37,38] attention turned to ovarian cancer. A phase I trial of IP dl1520 given on days 1–5 every 3 weeks in 16 women with relapsed ovarian cancer was performed. Doses of up to 1×10^{11} plaque-forming units (pfu) per injection (approximately 10^{12} viral particles) were administered, with one case of dose-limiting abdominal pain and diarrhoea at the 10^{10} pfu dose, although an overall maximum tolerated dose was not achieved. There were no objective or radiological responses, although there was some evidence of viral persistence within ascitic fluid for up to 10 days.[39]

There were several potential explanations for the poor result in this trial. Firstly, p53 sequence alone cannot explain the activity of dl1520, as Goodrum and Ornelles had suggested in 1998.[33] It was subsequently postulated that loss of p14^{Arf} was a better explanation for dl1520 selectivity,[40] although more recently it appears that loss of E1B-55K's ability to promote viral late mRNA export from the nucleus underlies the apparent tumour selectivity of the virus in pre-clinical models.[41] Many tumour cells are able to support viral mRNA export in the absence of E1B-55K, whereas normal cells are not. Secondly, the volume of saline used to deliver the virus (dl1520 was administered in 500 ml of normal saline), in an abdomen distorted by adhesions and scarring, might not be sufficient to allow full dispersal around the abdominal cavity. Thirdly, it was not possible to demonstrate definitively in these ovarian cancer trials whether tumour cells were infected with virus, and maximising infection of target cells is a key element in improving gene therapy approaches, not just in cancer. Finally, the presence of dose-limiting toxicity with abdominal pain following IP administration suggests that virus-induced acute inflammation is a potential barrier to therapy.

Mechanisms to improve selectivity

A series of strategies have been employed to address the shortcoming listed above. Together, these strategies involve analysis of all aspects of adenovirus biology and the most recent clinical trials have yielded more positive results.

Rb pathway targeting

Second-generation oncolytic adenovirus mutants target deficiencies in the Rb pathway and consequent G_1/S checkpoint, which are found in over 80% of human malignancies.[42] In ovarian cancer specifically, multiple different abnormalities in Rb pathway components have been described, which have prognostic significance as well as determining response to chemotherapy.[43–46]

Two adenovirus 5 (Ad5) mutants, dl922–947 and Δ24, have been described, both containing a 24 base pair deletion in the E1A CR2 region, between amino acids 122 and 129.[47,48] E1A CR2 contains an LxCxE motif that is present in a number of cellular proteins that bind to pRb with high affinity and weaken the pRb/E2F complex. As stated above, binding of E1A to pRb results in displacement of E2F, which is then capable of transactivating genes necessary for S phase entry and subsequent viral DNA replication. The net effect of the multiple Rb pathway abnormalities in malignant cells is a rise in free E2F, rendering the E1A CR2/pRb interaction redundant for viral replication. In addition, upregulation of E2F expression is a fundamental feature of many malignant cells,[49] yielding another mechanism by which E1A CR2-deleted viruses can achieve selectivity over normal cells.

In an initial assessment, dl922–947 was found to have greater activity against a range of tumour models than dl1520 and even Ad5 wild-type (WT), with significantly curtailed replication in quiescent normal cells.[50] In ovarian cancer, we have shown that dl922–947 has considerable activity.[49] In vitro, it induced S phase more rapidly than Ad5 WT and could do so in Go-arrested ovarian cancer cells. dl922–947 also has greater cytotoxicity than either Ad5 WT or dl1520 in ovarian cancer cells. In vivo, it significantly prolonged survival for mice treated bearing IP IGROV1 xenografts. In our initial assessment, at a ten-fold lower dose than the control virus, dl922–947 prolonged median survival from 26.5 to 49.5 days ($P<0.001$). At the higher dose, the survival advantage was such that median survival was not reached and 18 mice were still alive at day 125. At post-mortem, mice treated with dl922–947 showed the lowest tumour mass, especially those treated at a higher dose compared with control virus. Our subsequent data support these findings and have highlighted potential biomarkers for response to dl922–947 in ovarian cancer.[51] The initial data for Δ24 used glioblastoma models, but considerable activity was demonstrated.[11] Further development of Δ24 has employed a derivative in which the natural tropism of the virus was modified to ablate binding to the primary receptor CAR, which is discussed below.

Transductional targeting

Curiously for a virus that uses aerosol transmission as its primary mode of infection, most adenoviruses use CAR as the primary receptor, a molecule normally found in tight junctions,[4] where access for viruses might be more difficult. Although there are data suggesting that CAR expression can promote tumour formation and progression,[51] there is a body of data suggesting that CAR expression is downregulated in ovarian cancer.[52] However, careful examination of CAR, $\alpha v\beta 3$ and $\alpha v\beta 5$ expression in ovarian cancers suggests that the majority of tumours do express these receptors,[53] while primary ascitic cells can be infected with Ad5 vectors.[54] Nonetheless, efforts have been made to increase the infectivity of adenovirus in ovarian cancer by replacing the CAR-binding motif within the H1 loop of the knob domain of the adenovirus fibre protein with an RGD motif,[55] which increases infection of CAR-negative ovarian cancer cells with increased cell death both in vitro and in xenografts models.[56] Another strategy to bypass primary binding to CAR is to replace the fibre protein of Ad5 with that of Ad3 or Ad35, which are members of the group B adenoviruses that can utilise CD46 as a primary receptor.[6] Again, in ovarian cancer models with low CAR expression, chimeric Ad5/3 vectors had greater infectivity and greater efficacy than Ad5.[57] A further modification of this strategy has involved a mosaic fibre consisting of Ad5/3 and reovirus σ fibres, which again can improve infectivity with a consequent improvement in cell death.[58]

We have recently described another integrin retargeting strategy. The foot and mouth disease virus (FMDV) uses $\alpha v\beta 6$ as a primary receptor.[59] By incorporating an $\alpha v\beta 6$-selective peptide (A20FMDV2) into the H1 loop of the knob domain of Ad5, we were able to increase infection of CAR-negative tumour cells, with greater tumour uptake *in vivo* as well as reduced uptake in hepatic tissue.[60] The importance of hepatic uptake of adenovirus is described below.

Another strategy to redirect adenovirus infectivity is to ablate all natural receptor binding by 'cloaking' the adenovirus in a polymer into which ligands are then introduced to redirect binding to specific cell surface receptors, such as epidermal growth factor receptor (EGFR), that are overexpressed on malignant cells.[61] This has the advantage both of increasing specificity of adenovirus infection and of reducing adenovirus destruction mediated by neutralising antibodies, which are found in very high titre both in blood and ascites.[62]

Finally, all of these approaches only alter binding of the virus to cell surface receptors. However, the process of infection requires the subsequent steps to be functional (internalisation, endosome escape, microtubule-mediated trafficking and nuclear entry) and it is important to consider these steps in overall gene therapy efficacy. Recent data from our department has indicated that expression of CEACAM6, which is found in a wide range of malignant cells, blocks adenovirus trafficking within the cytoplasm to the nucleus by inhibiting Src signalling.[63] This novel finding suggests further that simple redirection of primary virus binding alone may not improve overall tumour cell infection.

Transcriptional targeting

By replacing key viral promoters with tumour- or tissue-specific promoters, it is possible to generate adenovirus vectors whose replication is restricted to specific cell types. This requires identification of genes whose expression is increased in tumours owing to increased transcription, rather than gene amplification, increased translation or altered protein turnover. Few such genes have been identified specifically in ovarian cancer. In prostate cancer, however, prostate-specific antigen (PSA) is transcriptionally upregulated. The vector CV706, which contains a PSA promoter/enhancer driving E1A expression, has shown some activity in phase I trials.[64] This strategy of cancer-specific transcriptional control was taken to the limit of feasibility with the Onyx-411 vector, which contained E2F-1 promoters driving both E1A (with a CR2 deletion as in dl922–947) and E4 expression. This vector demonstrated initial promising activity in a variety of cancer models.[65]

Increasing cytotoxicity

The ultimate goal of oncolytic viral gene therapy is the selective death of malignant cells following infection and replication. Although viruses are extremely potent inducers of cell death, multiple strategies have been employed to augment cytotoxicity. Because many oncolytic vectors contain deletions in non-essential gene regions, there is capacity within the genome to introduce a transgene with the aim of increasing toxicity. Many variations on this theme have been described, including tissue inhibitors of metalloproteinases,[66] prodrug activating enzymes,[67] short-hairpin RNA species,[68] wild-type p53[69] (rather counter-intuitively), cytokines and apoptosis inducers.[70] Although many positive pre-clinical data have been produced, it seems unlikely that these approaches represent a genuine step-change in the field.

We[71] and many others[72,73] have demonstrated that adenoviruses can synergise with a range of conventional chemotherapy drugs, including paclitaxel, cisplatin and gemcitabine, as well as with radiotherapy.[74] The origin of this synergy remains unclear, although expression of E1A alone sensitises cells to apoptosis-inducing agents. We have shown that dl922–947 can overcome multiple cell cycle checkpoints in ovarian cancer[75] and that this induces significant genomic DNA damage with activation of ATR-Chk1 signalling.[76] More significantly, inhibition of Chk1 with specific inhibitors and RNA interference significantly augments virus efficacy. This implies that synergy with DNA damaging agents at least (for example, cisplatin) may be explained by this mechanism. This is an area of much research currently.

Acute inflammation and hepatotoxicity

In 1999, an 18-year-old man, Jesse Gelsinger, with partial ornithine transcarbamylase (OTC) deficiency, died of multi-organ failure 98 hours after receiving a dose of 6×10^{11} particles/kg (over 10^{13} particles in total) of a non-replicating adenovirus vector encoding OTC via the right hepatic artery.[77] His clinical course was marked by an acute inflammatory reaction and jaundice that commenced shortly after the infusion. This was a most extreme demonstration that systemically administered adenovirus vectors can induce acute inflammatory responses, marked by production of multiple cytokines, especially tumour necrosis factor α (TNF-α), interleukin (IL)-6, IL-1 and IL-8,[78] as well as significant hepatotoxicity.[50] The origin of this toxicity is still under investigation but cytokine induction is seen within minutes of virus infusion,[79] implying that it is the mere presence of virus, rather than expression of individual viral genes, that is sufficient to induce the response. Although adenovirus can be found sequestered with hepatic macrophages (Kupffer cells) shortly following injection,[80] recent data suggest that it is splenic macrophages[81] that trigger a cytokine cascade led by IL-1α following binding of αvβ3 on the macrophage surface to penton base RGD motifs on the virus. In addition, there are also data to suggest that an inflammasome-mediated IL-1β response to double-stranded viral DNA within the cytoplasm occurs.[82] However, virus internalisation and release from the endosome occurs after binding of penton RGD motifs to αvβ3, suggesting that the splenic macrophage response may predominate in vivo. We have recently demonstrated that the acute inflammatory response to adenovirus acts to reduce virus efficacy: inhibition of TNF-α using both RNA interference and inhibitory monoclonal antibodies augmented virus efficacy in models of ovarian cancer by suppression of cellular inhibitors of apoptosis 1 and 2 (cIAP1/2) and consequent increase in caspase-mediated apoptosis.[78]

Recent data have also revealed that the hepatic uptake of adenovirus is mediated indirectly via coagulation factors. Initial results suggested that factor (F) IX and complement C4-binding protein interacted with the fibre protein, which in turn promoted Kupffer cell uptake.[83] However, more recent publications suggest that FX is the principal factor involved and that it binds directly to the more abundant hexon protein to mediate uptake within the liver.[84] Interestingly, our data on the A20FMDV2-retargeted virus that differs from Ad5 WT only in its fibre knob H1 loop indicate that there is reduced hepatic uptake compared with wild-type viruses, implying that fibre protein motifs can still influence whether virus is sequestered within the liver.[60] In addition, ablating the FX-binding motifs on hexon did not alter the inflammatory profile of systemically administered adenovirus at low and intermediate doses and actually increased cytokine release at high dose,[85] implying that there is a separation between induction of inflammation and hepatic sequestration. This is supported by our data whereby blockade of TNF-α had no effect on hepatic toxicity in nude female mice.[78]

Clinical trial update and conclusions

The history of viral gene therapy trials in ovarian cancer is not a very happy one. However, there was considerable excitement with the presentation and publication of a recent phase I trial of IP Ad5 Δ24-RGD in women with relapsed gynaecological cancers, the majority of whom had ovarian cancer.[86] As stated above, Ad5 Δ24-RGD contains a 24 base pair deletion in E1A CR2 and an integrin-bindng RGD motif in the H1 loop of the fibre knob domain to redirect primary virus binding away from CAR to αvβ3 and αvβ5 integrins. Doses of up to 1×10^{12} particles/day were administered without dose-limiting toxicity, although grade 1–2 abdominal pain and fever were experienced. Rising titres of virus in ascites beyond day 3 were suggestive of active virus replication and 71% of patients had stable disease 1 month post-treatment. Although highly preliminary, this is the first significant gene therapy clinical trial in ovarian cancer for 8 years. It is hoped that this will be followed by phase II and even phase III studies.

These future trials will have multiple questions to address, the most pressing of which are the role of acute inflammatory responses and hepatic uptake – abdominal pain is a universal feature in gene therapy trials that include IP administration of adenovirus and is likely to be the dose-limiting toxicity. In addition, as with many novel targeted agents, the optimum therapeutic approach is likely to involve administration with or following conventional chemo- or radiotherapy, but the timing, dosing and scheduling of these combinations will take many trials to optimise. Most importantly, there remain many questions about the biology of adenoviruses that are unanswered – many of these relate to the role of host cell factors in determining cell fate following infection and the potential role of immune responses in cell death in whole organisms. The next few years will be crucial in answering these questions and it remains essential that clinical trials continue to allow further progress.

References

1. Everts B, van der Poel HG. Replication-selective oncolytic viruses in the treatment of cancer. *Cancer Gene Ther* 2005;12:141–61.
2. Zygiert Z. Hodgkin's disease: remissions after measles. *Lancet* 1971;i:593.
3. Bergelson JM, Cunningham JA, Droguett G, Kurt-Jones EA, Krithivas A, Hong JS, *et al.* Isolation of a common receptor for Coxsackie B viruses and adenoviruses 2 and 5. *Science* 1997;275:1320–3.
4. Raschperger E, Thyberg J, Pettersson S, Philipson L, Fuxe J, Pettersson RF. The coxsackie- and adenovirus receptor (CAR) is an *in vivo* marker for epithelial tight junctions, with a potential role in regulating permeability and tissue homeostasis. *Exp Cell Res* 2006;312:1566–80.
5. Lim BK, Xiong D, Dorner A, Youn TJ, Yung A, Liu TI, *et al.* Coxsackievirus and adenovirus receptor (CAR) mediates atrioventricular-node function and connexin 45 localization in the murine heart. *J Clin Invest* 2008;118:2758–70.
6. Segerman A, Atkinson JP, Marttila M, Dennerquist V, Wadell G, Arnberg N. Adenovirus type 11 uses CD46 as a cellular receptor. *J Virol* 2003;77:9183–91.
7. Wang H, Li ZY, Liu Y, Persson J, Beyer I, Möller T, *et al.* Desmoglein 2 is a receptor for adenovirus serotypes 3, 7, 11 and 14. *Nat Med* 2011;17:96–104.
8. Kelkar SA, Pfister KK, Crystal RG, Leopold PL. Cytoplasmic dynein mediates adenovirus binding to microtubules. *J Virol* 2004;78:10122–32.
9. Mabit H, Nakano MY, Prank U, Saam B, Döhner K, Sodeik B, *et al.* Intact microtubules support adenovirus and herpes simplex virus infections. *J Virol* 2002;76:9962–71.
10. Saphire AC, Guan T, Schirmer EC, Nemerow GR, Gerace L. Nuclear import of adenovirus DNA *in vitro* involves the nuclear protein import pathway and hsc70. *J Biol Chem* 2000;275:4298–304.
11. Flak MB, Connell CM, Chelala C, Archibald K, Salako MA, Pirlo KJ, *et al.* p21 Promotes oncolytic adenoviral activity in ovarian cancer and is a potential biomarker. *Mol Cancer* 2010;9:175.
12. White E. Regulation of the cell cycle and apoptosis by the oncogenes of adenovirus. *Oncogene* 2001;20:7836–46.
13. Madhusudan S, Tamir A, Bates N, Flanagan E, Gore ME, Barton DP, *et al.* A multicenter Phase I gene therapy clinical trial involving intraperitoneal administration of E1A-lipid complex in patients with recurrent epithelial ovarian cancer overexpressing HER-2/*neu* oncogene. *Clin Cancer Res* 2004;10:2986–96.
14. Martin ME, Berk AJ. Adenovirus E1B 55K represses p53 activation *in vitro*. *J Virol* 1998;72:3146–54.
15. Wold WS, Gooding LR. Region E3 of adenovirus: a cassette of genes involved in host immunosurveillance and virus-cell interactions. *Virology* 1991;184:1–8.
16. Shtrichman R, Sharf R, Kleinberger T. Adenovirus E4orf4 protein interacts with both Balpha and B′ subunits of protein phosphatase 2A, but E4orf4-induced apoptosis is mediated only by the interaction with Balpha. *Oncogene* 2000;19:3757–65.
17. Carson CT, Orazio NI, Lee DV, Suh J, Bekker-Jensen S, Araujo FD, *et al.* Mislocalization of the MRN complex prevents ATR signaling during adenovirus infection. *EMBO J* 2009;28:652–62.
18. Karen KA, Hoey PJ, Young CS, Hearing P. Temporal regulation of the Mre11-Rad50-Nbs1 complex during adenovirus infection. *J Virol* 2009;83:4565–73.
19. Huang JT, Schneider RJ. Adenovirus inhibition of cellular protein synthesis involves inactivation of cap-binding protein. *Cell* 1991;65:271–80.
20. Branton PE, Roopchand DE. The role of adenovirus E4orf4 protein in viral replication and cell killing. *Oncogene* 2001; 20: 7855–65.
21. Lavoie JN, Nguyen M, Marcellus RC, Branton PE, Shore GC. Lavoie E4orf4, a novel adenovirus death factor that induces p53-independent apoptosis by a pathway that is not inhibited by zVAD-fmk. *J Cell Biol* 1998;140:637–45.

22. Tollefson AE, Ryerse JS, Scaria A, Hermiston TW, Wold WS. The E3-11.6-kDa adenovirus death protein (ADP) is required for efficient cell death: characterization of cells infected with adp mutants. *Virology* 1996;220:152–62.
23. Tollefson AE, Scaria A, Hermiston TW, Ryerse JS, Wold LJ, Wold WS. The adenovirus death protein (E3-11.6K) is required at very late stages of infection for efficient cell lysis and release of adenovirus from infected cells. *J Virol* 1996;70:2296–306.
24. Baird SK, Aerts JL, Eddaoudi A, Lockley M, Lemoine NR, McNeish IA. Oncolytic adenoviral mutants induce a novel mode of programmed cell death in ovarian cancer. *Oncogene* 2008;27:3081–90.
25. Ito H, Aoki H, Kuhnel F, Kondo Y, Kubicka S, Wirth T, *et al.* Autophagic cell death of malignant glioma cells induced by a conditionally replicating adenovirus. *J Natl Cancer Inst* 2006;98:625–36.
26. Jiang H, Gomez-Manzano C, Aoki H, Alonso MM, Kondo S, McCormick F, *et al.* Examination of the therapeutic potential of Delta-24-RGD in brain tumor stem cells: role of autophagic cell death. *J Natl Cancer Inst* 2007;99:1410–14.
27. Ahmed AA, Etemadmoghadam D, Temple J, Lynch AG, Riad M, Sharma R, *et al.* Driver mutations in *TP53* are ubiquitous in high grade serous carcinoma of the ovary. *J Pathol* 2010;221:49–56.
28. Buller RE, Runnebaum IB, Karlan BY, Horowitz JA, Shahin M, Buekers T, *et al.* A phase I/II trial of rAd/p53 (SCH 58500) gene replacement in recurrent ovarian cancer. *Cancer Gene Ther* 2002;9:553–66.
29. Wen SF, Mahavni V, Quijano E, Shinoda J, Grace M, Musco-Hobkinson ML, *et al.* Assessment of p53 gene transfer and biological activities in a clinical study of adenovirus-p53 gene therapy for recurrent ovarian cancer. *Cancer Gene Ther* 2003;10:224–38.
30. Zeimet AG, Marth C. Why did p53 gene therapy fail in ovarian cancer? *Lancet Oncol* 2003;4:415–22.
31. Heise C, Sampson-Johannes A, Williams A, McCormick F, Von Hoff DD, Kirn DH. ONYX-015, an E1B gene-attenuated adenovirus, causes tumor-specific cytolysis and antitumoral efficacy that can be augmented by standard chemotherapeutic agents. *Nat Med* 1997;3:639–45.
32. Heise C, Ganly I, Kim YT, Sampson-Johannes A, Brown R, Kirn D. Efficacy of a replication-selective adenovirus against ovarian carcinomatosis is dependent on tumor burden, viral replication and p53 status. *Gene Ther* 2000;7:1925–9.
33. Goodrum FD, Ornelles DA. p53 status does not determine outcome of E1B 55-kilodalton mutant adenovirus lytic infection. *J Virol* 1998;72:9479–90.
34. Harada JN, Berk AJ. p53-Independent and -dependent requirements for E1B-55K in adenovirus type 5 replication. *J Virol* 1999;73:5333–44.
35. Nemunaitis J, Ganly I, Khuri F, Arseneau J, Kuhn J, McCarty T, *et al.* Selective replication and oncolysis in p53 mutant tumors with ONYX-015, an E1B-55KD gene-deleted adenovirus, in patients with advanced head and neck cancer: a phase II trial. *Cancer Res* 2000;60:6359–66.
36. Mulvihill S, Warren R, Venook A, Adler A, Randlev B, Heise C, *et al.* Safety and feasibility of injection with an E1B-55 kDa gene-deleted, replication-selective adenovirus (ONYX-015) into primary carcinomas of the pancreas: a phase I trial. *Gene Ther* 2001;8:308–15.
37. Nemunaitis J, Cunningham C, Buchanan A, Blackburn A, Edelman G, Maples P, *et al.* Intravenous infusion of a replication-selective adenovirus (ONYX-015) in cancer patients: safety, feasibility and biological activity. *Gene Ther* 2001;8:746–59.
38. Reid T, Galanis E, Abbruzzese J, Sze D, Andrews J, Romel L, Hatfield M, Rubin J, Kirn D. Intra-arterial administration of a replication-selective adenovirus (dl1520) in patients with colorectal carcinoma metastatic to the liver: a phase I trial. *Gene Ther* 2001;8:1618–26.
39. Vasey PA, Shulman LN, Campos S, Davis J, Gore M, Johnston S, *et al.* Phase I trial of intraperitoneal injection of the E1B-55-kd-gene-deleted adenovirus ONYX-015 (*dl*1520) given on days 1 through 5 every 3 weeks in patients with recurrent/refractory epithelial ovarian cancer. *J Clin Oncol* 2002;20:1562–9.
40. Ries SJ, Brandts CH, Chung AS, Biederer CH, Hann BC, *et al.* Loss of $p14^{ARF}$ in tumor cells facilitates replication of the adenovirus mutant dl1520 (ONYX-015). *Nat Med* 2000;6:1128–33.
41. O'Shea CC, Johnson L, Bagus B, Choi S, Nicholas C, Shen A, *et al.* Late viral RNA export, rather than p53 inactivation, determines ONYX-015 tumor selectivity. *Cancer Cell* 2004;6:611–23.
42. Sherr CJ, McCormick F. The RB and p53 pathways in cancer. *Cancer Cell* 2002;2:103–12.

43. Barboule N, Baldin V, Jozan S, Vidal S, Valette A. Increased level of p21 in human ovarian tumors is associated with increased expression of cdk2, cyclin A and PCNA. *Int J Cancer* 1998;76:891–6.
44. Plisiecka-Hałasa J, Karpińska G, Szymańska T, Ziółkowska I, Madry R, Timorek A, *et al.* $P21^{WAF1}$, $P27^{KIP1}$, TP53 and C-MYC analysis in 204 ovarian carcinomas treated with platinum-based regimens. *Ann Oncol* 2003;14:1078–85.
45. Bali A, O'Brien PM, Edwards LS, Sutherland RL, Hacker NF, Henshall SM. Cyclin D1, p53, and $p21^{Waf1/Cip1}$ expression is predictive of poor clinical outcome in serous epithelial ovarian cancer. *Clin Cancer Res* 2004;10:5168–77.
46. Etemadmoghadam D, deFazio A, Beroukhim R, Mermel C, George J, Getz G, *et al*; AOCS Study Group. Integrated genome-wide DNA copy number and expression analysis identifies distinct mechanisms of primary chemoresistance in ovarian carcinomas. *Clin Cancer Res* 2009;15:1417–27.
47. Fueyo J, Gomez-Manzano C, Alemany R, Lee PS, McDonnell TJ, Mitlianga P, *et al.* A mutant oncolytic adenovirus targeting the Rb pathway produces anti-glioma effect *in vivo*. *Oncogene* 2000;19:2–12. Erratum in: *Oncogene* 2000;19:5038.
48. Heise C, Hermiston T, Johnson L, Brooks G, Sampson-Johannes A, Williams A, *et al.* An adenovirus E1A mutant that demonstrates potent and selective systemic anti-tumoral efficacy. *Nat Med* 2000;6:1134–9. Erratum in: *Nat Med* 2000;6:1412.
49. Johnson DG, Cress WD, Jakoi L, Nevins JR. Oncogenic capacity of the E2F1 gene. *Proc Natl Acad Sci U S A* 1994;91:12823–7.
50. Lockley M, Fernandez M, Wang Y, Li NF, Conroy S, Lemoine N, *et al.* Activity of the adenoviral E1A deletion mutant dl922-947 in ovarian cancer: comparison with E1A wild-type viruses, bioluminescence monitoring, and intraperitoneal delivery in icodextrin. *Cancer Res* 2006;66:989–98.
51. Qin M, Escuadro B, Dohadwala M, Sharma S, Batra RK. A novel role for the coxsackie adenovirus receptor in mediating tumor formation by lung cancer cells. *Cancer Res* 2004;64:6377–80.
52. Kim M, Zinn KR, Barnett BG, Sumerel LA, Krasnykh V, Curiel DT, *et al.* The therapeutic efficacy of adenoviral vectors for cancer gene therapy is limited by a low level of primary adenovirus receptors on tumour cells. *Eur J Cancer* 2002;38:1917–26.
53. Zeimet AG, Muller-Holzner E, Schuler A, Hartung G, Berger J, Hermann M, *et al.* Determination of molecules regulating gene delivery using adenoviral vectors in ovarian carcinomas. *Gene Ther* 2002;9:1093–100.
54. Kelly FJ, Miller CR, Buchsbaum DJ, Gomez-Navarro J, Barnes MN, Alvarez RD, *et al.* Selectivity of TAG-72-targeted adenovirus gene transfer to primary ovarian carcinoma cells versus autologous mesothelial cells *in vitro*. *Clin Cancer Res* 2000;6:4323–33.
55. Reynolds P, Dmitriev I, Curiel D. Insertion of an RGD motif into the HI loop of adenovirus fiber protein alters the distribution of transgene expression of the systemically administered vector. *Gene Ther* 1999;6:1336–9.
56. Bauerschmitz GJ, Lam JT, Kanerva A, Suzuki K, Nettelbeck DM, Dmitriev I, *et al.* Treatment of ovarian cancer with a tropism modified oncolytic adenovirus. *Cancer Res* 2002;62:1266–70.
57. Kanerva A, Zinn KR, Chaudhuri TR, Lam JT, Suzuki K, Uil TG, *et al.* Enhanced therapeutic efficacy for ovarian cancer with a serotype 3 receptor-targeted oncolytic adenovirus. *Mol Ther* 2003;8:449–58.
58. Tsuruta Y, Pereboeva L, Glasgow JN, Rein DT, Kawakami Y, Alvarez RD, *et al.* A mosaic fiber adenovirus serotype 5 vector containing reovirus sigma 1 and adenovirus serotype 3 knob fibers increases transduction in an ovarian cancer *ex vivo* system via a coxsackie and adenovirus receptor-independent pathway. *Clin Cancer Res* 2007;13:2777–83.
59. Jackson T, Sheppard D, Denyer M, Blakemore W, King AM. The epithelial integrin alphavbeta6 is a receptor for foot-and-mouth disease virus. *J Virol* 2000;74:4949–56.
60. Coughlan L, Vallath S, Saha A, Flak M, McNeish IA, Vassaux G, Marshall JF, Hart IR, Thomas GJ. *In vivo* retargeting of adenovirus type 5 to alphavbeta6 integrin results in reduced hepatotoxicity and improved tumor uptake following systemic delivery. *J Virol* 2009;83:6416–28.
61. Fisher KD, Stallwood Y, Green NK, Ulbrich K, Mautner V, Seymour LW. Polymer-coated adenovirus permits efficient retargeting and evades neutralising antibodies. *Gene Ther* 2001;8:341–8.
62. Stallwood Y, Fisher KD, Gallimore PH, Mautner V. Neutralisation of adenovirus infectivity by ascitic fluid from ovarian cancer patients. *Gene Ther* 2000;7:637–43.

63. Wang Y, Gangeswaran R, Zhao X, Wang P, Tysome J, Bhakta V, *et al.* CEACAM6 attenuates adenovirus infection by antagonizing viral trafficking in cancer cells. *J Clin Invest* 2009;119:1604–15.
64. DeWeese TL, van der Poel H, Li S, Mikhak B, Drew R, Goemann M, *et al.* A phase I trial of CV706, a replication-competent, PSA selective oncolytic adenovirus, for the treatment of locally recurrent prostate cancer following radiation therapy. *Cancer Res* 2001;61:7464–72.
65. Johnson L, Shen A, Boyle L, Kunich J, Pandey K, Lemmon M, *et al.* Selectively replicating adenoviruses targeting deregulated E2F activity are potent, systemic antitumor agents. *Cancer Cell* 2002;1:325–37.
66. Yang SW, Cody JJ, Rivera AA, Waehler R, Wang M, Kimball KJ, *et al.* Conditionally replicating adenovirus expressing TIMP2 for ovarian cancer therapy. *Clin Cancer Res* 2011;17:538–49.
67. Chen MJ, Green NK, Reynolds GM, Flavell JR, Mautner V, Kerr DJ, *et al.* Enhanced efficacy of *Escherichia coli* nitroreductase/CB1954 prodrug activation gene therapy using an E1B-55K-deleted oncolytic adenovirus vector. *Gene Ther* 2004;11:1126–36.
68. Höti N, Chowdhury WH, Mustafa S, Ribas J, Castanares M, Johnson T, *et al.* Armoring CRAds with p21/Waf-1 shRNAs: the next generation of oncolytic adenoviruses. *Cancer Gene Ther* 2010;17:585–97.
69. He X, Liu J, Yang C, Su C, Zhou C, Zhang Q, *et al.* 5/35 Fiber-modified conditionally replicative adenovirus armed with p53 shows increased tumor-suppressing capacity to breast cancer cells. *Hum Gene Ther* 2011;22:283–92.
70. Ren XW, Liang M, Meng X, Ye X, Ma H, Zhao Y, *et al.* A tumor-specific conditionally replicative adenovirus vector expressing TRAIL for gene therapy of hepatocellular carcinoma. *Cancer Gene Ther* 2006;13:159–68.
71. Ingemarsdotter CK, Baird SK, Connell CM, Öberg D, Halldén G, McNeish IA. Low-dose paclitaxel synergizes with oncolytic adenoviruses via mitotic slippage and apoptosis in ovarian cancer. *Oncogene* 2010;29:6051–63.
72. Hecht JR, Bedford R, Abbruzzese JL, Lahoti S, Reid TR, Soetikno RM, *et al.* A phase I/II trial of intratumoral endoscopic ultrasound injection of ONYX-015 with intravenous gemcitabine in unresectable pancreatic carcinoma. *Clin Cancer Res* 2003;9:555–61.
73. Cheong SC, Wang Y, Meng JH, Hill R, Sweeney K, Kirn D, *et al.* E1A-expressing adenoviral E3B mutants act synergistically with chemotherapeutics in immunocompetent tumor models. *Cancer Gene Ther* 2008;15:40–50.
74. Rogulski KR, Freytag SO, Zhang K, Gilbert JD, Paielli DL, Kim JH, *et al.* *In vivo* antitumor activity of ONYX-015 is influenced by p53 status and is augmented by radiotherapy. *Cancer Res* 2000;60:1193–6.
75. Connell CM, Wheatley SP, McNeish IA. Nuclear survivin abrogates multiple cell cycle checkpoints and enhances viral oncolysis. *Cancer Res* 2008;68):7923–31.
76. Connell CM, Shibata A, Tookman LA, Archibald KM, Flak MB, Pirlo KJ, Lockley M, Wheatley SP, McNeish IA. Genomic DNA damage and ATR-Chk1 signaling determine oncolytic adenoviral efficacy in human ovarian cancer cells. *J Clin Invest* 2011 [Epub ahead of print].
77. Raper SE, Chirmule N, Lee FS, Wivel NA, Bagg A, Gao GP, *et al.* Fatal systemic inflammatory response syndrome in a ornithine transcarbamylase deficient patient following adenoviral gene transfer. *Mol Genet Metab* 2003;80:148–58.
78. Salako MA, Kulbe H, Ingemarsdotter CK, Pirlo KJ, Williams SL, Lockley M, *et al.* Inhibition of the inflammatory cytokine TNF-α increases adenovirus activity in ovarian cancer via modulation of cIAP1/2 expression. *Mol Ther* 2011;19:490–9.
79. Lieber A, He CY, Meuse L, Schowalter D, Kirillova I, Winther B, *et al.* The role of Kupffer cell activation and viral gene expression in early liver toxicity after infusion of recombinant adenovirus vectors. *J Virol* 1997;71:8798–807.
80. Shayakhmetov DM, Li ZY, Ni S, Lieber A. Analysis of adenovirus sequestration in the liver, transduction of hepatic cells, and innate toxicity after injection of fiber-modified vectors. *J Virol* 2004;78:5368–81.
81. Di Paolo NC, Miao EA, Iwakura Y, Murali-Krishna K, Aderem A, Flavell RA, *et al.* Virus binding to a plasma membrane receptor triggers interleukin-1 alpha-mediated proinflammatory macrophage response *in vivo*. *Immunity* 2009;31:110–21.

82. Muruve DA, Pétrilli V, Zaiss AK, White LR, Clark SA, Ross PJ, *et al.* The inflammasome recognizes cytosolic microbial and host DNA and triggers an innate immune response. *Nature* 2008;452:103–7.
83. Shayakhmetov DM, Gaggar A, Ni S, Li ZY, Lieber A. Adenovirus binding to blood factors results in liver cell infection and hepatotoxicity. *J Virol* 2005;79:7478–91.
84. Waddington SN, McVey JH, Bhella D, Parker AL, Barker K, Atoda H, *et al.* Adenovirus serotype 5 hexon mediates liver gene transfer. *Cell* 2008;132:397–409.
85. Alba R, Bradshaw AC, Coughlan L, Denby L, McDonald RA, Waddington SN, *et al.* Biodistribution and retargeting of FX-binding ablated adenovirus serotype 5 vectors. *Blood* 2010;116:2656–64.
86. Kimball KJ, Preuss MA, Barnes MN, Wang M, Siegal GP, Wan W, *et al.* A phase I study of a tropism-modified conditionally replicative adenovirus for recurrent malignant gynecologic diseases. *Clin Cancer Res* 2010;16:5277–87.

12

Chapter 12

Endometrial cancer: what have the clinical trials taught us?

Andrew Clamp

Introduction

Endometrial cancer is the fourth most common female malignancy in the UK, with 7536 cases diagnosed in 2007.[1] Notably, the age-standardised incidence of endometrial cancer rose by 40% between 1993 and 2007, which was related to several factors but most importantly the rising epidemic of obesity.[2] Owing to the early warning symptom of postmenopausal bleeding, 75% of cases present at an early stage (International Federation of Gynecology and Obstetrics [FIGO] stage I) and in most cases can be managed by surgery alone. However, 25% of patients, particularly those with cancers of high histological grade (type II endometrial cancer) present with more advanced disease. These women are candidates for adjuvant treatment strategies and are at significant risk of disease recurrence. Indeed, there were 1741 deaths due to advanced/recurrent endometrial cancer in the UK in 2008.[1]

In the past decade, a large number of clinical trials have been conducted that have attempted to address several important issues with respect to improving the outcomes in women with endometrial cancer. In this chapter I provide a synopsis of the published and continuing clinical research in several controversial areas, from initial surgical management through adjuvant systemic therapy to the management of recurrent disease.

Surgery at first presentation

In most cases, the initial management of endometrial cancer confined to the uterus should be surgical and consist of total abdominal hysterectomy (TAH), bilateral salpingo-oophorectomy (BSO) and inspection of the abdominal cavity with peritoneal washings.[3] While the complication rate from abdominal hysterectomy is low, many women with endometrial cancer are elderly and have significant comorbidities. Alternative surgical strategies have therefore been investigated.

Laparoscopic surgery

Laparoscopic hysterectomy is an attractive approach as it may potentially reduce some of the morbidity associated with an open procedure.[4] Three phase III randomised controlled trials have now been published that compared a laparoscopic approach with abdominal surgery in a total of 3260 women with early-stage endometrial cancer.[5–7] The LAP2 trial[5] included 2616 women who underwent hysterectomy, BSO and routine pelvic and para-aortic lymphadenectomy either by a laparoscopic or an open approach. Laparoscopic surgery was associated with a lower risk of postoperative complications (14% versus 21%; $P < 0.001$), shorter hospitalisation (52% versus 94% stayed more than 2 days; $P < 0.0001$) and improved quality of life for at least 6 weeks after surgery[8] although the magnitude of the improvement demonstrated may not have great clinical significance. However, 26% of the women initially randomised to the laparoscopic approach required conversion to a laparotomy. Smaller Dutch[6] and Australasian[7] studies have largely confirmed these findings and reassuringly reported much lower rates of conversion to open surgery. However, while the reduced morbidity of laparoscopic hysterectomy has clearly been demonstrated, data on recurrence rates and survival outcomes have not yet been reported and it is therefore too early to consider laparoscopic surgery as a new standard of care.

Systematic lymphadenectomy

The role of lymphadenectomy as part of routine surgical staging is hotly debated (Table 10.1). While this procedure may allow accurate staging and potentially allow planning of adjuvant treatment strategies, it is becoming clear that it has no therapeutic role in women with low-risk endometrial cancer but increases postoperative morbidity, in particular the rate of lymphoedema. In a randomised trial conducted by Benedetti-Panici *et al*,[9] 514 women with clinical stage I endometrial cancer and myometrial invasion documented intraoperatively were randomised to undergo TAH/BSO with or without systematic pelvic lymphadenectomy. In the lymphadenectomy arm, 13.3% of the women had histologically involved lymph nodes compared with 3.3% of those who did not undergo systematic lymph node dissection. After a median follow-up of 49 months, no differences in disease-free survival or overall survival (OS) were noted between the two arms. The ASTEC trial[10] conducted the same randomisation in 1408 women with histologically proven endometrial cancer thought preoperatively to be confined to the uterus. In the lymphadenectomy arm, 9% of the women had pathological nodal involvement. Again, after 37 months median follow-up, no differences in disease-free survival or OS were detectable.

Although these studies clearly do not support the routine use of pelvic lymphadenectomy, they have been heavily criticised. The surgical yield of lymph nodes in the ASTEC trial was low with a median of 12 lymph nodes removed and retrospective studies suggest improved outcomes with more extensive lymph node resections[11] – however, sensitivity analysis of the ASTEC data does not show a trend towards better outcomes in women in whom more lymph nodes were removed. While postoperative therapy was controlled in the ASTEC trial owing to a subsequent randomisation to adjuvant pelvic irradiation, this was left to the investigator's discretion in the Italian study, resulting in an imbalance in postoperative treatment between the two arms that may have affected outcome. However, it was notable that adjuvant chemotherapy was used more frequently in women who underwent lymphadenectomy.

Importantly, however, both trials only included women at low risk of nodal involvement and it is perhaps therefore unsurprising that no survival benefit was detected. The therapeutic role of lymphadenectomy in women with higher risk endometrial cancer is still undefined. The retrospective analysis in the SEPAL study[12]

Table 10.1 Studies exploring the role of systematic lymphadenectomy in endometrial cancer

Study	Inclusion criteria	Arm	Women (*n*)	LNs sampled (median)	% LN involvement	5 year DFS (%)	5 year OS (%)
Randomised controlled trials							
ASTEC trial (2009)[10]	Histologically proven endometrial cancer preoperatively thought to be confined to uterus	Lymphadenectomy	704	12	9	73	80
		No lymphadenectomy	704	0	1	79	81
Benedetti-Panici *et al.* (2008)[9]	Clinical stage I endometrial cancer with intraoperative documentation of myometrial invasion	Lymphadenectomy	264	30	13.3	81.0	85.9
		No lymphadenectomy	250	0	3.2	81.7	90.0
Retrospective analysis							
SEPAL, low risk (2010)[12]	Stage IA grade 1–2 endometrioid cancer. LVSI negative	Pelvic lymphadenectomy	131	34	0	92.7	94.2
		Para-aortic lymphadenectomy	133	82	0	95.3	96.2
SEPAL, intermediate–high risk (2010)[12]	All other endometrial cancers	Pelvic lymphadenectomy	194	34	24	64.8	72.6
		Para-aortic lymphadenectomy	213	82	29	80.3	83.2

DFS = disease-free survival; LN = lymph node; LVSI = lymphovascular space invasion; OS = overall survival provides intriguing data to indicate that further clinical trial evaluation of systematic pelvic and para-aortic lymphadenectomy is warranted in this group. The SEPAL study included 671 women with endometrial cancer who were treated over an 18 year period at two neighbouring Japanese specialist centres. One centre routinely performed systematic pelvic and para-aortic nodal dissection and the other performed only pelvic lymphadenectomy. In women at intermediate to high risk of disease recurrence, a significant difference in OS was noted in favour of the group undergoing more radical nodal dissection (5 year OS 83% versus 73%; $P = 0.0009$). While the two groups were balanced for age and histopathological factors, the two centres had differing policies for adjuvant treatment, resulting in more women in the para-aortic lymphadenectomy group receiving postoperative chemotherapy. Indeed, both para-aortic lymphadenectomy (hazard ratio [HR] 0.48; 95% CI 0.29–0.83) and use of chemotherapy (HR 0.59; 95% CI 0.37–1.00) were significant independent factors associated with improved OS in multivariate analysis. Even taking into account the inherent weaknesses of retrospective analyses and the lack of surgical morbidity data, these results provide support for further randomised controlled trials, such as the proposed LYTEC study of lymphadenectomy in intermediate- to high-risk endometrial cancer (Figure 10.1).

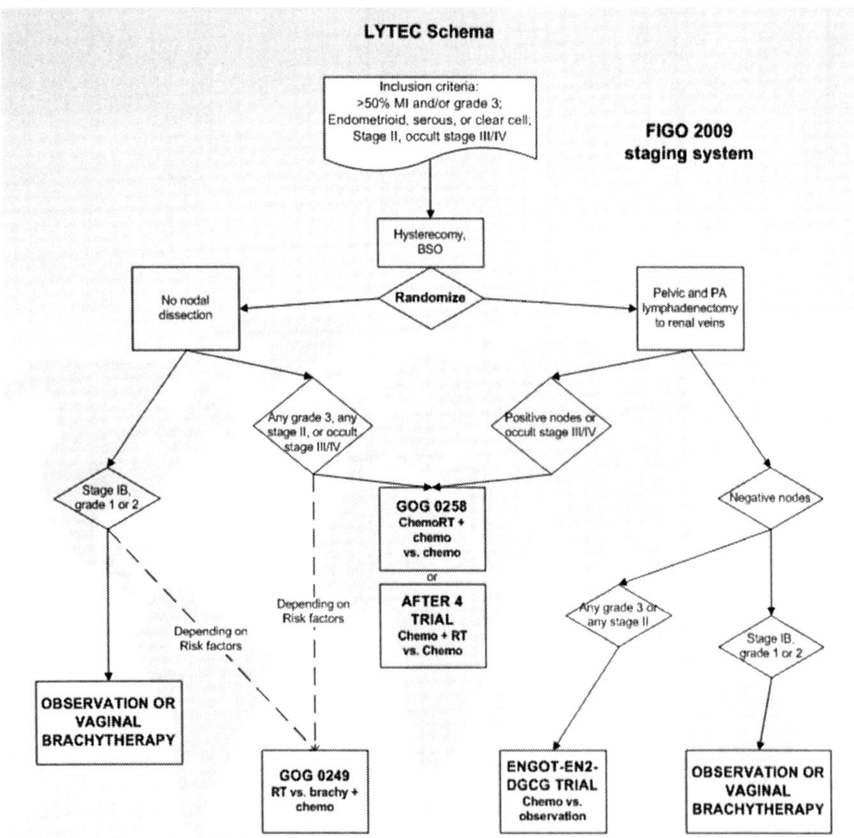

Figure 10.1 The schema for the proposed LYTEC study of lymphadenectomy in intermediate- to high-risk endometrial cancer

Adjuvant therapy for endometrial cancer

While surgery alone is adequate treatment for many women with low-risk endometrial cancers, it is clear that a substantial minority of cases are at significant risk of disease recurrence. Indeed, in a retrospective case series of 915 women treated at the Mayo Clinic between 1984 and 1996, 21% developed recurrent disease.[13] The authors defined a high-risk subgroup that had a 46% risk of disease recurrence at 5 years as those women who had one or more of the following:

- outer third myometrial invasion
- cervical stromal involvement
- nodal involvement
- peritoneal disease at presentation.

Adjuvant radiotherapy

Adjuvant pelvic external beam radiotherapy (EBRT) has traditionally been offered to up to one-third of women felt to be at elevated risk of disease recurrence based on evidence from randomised trials.[14–16] Although this modality reduces the risk of local pelvic recurrence by up to 18% in selected patient groups (those with at least two risk factors from: age older than 60 years; histologic grade 3; more than 50% myometrial invasion),[17] the absolute benefit for an unselected population is significantly smaller and it has not been shown to affect OS. EBRT is also associated with a 3–4% risk of significant long-term, predominantly gastrointestinal, toxicity.

The results of the PORTEC-2 trial[18] published in 2010 demonstrate that vaginal brachytherapy (VBT) is as effective as EBRT in reducing the risk of vaginal relapse in women with endometrial cancer of high-intermediate risk (age above 60 years and stage IB grade 1–2 or stage IA grade 3 with myometrial invasion; any age and stage II grade 1–2 or grade 3 with less than 50% myometrial invasion). Although there was a slightly higher rate of pelvic nodal relapse in women receiving VBT, this generally occurred in the presence of more disseminated metastatic disease and the OS was not significantly different between the two arms. Importantly, VBT was associated with lower acute toxicity and clinically significant better quality of life than EBRT.[19] VBT should therefore be considered as a new standard of care for this particular patient group.[20]

Adjuvant chemotherapy

In women with high-risk endometrial cancer, there is a significant risk of disease relapse despite adjuvant pelvic irradiation. Long-term prospective follow-up of women with stage IB grade 3 endometrioid endometrial carcinoma treated by surgery followed by EBRT as part of the PORTEC study demonstrated that 5 year OS was only 58%, and 31% of the women developed distant metastatic disease.[21] Such data clearly provide the rationale for evaluating systemic adjuvant therapy. Chemotherapy has now been evaluated in several randomised studies with conflicting results (Table 10.2). All these trials have been relatively underpowered and hampered by long recruitment periods. They all evaluated chemotherapy regimens based on doxorubicin and cisplatin. This doublet was the historical standard of care in advanced/recurrent disease as it had been demonstrated to have a higher response rate (42% versus 25%) and superior progression-free survival (PFS) to single-agent doxorubicin.[22,23]

Table 10.2 Randomised trials evaluating adjuvant chemotherapy in endometrial cancer

Trial		Women (*n*)	5 year PFS (%)	5 year OS (%)
Gynecologic Oncology Group GOG122 – Randall *et al.* (2003)[24]				
Radiotherapy	Whole abdominal irradiation 30 Gy in 20 fractions, 15 Gy pelvic boost	202	38	42
Chemotherapy	7 × (doxo 60 mg/m² + cis 50 mg/m²) q3w + 1 × cis 50 mg/m²	194	50	55
Maggi *et al.* (2006)[25]				
Radiotherapy	Pelvic EBRT 45–50 Gy	168	63	69
Chemotherapy	5 × (doxo 45 mg/m² + cis 50 mg/m² + cyclo 600 mg/m²) q4w	177	63	66
Japanese Gynecologic Oncology Group – Susumu *et al.* (2008)[26]				
Radiotherapy	Pelvic EBRT 40 Gy	193	84	85
Chemotherapy	3 × (doxo 40 mg/m² + cis 50 mg/m² + cyclo 333 mg/m²) q4w	192	82	87
NSGO/EORTC – Hogberg *et al.* (2010)[27]				
Radiotherapy	EBRT 44 Gy	191	72	76
Sequential	EBRT 44 Gy – 4 × (doxo 50 mg/m² + cis 50 mg/m²) q4w (recommended)	187	79	83
ILIADE-III – Hogberg *et al.* (2010)[27]				
Radiotherapy	EBRT 45 Gy	76	61	73
Sequential	3 × (doxo 60 mg/m² + cis 50 mg/m²) q3w – EBRT 45 Gy	80	74	78

cis = cisplatin; cyclo = cyclophosphamide; doxo = doxorubicin; EBRT = external beam radiotherapy; OS = overall survival; PFS = progression-free survival; q3w = every 3 weeks; q4w = every 4 weeks; WAI = whole abdominal irradiation

Initial trials compared chemotherapy against radiotherapy. The GOG122 trial[24] compared eight cycles of chemotherapy (seven doxorubicin–cisplatin and one single-agent cisplatin) with whole abdominal irradiation and pelvic boost in 396 women with stage III/IV endometrial carcinoma of all histological sub-types and less than 2 cm diameter residual disease after surgery. The stage-adjusted hazard ratios for both death and recurrence favoured systemic treatment (HR for death 0.68; 95% CI 0.52–0.89; $P<0.01$) although this was associated with more acute toxicity and treatment-related deaths (4% versus 2%). This study has been criticised both for including patients with macroscopic residual disease and for using whole abdominal irradiation, which was not generally considered to be a worldwide standard, as the control regimen. Maggi *et al.*[25] randomised 345 women with stage IB/II grade 3 or stage III endometrioid endometrial carcinoma to five cycles of CAP chemotherapy (cyclophosphamide–Adriamycin® [doxorubicin]–cisplatin) or pelvic EBRT. After a median 95.5 months follow-up there was no significant difference in OS between the two arms, with HR for death of 0.95 (95% CI 0.66–1.36; $P=0.76$). Notably, however, most distant relapses (44 versus 35) and fewer pelvic relapses (20 versus 27) occurred in women receiving EBRT, suggesting that the two treatment modalities could be complementary in their adjuvant effects. The Japanese Gynecologic Oncology Group compared three cycles of low-dose CAP chemotherapy with pelvic EBRT in 385 evaluable women with intermediate- to high-risk endometrial cancer.[26] Again, no difference in recurrence rates or OS was seen in the whole trial population between the two treatment strategies. However, a post-hoc analysis indicated that a subset of women with a high-intermediate risk of recurrence (stage IB disease if aged over 70 years or with grade 3 disease; stage II disease; stage I/II disease with positive ascitic cytology) may gain benefit from adjuvant chemotherapy with a hazard ratio for OS of 0.24 (95% CI 0.09–0.69; $P=0.006$). Nevertheless, the fact that no benefit from chemotherapy was demonstrated in women with stage III disease means that this analysis needs to be viewed with considerable caution. It should be noted that this study used what is generally considered to be a suboptimally dosed chemotherapy regimen of short duration (three cycles) and also included 190 women (49% of the total) with stage IB grade 1/2 cancers who have a low risk of systemic recurrence and are unlikely to gain benefit from adjuvant chemotherapy.

As radiotherapy has a proven role in preventing loco-regional relapse while chemotherapy may reduce systemic recurrence, the potential role of sequential combined therapy has also been evaluated. The full results of a combined analysis of two trials exploring this regimen were published in 2010.[27] The NSGO-EC-9501/EORTC-55991 study randomised 378 women with endometrial cancer of all histological sub-types felt to be at high risk of micrometastatic disease to four cycles of sequential chemotherapy (83% doxorubicin/epirubicin–cisplatin) and pelvic EBRT or pelvic EBRT alone. While the sequence of treatment was left to the investigators' discretion, only 17% received initial chemotherapy. This administration of chemotherapy post-EBRT may have affected its tolerability as only 72% of the women completed four cycles. The MaNGO-ILIADE III trial included 156 women with stage II–IIIC endometrioid cancers who were randomised to pelvic EBRT or three cycles of doxorubicin–cisplatin before EBRT. Combined analysis of the survival data showed statistically significant improvements in favour of the sequential treatment arms for both PFS (HR 0.63; 95% CI 0.44–0.89; $P=0.009$) and cancer-specific survival (HR 0.55; 95% CI 0.35–0.88; $P=0.01$), although the difference in OS failed to reach statistical significance (HR 0.69; 95% CI 0.46–1.03; $P=0.07$). This translated into 9% improvements in 5 year PFS and cancer-specific survival. Interestingly, the benefit from chemotherapy appeared to be confined to patients with endometrioid cancers and in this group significant improvement in OS was noted (5 year OS 74% versus 84%; $P = 0.05$). However, women with serous and clear-cell cancers only made up 26% of the trial population. Although this analysis can be criticised because of the heterogeneous nature of the patients included in terms of disease stage and histological sub-types and the permissive nature of the experimental arm in the NSGO/EORTC trial, sensitivity analyses did not demonstrate heterogeneity in treatment effect with regard to any of these parameters.

In summary, the results of these five randomised trials suggest that adjuvant chemotherapy may have a survival benefit in the treatment of high-risk endometrial cancer but the optimal treatment strategy and the selection of appropriate subsets of patients are not clear. Further well-designed clinical trials are clearly required. This is reflected in current European guidance[3] which recommends that adjuvant chemotherapy preferably within the context of a clinical trial should be discussed with suitable patients who have undergone surgery for high-grade cancers of stage IB or higher.

Current adjuvant chemotherapy trials

Rather than using doxorubicin–cisplatin chemotherapy, continuing adjuvant chemotherapy trials are evaluating paclitaxel-based regimens based on the results of a phase III Gynecologic Oncology Group (GOG) trial that demonstrated a 3 month improvement in OS when paclitaxel was added to doxorubicin–cisplatin in chemotherapy-naïve patients with advanced/recurrent disease.[28] The considerable toxicity associated with this triplet regimen and the results of several phase II studies[29,30] investigating carboplatin–paclitaxel have led to the adoption of the latter combination as the current de facto standard of care although the results of formal phase III trial comparison in GOG-0209 are awaited.

Based on encouraging phase II data demonstrating promising efficacy and the safety of adjuvant concurrent chemoradiotherapy,[31] the PORTEC-3 study is currently randomising women with high-risk endometrial cancer (endometrioid stage IA grade 3 with myometrial and lymphovascular invasion; stage IB grade 3, stage II, stage IIIA, stage IIIC, or stage IIIB with parametrial involvement only; serous/clear-cell carcinomas stages IA with myometrial involvement to stage IIIC) to pelvic EBRT alone or pelvic EBRT with two cycles of concurrent cisplatin 50 mg/m^2 followed by four cycles of sequential 3-weekly carboplatin–paclitaxel. This international trial aims to recruit 670 women and is powered to detect a 10% improvement in 5 year OS from 65% to 75%. Concurrent cisplatin-based chemoradiotherapy is also being explored in the GOG-0258 study in which women with optimally debulked stage III–IVA endometrial cancer are randomised to either six cycles of carboplatin–paclitaxel as standard of care or an experimental arm similar to that employed in PORTEC-3.

Adjuvant chemotherapy alone is currently under investigation in the ENGOT-DCCG-EN2 trial, which is comparing six cycles of adjuvant carboplatin–paclitaxel versus observation alone in women with node-negative early-stage high-risk endometrial cancer. Systematic pelvic lymphadenectomy is a mandatory requirement for entry into this study, which is powered to detect a 12% improvement in 5 year OS from 74% to 86% and thus needs to recruit 678 women. It is also proposed to compare carboplatin–paclitaxel alone versus sequential pelvic EBRT–chemotherapy in the NSGO After4 trial.

The proposed LYTEC trial (see Figure 10.1) is an important attempt to address the therapeutic role of systematic pelvic and para-aortic lymphadenectomy in the context of the current adjuvant studies discussed above. It aims to randomise women with endometrial cancer with more than 50% myometrial invasion, high-grade histological sub-type or stage II/occult stage III/IV disease to TAH/BSO with or without lymphadenectomy with subsequent adjuvant treatment conducted within phase III clinical trials based on histopathological findings. Such an approach would avoid many of the drawbacks of previous surgical/adjuvant studies and allow the most efficient use of potential clinical trial participants to increase the evidence base we have to decide on the first-line management of endometrial cancer.

Management of recurrent endometrial cancer

The management of recurrent endometrial cancer can be complex and requires the assessment of several factors including the site(s) of disease recurrence, histological grade and the patient's performance status, comorbidities and wishes. Prior treatment history is also becoming increasingly relevant owing to the evolving role of adjuvant therapies as discussed above.

Isolated vaginal recurrence can occur in up to 18% of women presenting with recurrent disease and can often be salvaged by pelvic radiotherapy if this has not been used in the adjuvant setting, with 5 year OS of 60% reported.[13,14] If isolated pelvic recurrence occurs after adjuvant pelvic EBRT, exenterative surgery can be considered in selected patients, with 5 year OS of 20–30% reported.

In the majority of patients, however, recurrence will be manifest at multiple disease sites and systemic treatment will be necessary. In selected cases with hormone receptor-positive or low-grade endometrioid cancers, hormonal therapy with oral progestogens is appropriate and durable responses in 37% of women with grade 1 or progesterone receptor-positive cancers have been reported in the phase III setting.[32] Women with recurrent high-grade cancers are, however, unlikely to respond to hormonal manipulation, and chemotherapy is appropriate. As discussed above, the current standard of care is carboplatin–paclitaxel, which is associated with response rates of 50–60% and median OS of 25–26 months in phase II trials.[29,30] However, retrospective institutional studies indicate somewhat lower response rates and shorter OS, particularly in women with poor performance status or who have received prior chemotherapy.[33]

While first-line chemotherapy is now relatively well defined, options at disease progression are not clear and the benefit in terms of survival and symptom control/quality of life from second-line treatment is uncertain. Although there appears to be a subset of patients who may gain benefit from re-challenge from carboplatin–paclitaxel chemotherapy, the concept of a platinum-free interval as in ovarian cancer has not been proven. However, a small retrospective series of 31 women re-treated with carboplatin–paclitaxel after benefit in the first-line setting suggested that response rates were related to treatment-free interval (TFI): 65% of those with a more than 12 month TFI responded to re-challenge compared with 25% of those with a less than 12 month TFI.[34] This population clearly reflects only a small subset of patients with disease progression after first-line therapy, however.

Response rates to novel cytotoxic agents including PEGylated liposomal doxorubicin, topotecan, trabectedin and ixabepilone have been disappointingly low (generally under 10%) in the second-line setting, with median OS of 9 months.[35,36] Although ixabepilone is currently being explored in the phase III setting in this indication against either doxorubicin or paclitaxel, it is likely that we have reached a ceiling with the use of cytotoxics and that research into molecularly targeted agents should be actively pursued.

Targeted therapies in recurrent endometrial cancer

Markers of angiogenesis and in particular high VEGF expression have been shown to be associated with poor prognosis in endometrial cancer[37,38] and anti-angiogenic treatment strategies have been explored in recurrent endometrial cancer in phase II studies. While both oral VEGFR tyrosine kinase inhibitors and bevacizumab have demonstrated clinical activity, only the efficacy of the latter merits further investigation. In a study of 53 women whose endometrial cancer had progressed despite one or two prior chemotherapy regimens, responses to bevacizumab were seen in 15% of the patients, with a 6 month PFS of 36%, almost twice that seen with cytotoxic agents in a similar patient population.[39]

The phosphatidylinositol 3-kinase (PI3K)-AKT-mTOR signalling pathway plays a key role in endometrial carcinogenesis and is important for several processes essential for cancer progression, including cell growth, survival and motility.[40] Loss of PTEN, a lipid phosphatase that normally terminates PI3K-dependent signalling, is seen in 37–61% of endometrial cancers, while activating mutations of the PI3K catalytic subunit are found in 36%.[41] Several drug classes have been developed that inhibit this signalling pathway. The mTOR inhibitors are at the most advanced stage of clinical development and phase II trials of several of these agents have been reported in endometrial cancer.[42–44] All of these studies have demonstrated modest clinical activity in chemotherapy-pretreated endometrial cancer although this does not consistently correlate with markers of PI3K pathway activation. Further phase II clinical trials are continuing exploring combinations of mTOR inhibitors and chemotherapy/hormonal therapy. There are also advanced plans for a phase III trial (NCIC-EN.8) of oral ridaforolimus compared with either chemotherapy or oral progestogens as second-line treatment for advanced/recurrent disease. However, the toxicities of PI3K inhibition, in particular glucose intolerance and hyperlipidaemia, need to be borne in mind in women who are often elderly and obese and so predisposed to these problems.

In summary, the second-line management of patients with advanced/recurrent endometrial cancer is currently undefined and all patients should be encouraged to participate in clinical trials if these are available.

Uncommon histological sub-types

Three uncommon histological sub-types account for 10–15% of all endometrial carcinomas. Serous carcinomas, clear-cell carcinomas and carcinosarcomas differ in their clinical behaviour from endometrioid carcinomas as they are more likely to present at an advanced stage and consequently have poorer prognosis.[45–47] It is also apparent that, although all these cancers derive from the endometrium, the molecular drivers of carcinogenesis are distinct. For instance, serous carcinomas are characterised by p53 (*TP53*) mutations and often *HER2* gene amplification rather than the *PTEN* loss and mismatch repair gene abnormalities seen in endometrioid cancers.[41,47] Gene expression profiling also indicates that these three sub-types are molecularly distinct from endometrioid carcinomas and from each other. It is also intriguing that serous endometrial cancers express a distinct genetic profile to that of serous ovarian cancers although a clinical propensity for peritoneal spread is shared by these cancers whereas clear-cell carcinomas of ovarian and endometrial origin have similar expression profiles.[48,49]

Carcinosarcomas have traditionally been excluded from endometrial cancer trials and attempts have been made to perform carcinosarcoma-specific clinical studies.[50] These have demonstrated similar response rates to carboplatin–paclitaxel chemotherapy, although perhaps with shorter OS compared with endometrioid cancers,[50] and have hinted at a benefit from adjuvant chemotherapy.[51]

Serous and clear-cell carcinomas are, however, managed similarly to endometrioid carcinomas although many centres apply a lower threshold for employing adjuvant chemotherapy. While response rates to chemotherapy in the advanced setting appear similar across sub-types, a retrospective analysis of the phase III GOG studies performed indicates that clear-cell carcinomas have a worse prognosis with a hazard ratio for OS of 1.51 compared with endometrioid cancers.[52] Similar analyses of the GOG122 and NSGO/EORTC adjuvant chemotherapy trials[24,27] fail to show any significant survival benefit in women with serous and clear-cell carcinomas, although numbers participating in both studies were small. These data indicate that consideration should be given to designing histological sub-type-specific trials in endometrial cancer or at least considering stratification by histology with sufficient statistical power to allow meaningful comparisons to be made between study arms in each group. This would need international collaboration although the relative over-representation of serous and clear-cell carcinoma in the advanced/recurrent endometrial cancer population may make this feasible.

Conclusion

The increasing incidence of endometrial cancer has led to revitalised efforts to improve outcomes and to apply risk-based management strategies appropriately. For women at intermediate to high risk of disease recurrence, this has led to increased complexity and intensity of management driven particularly by the realisation that endometrial cancer is a relatively chemosensitive disease. While results of randomised studies point towards a survival benefit with adjuvant chemotherapy, the appropriate scheduling of this and the subgroup of patients likely to benefit has not been properly elucidated and this is a key area for future research, together with the role of systematic pelvic and para-aortic lymphadenectomy in high-risk patients.

It has also become clear that women with low- to intermediate-risk early-stage disease do not require intensive management. Lymphadenectomy is not required in these women and, if radiotherapy is appropriate, this should be administered by VBT rather than by EBRT.

However, the management of recurrent disease after failure of first-line chemotherapy is undefined and further clinical research is required to define how new molecularly targeted approaches can be incorporated into treatment algorithms. This is particularly apposite as it is becoming clear that the uncommon histological sub-types – serous, clear-cell and carcinosarcoma – arise through different molecular pathways and may therefore need different treatment strategies.

References

1. Cancer Research UK. Uterine (womb) cancer statistics – UK [info.cancerresearchuk.org/cancerstats/types/uterus].
2. Lindemann K, Vatten LJ, Ellstrøm-Engh M, Eskild A. Body mass, diabetes and smoking and endometrial cancer risk: a follow-up study. *Br J Cancer* 2008;98:1582–5.
3. Plataniotis G, Castiglione M. Endometrial cancer: ESMO clinical practice guidelines for diagnosis, treatment and follow-up. *Ann Oncol* 2010;21(suppl 5):v41–v45.
4. Vergote I, Amant F, Neven P. Laparoscopic hysterectomy for early endometrial cancer. *Lancet Oncol* 2010;11:707–8.

5. Walker JL, Piedmonte MR, Spirtos NM, Eisenkop SM, Schlaerth JB, Mannel RS, *et al.* Randomized trial of laparoscopy versus laparotomy for comprehensive surgical staging of endometrial cancer. A Gynecologic Oncology Group Study (LAP2). *J Clin Oncol* 2009;27:5331–6.
6. Mourits MJE, Bijen CB, Arts HJ, ter Brugge HG, van der Sijde R, Paulsen L, *et al.* Safety of laparoscopy versus laparotomy in early stage endometrial cancer. A randomized trial. *Lancet Oncol* 2010;11:763–71.
7. Janda M, Gebski V, Brand A, Hogg R, Jobling TW, Land R, *et al.* Quality of life after total laparoscopic hysterectomy versus total abdominal hysterectomy for stage I endometrial cancer (LACE). A randomised trial. *Lancet Oncol* 2010;11:772–80.
8. Kornblith AB, Huang HQ, Walker JL, Spirtos NM, Rotmensch J, Cella D. Quality of life in patients with endometrial cancer undergoing laparoscopic FIGO staging compared to laparotomy: A Gynecologic Oncology Group Study *J Clin Oncol* 2009;27:5337–42.
9. Benedetti-Panici P, Basile S, Maneschi F, Alberto Lissoni A, Signorelli M, Scambia G, *et al.* Systematic pelvic lymphadenectomy versus no lymphadenectomy in early-stage endometrial cancer. Randomized clinical trial. *J Natl Cancer Inst* 2008;101:1707–16.
10. ASTEC Study Group. Efficacy of systematic pelvic lymphadenectomy in endometrial cancer (MRC ASTEC trial): a randomised study. *Lancet* 2009;373:125–36.
11. Chan JK, Cheung MK, Huh WK, Osann K, Husain A, Teng NN, *et al.* Therapeutic role of lymph node resection in endometrioid corpus cancer: a study of 12,333 patients. *Cancer* 2006;107:1823–30.
12. Todo Y, Koto H, Kaneuchi M, Watari H. Takeda M, Sakuragi N. Survival effect of para-aortic lymphadenectomy in endometrial cancer (SEPAL study): a retrospective cohort analysis. *Lancet* 2010;375:1165–72.
13. Mariani A, Dowdy SC, Keeney GL, Long HJ, Lesnick TG, Podratz KC. High-risk endometrial cancer subgroups: candidates for target-based adjuvant therapy. *Gynecol Oncol* 2004;95:120–6.
14. Creutzberg CL, van Putten WLJ, Koper PCM, Lybeert ML, Jobsen JJ, Wárlám-Rodenhuis CC, *et al.* Surgery and postoperative radiotherapy versus surgery alone for patients with stage I endometrial carcinoma: multicentre randomised trial. *Lancet* 2000;355:1404–11.
15. Keys HM, Roberts JA, Brunetto VL, Zaino RJ, Spirtos NM, Bloss JD, *et al.* A phase III trial of surgery with or without adjunctive external pelvic radiation therapy in intermediate endometrial adenocarcinoma. *Gynecol Oncol* 2004;92:744–51.
16. ASTEC/EN.5 Study Group, Blake P, Swart AM, Orton J, Kitchener H, Whelan T, Lukka H, *et al.* Adjuvant external beam radiotherapy in the treatment of endometrial cancer (MRC ASTEC and NCICCTG EN.5 randomised trials): pooled trial results, systematic review, and meta-analysis. *Lancet* 2009;373:137–46.
17. Scholten AN, van Putten WLJ, Beerman H, Smit VT, Koper PC, Lybeert ML, *et al.* Postoperative radiotherapy for stage I endometrial carcinoma: long-term follow-up of the randomized PORTEC trial with centralized pathology review. *Int J Radiat Oncol Biol Phys* 2005;63:834–8.
18. Nout RA, Smit VT, Putter H, Jürgenliemk-Schulz IM, Jobsen JJ, Lutgens LC, *et al.* Vaginal brachytherapy versus pelvic external beam radiotherapy for patients with endometrial cancer of high-intermediate risk (PORTEC-2): an open-label non-inferiority randomised trial. *Lancet* 2010;375:816–23.
19. Nout RA, Putter H, Jürgenliemk-Schulz IM, Jobsen JJ, Lutgens LC, van der Steen-Banasik EM, *et al.* Quality of life after pelvic radiotherapy or vaginal brachytherapy for endometrial cancer: first results of the randomized PORTEC-2 trial. *J Clin Oncol* 2009;27:3547–56.
20. Kitchener HC, Powell M. Radiotherapy for endometrial cancer: a key piece of the jigsaw. *Lancet* 2010;375:781–2.
21. Creutzberg CL, van Putten WL, Warlam-Rodenhuis CC, van den Bergh AC, de Winter KA, Koper PC, *et al.* Outcome of high-risk stage IC, grade 3 compared with stage I endometrial carcinoma patients: The Postoperative Radiation Therapy in Endometrial Cancer Trial. *J Clin Oncol* 2004;22:1234–41.
22. Thigpen JT, Brady MF, Homesley HD, Malfetano J, DuBeshter B, Burger RA, *et al.* Phase III trial of doxorubicin with or without cisplatin in advanced endometrial carcinoma: a Gynaecologic Oncology Group study. *J Clin Oncol* 2004;22:3902–8.

23. Aapro MS, van Wijk FH, Bolis G, Chevallier B, van der Burg ME, Poveda A, *et al.* Doxorubicin vs doxorubicin-cisplatin in endometrial carcinoma: definitive results of a randomised study (55872) by the EORTC Gynaecological Cancer Group. *Ann Oncol* 2003;14:441–8.
24. Randall ME, Filiaci VL, Muss H, Spirtos NM, Mannel RS, Fowler J, *et al.* Randomized phase III trial of whole abdominal irradiation versus doxorubicin and cisplatin chemotherapy in advanced endometrial carcinoma: A Gynecologic Oncology Group study. *J Clin Oncol* 2006;24:36–44.
25. Maggi R, Lissoni A, Spina F, Melpignano M, Zola P, Favalli G, *et al.* Adjuvant chemotherapy versus radiotherapy in high-risk endometrial carcinoma: results of a randomised trial. *Br J Cancer* 2006;95:266–71.
26. Susumu N, Sagae S, Udagawa Y, Niwa K, Kuramoto H, Satoh S, *et al.* Randomized phase III trial of pelvic radiotherapy versus cisplatin-based combined chemotherapy in patients with intermediate and high-risk endometrial cancer: A Japanese Gynecologic Oncology Group Study. *Gynecol Oncol* 2008;108:226–33.
27. Hogberg T, Signorelli M, de Oliveira CF, Fossati R, Lissoni AA, Sorbe B, *et al.* Sequential adjuvant chemotherapy and radiotherapy in endometrial cancer: results from two randomised studies. *Eur J Cancer* 2010;46:2422–31.
28. Fleming GF, Brunetto VL, Cella D, Look KY, Reid GC, Munkarah AR, *et al.* Phase III trial of doxorubicin and cisplatin with or without paclitaxel plus filgrastim in advanced endometrial carcinoma: A Gynecologic Oncology Group Study. *J Clin Oncol* 2004;22:2159–66.
29. Hoskins PJ, Swenerton KD, Pike JA, Wong F, Lim P, Acquino-Parsons C, *et al.* Paclitaxel and carboplatin, alone or with irradiation in advanced or recurrent endometrial cancer: a phase II study. *J Clin Oncol* 2001;19:4048–53.
30. Sorbe B, Andersson H, Boman K, Rosenberg P, Kalling M. Treatment of primary advanced or recurrent endometrial carcinoma with a combination of carboplatin and paclitaxel – long-term follow-up. *Int J Gynecol Cancer* 2008;18:803–8.
31. Greven K, Winter K, Underhill K, Fontenesci J, Cooper J, Burke T. Final analysis of RTOG9708: adjuvant postoperative irradiation combined with cisplatin/paclitaxel chemotherapy following surgery for patients with high-risk endometrial cancer. *Gynecol Oncol* 2006;103:155–9.
32. Thigpen JT, Brady MF, Alvarez RD, Adelson MD, Homesley HD, Manetta A, *et al.* Oral medroxyprogesterone acetate in the treatment of advanced or recurrent endometrial carcinoma: a dose–response study of the gynecologic oncology group. *J Clin Oncol* 1999;17:1736–44.
33. Sovak MA, Dupont J, Hensley ML, Ishill N, Gerst S, Abu-Rustum N, *et al.* Paclitaxel and carboplatin in the treatment of advanced or recurrent endometrial cancer: a large retrospective study. *Int J Gynecol Cancer* 2007;17:197–203.
34. Mazgani M, Le N, Hoskins PJ; British Columbia Cancer Agency. Reuse of carboplatin and paclitaxel in patients with relapsed endometrial cancer: The British Columbia Cancer Agency experience. *Gynecol Oncol* 2008;111:474–7.
35. Moore KN, Tian C, McMeekin DS, Thigpen JT, Randall ME, Gallion HH. Does the progression-free interval after primary chemotherapy predict survival after salvage chemotherapy in advanced and recurrent endometrial cancer? *Cancer* 2010;116:5407–14.
36. Dizon D, Blessing JA, McMeekin DS, Sharma SK, Disilvestro P, Alvarez RD. Phase II trial of ixabepilone as second-line treatment in advanced endometrial cancer: Gynecologic Oncology Group Trial 129P. *J Clin Oncol* 2009;27:3104–8.
37. Kamat AA, Merritt WM, Coffey D, Lin YG, Patel PR, Broaddus R, *et al.* Clinical and biological signficance of vascular endothelial growth factor in endometrial cancer. *Clin Cancer Res* 2007;13:7487–95.
38. Stefansson IM, Salvesen HB, Akslen LA. Vascular proliferation is important for clinical progress of endometrial cancer. *Cancer Res* 2006;66:3303–9.
39. Aghajanian C, Sill MW, Darcy K, Greer B, McMeekin DS, Rose PG, *et al.* A phase II evaluation of bevacizumab in the treatment of recurrent or persistent endometrial cancer: a Gynecologic Oncology Group study. *J Clin Oncol* 2009;27(15s):abstr 5531.
40. Courtney KD, Corcoran RB, Engelmann JE. The PI3K pathway as a drug target in human cancer. *J Clin Oncol* 2010;28:1075–83.
41. Hecht JL, Mutter GL. Molecular and pathological aspects of endometrial carcinogenesis. *J Clin Oncol* 2006;24:4783–91.

42. Slomovitz BM, Lu KH, Johnston T, Coleman RL, Munsell M, Broaddus RR, *et al.* A Phase 2 study of the oral mammalian target of rapamycin inhibitor everolimus in patients with recurrent endometrial carcinoma. *Cancer* 2010;116:5415–19.
43. Oza AM, Elit L, Provencher D, Biagi JJ, Panasci L, Sederias J, *et al.* A phase II study of temsirolimus (CCI-779) in patients with metastatic and/or locally advanced recurrent endometrial cancer previously treated with chemotherapy: NCIC CTG IND 160b. *J Clin Oncol* 2008;26(15s):abstr 5516.
44. Colombo N, McMeekin DS, Schwartz P, J. Kostka, C. Sessa, P. Gehrig, *et al.* A phase II trial of the mTOR inhibitor AP23573 as a single agent in advanced endometrial cancer. *J Clin Oncol* 2007;25(18s):abstr 5516.
45. Amant F, Cadron I, Fuso L, Berteloot P, de Jonge E, Jacomen G, *et al.* Endometrial carcinosarcomas have a different prognosis and pattern of spread compared to high-risk epithelial endometrial cancer. *Gynecol Oncol* 2005;98:274–80.
46. Olawaiye AB, Boruta DM. Management of women with clear cell endometrial cancer: a Society of Gynecologic Oncology (SGO) review. *Gynecol Oncol* 2009;113:277–83.
47. Boruta DM, Gehrig PA, Fader AN, Olawaiye AB. Management of women with uterine papillary serous cancer: a Society of Gynecologic Oncology (SGO) review. *Gynecol Oncol* 2009;113:142–53.
48. Zom KK, Bonome T, Gangi L, Chandramouli GV, Awtrey CS, Gardner GJ, *et al.* Gene expression profiles of serous, endometrioid and clear cell subtypes of ovarian and endometrial cancer. *Clin Cancer Res* 2005;11:6422–30.
49. Maxwell GL, Chandramouli GLR, Dainty L, Litzi TJ, Berchuck A, Barrett JC, *et al.* Microarray analysis of endometrial carcinomas and mixed Mullerian tumors reveals distinct gene expression profiles associated with different histologic types of uterine cancer. *Clin Cancer Res* 2005;11:4056–66.
50. Powell MA, Filiaci VL, Rose PG, Mannel RS, Hanjani P, Degeest K, *et al.* Phase II evaluation of paclitaxel and carboplatin in the treatment of carcinosarcoma of the uterus: a Gynecologic Oncology Group study. *J Clin Oncol* 2010;28:2727–31.
51. Wolfson AH, Brady MF, Rocereto T, Mannel RS, Lee YC, Futoran RJ, *et al.* A gynaecologic oncology group randomized phase III trial of whole abdominal irradiation (WAI) vs. cisplatin-ifosfamide and mesna (CIM) as post-surgical therapy in stage I–IV carcinosarcoma of the uterus. *Gynecol Oncol* 2007;107:177–85.
52. McMeekin DS, Filiaci VL, Thigpen JT, Gallion HH, Fleming GF, Rodgers WH; Gynecologic Oncology Group study. The relationship between histology and outcome in advanced and recurrent endometrial cancer patients participating in first-line chemotherapy trials: a Gynecologic Oncology Group study. *Gynecol Oncol* 2007;106:16–22.

13

Chapter 13

Targeting therapies in cancer: opportunities in ovarian cancer

Ahmed Ashour Ahmed, Stefan Knapp, Anil K Sood and Robert C Bast Jr

Introduction

In 2008, 225 000 women worldwide were diagnosed with ovarian cancer and an estimated 140 000 died of the disease.[1] This makes ovarian cancer the most lethal gynaecological malignancy. In spite of the increased overall 5 year survival, the mortality rate from the disease has shown either a slight decrease or even an increase in certain age groups. For example, in the UK, the 5 year survival increased from 21% in 1971–75 to 38.9% in 2001–06 but the mean mortality rate only decreased by 10% over the same period (from 12.02 per 100 000 to 10.77 per 100 000, respectively), with a paradoxical increase in mean mortality rate in the over-65 age group over the same period of 37% (from 40.8 per 100 000 to 55.8 per 100 000, respectively).[2] A similar trend has been observed in the USA, where the 5 year survival increased from 37% in 1975–77 to 45% in 1999–2006 ($P < 0.05$). However, the mean mortality rate only decreased by 11.4% over the same time period (from 9.8 per 100 000 to 8.8 per 100 000, respectively). Similarly, the mean mortality rate in the over-65 age group increased by 15.7% (from 38.4 per 100 000 to 44.5 per 100 000, respectively).[3] Improved progression-free survival (PFS) and overall survival (OS) in developed countries possibly relates to the more consistent use of cytoreductive surgery and to the development of combination chemotherapy for primary and recurrent disease. The inconsistencies between the sharp increase in the overall 5 year survival and a modest improvement in cancer-specific mortality is presumably because of the disproportionately high percentage of women diagnosed with late-stage ovarian cancer, for whom treatment still remains a challenge.

In spite of the high overall initial response rate of more than 70% to platinum- and taxane-based regimens,[4] the majority of patients die from the progressive growth of recurrent, chemotherapy-resistant disease. Several other agents have demonstrated activity against recurrent ovarian cancer individually and in combinations, including PEGylated liposomal doxorubicin, gemcitabine and topotecan.[5–8] Inclusion of such drugs in empirical combinations with carboplatin and paclitaxel for primary chemotherapy has not improved outcomes over those observed with carboplatin and paclitaxel alone.[9–11] However, the development of targeted therapy and an increasing understanding of the molecular subclasses of ovarian cancer, as well as our emerging knowledge of key drivers of ovarian cancer progression, offer great opportunities for improving therapies in ovarian cancer.[12] One important concept that has been re-emphasised by recent genomic discoveries is personalisation of therapies, matching activated signalling or damaged repair pathways with drugs that inhibit relevant targets.

This chapter outlines the recent advances in the molecular classification of ovarian cancer and the efforts for rationalised targeted therapies of molecular drivers of individual cancers with a particular emphasis on kinases and their inhibitors. We highlight the challenges that face targeting strategies, particularly at the interface between target discovery and validation that leads to the development of targeting agents.

Ovarian cancer: one name, many diseases

Similar to most cancer types, ovarian cancer is a heterogeneous disease comprising a diversity of histological sub-types that could be broadly classified into epithelial, germ cell and mesenchymal tumours. Epithelial ovarian cancers represent some 90% of ovarian cancers and consist of many histotypes, including serous, endometrioid, mucinous and clear-cell cancers. It is important to note that, while the standard management of epithelial ovarian cancer is debulking surgery combined with carboplatin and paclitaxel, such chemotherapies are not equally effective for all histotypes of epithelial ovarian cancer. For example, clear-cell and mucinous ovarian cancers are resistant to standard therapies and alternative approaches are required.[13,14] In addition to the histotypes, recent work has shown that it is possible to subclassify individual histological types of ovarian cancers using profiling methods.[15] Such molecular subclasses have distinct biological, clinical and prognostic features. Therefore, personalised therapies that are based on the identification of molecular drivers of individual cancers are required for optimal management of ovarian cancer.

Molecular drivers of ovarian cancer as targets for therapy

Recent insights into the molecular drivers of the major histotypes of epithelial ovarian cancers have resulted in the classification of these tumours into two major molecular sub-types depending on whether such cancers contain *KRAS/BRAF* or *TP53* mutations.[16] This classification may become highly valuable in clinical management by enabling the selection of patients for targeted therapies.[17]

Type I cancers include borderline serous, low-grade serous, low-grade mucinous, endometrioid and clear-cell cancers. In this type, DNA copy number abnormalities are relatively uncommon. Activating mutations in *KRAS* or *BRAF* represent a substantial minority of borderline serous tumours and low-grade serous cancer.[18] *KRAS* mutations are also common and occur in up to 50% of mucinous cancers[19] and in about 10% of endometrioid and clear-cell cancers.[20] Mutations of *PTEN* are also observed, particularly in endometrioid cancers.

RAS proteins are a family of GTPases that includes KRAS, HRAS and NRAS and which act as molecular switches for relaying signalling information from activated receptors.[21] KRAS circulates between aguanosine 5′-triphosphate (GTP)-bound active state and a guanosine diphosphate (GDP)-bound inactive state. Growth factors binding to cell surface receptors, such as epidermal growth factor receptor (EGFR), activate guanine nucleotide exchange factors (GEFs) that are capable of displacing GDP from KRAS with GTP. Inactivation of KRAS is mediated via GTPase-activating proteins (GAPs) that leads to the hydrolysis of KRAS-bound GTP.[21] Activating mutations in

KRAS lead to resistance to GAPs and the accumulation of active KRAS.[22] Activated KRAS is capable of binding and activating a wide variety of effectors, most notably the following KRAS targets:

- the PI3K/AKT pathway, leading to enhanced survival
- the BRAF/mitogen-activated protein kinase kinase (MEK)/extracellular signal-regulated kinase (ERK) cascade, leading to enhanced proliferation through phosphorylation of cyclin D1
- the RAL and RAC exchange factors RALGDS and TIAM1, leading to regulation of vesicle transport and actin organisation, respectively.

While *KRAS* mutations represent a common feature of these cancers, mouse models have shown that *KRAS* mutations (G12D) alone induce endometriosis-like lesions and are thus insufficient to induce ovarian cancer,[23] unlike the case for lung cancer and T cell lymphomas where conditional expression of *KRAS* (G12D) alone is capable of establishing such tumours.[24] A search for a second 'hit' in tumours bearing *KRAS* mutations will be important to gain further insights into the pathogenesis of such tumours.

The second group, collectively called type II ovarian cancer, is genetically defined by mutations in the DNA repair mediator *TP53*. These tumours are characterised by frequent nuclear and architectural atypias, high-grade lesions and high levels of genomic copy number alterations. We have shown that mutations in *TP53* are present in almost all high-grade advanced stage ovarian cancers.[25] These tumours are characterised by their high response rate to carboplatin-based therapy, frequent mutations or dysfunction of the *BRCA* homologous DNA repair genes and aberrations of a wide variety of signalling pathways that offer broad opportunities for targeted therapies.

Challenges for drug discovery and development: the story of targeting kinases

Once a plausible target for therapy has been identified and validated, the next challenge is the discovery of chemical inhibitors that can be tested for efficacy in pre-clinical and clinical studies. This process is often difficult and time-consuming. In general, the process of inhibitor discovery involves:

1. screening and lead identification
2. lead optimisation and clinical candidate identification
3. toxicology and pharmacology studies, including scale-up for clinical development and CMC (chemistry, manufacturing and controls)
4. phase I studies that assess toxicology
5. phase II studies that assess early efficacy
6. phase III studies that study the efficacy and benchmarking of the identified inhibitor, usually with a large patient population.

As an example of this process, we briefly discuss efforts in kinase inhibitor identification.

Targeting kinases with an established biological role in ovarian cancer

In the human genome, 518 kinases have been identified.[26] The structure of the kinase catalytic domain is characterised by a bi-lobal domain arrangement and the presence of a number of conserved regulatory elements such as the ATP/Mg^{2+} binding motif VIAK and DFG, the catalytic loop HRD motif and the activation segment.[26] The ATP binding site is located in a deep cleft between both kinase lobes. Most kinase inhibitors that have been developed to date target the ATP binding sites. ATP-competitive kinase inhibitors can be generally classified into type I inhibitors that bind to the active state of the kinase and type II inhibitors that bind to the inactive state of the kinase.[27] The kinase active state is highly conserved while inactive kinase conformations are structurally more diverse, making type II inhibitors an interesting strategy for the development of ATP-competitive compounds with increase selectivity. However, type II inhibitors also often cross-react with a large number of diverse kinases, which may result in adverse effects during therapy and potentially increased toxicity. Structure-aided design is, therefore, an important component for optimisation of inhibitor specificity.[27] The inactive states to which type II inhibitors bind are characterised by an open and outward-oriented DFG motif. This movement opens an allosteric binding site that increases the size of the ATP pocket that can be targeted, and sequence diversity in that pocket may allow the design of inhibitors with increase selectivity.[28,29] Indeed, the first kinase inhibitor to be approved was the the type II ABL kinase inhibitor imatinib,[30] which is, however, still not entirely specific. Further rationalised modifications of the inhibitor by exploiting unique molecular properties of the target, such as non-conserved dehydration propensities, have proven effective in improving specificity and reducing toxicity.[31] A third approach is through the use of allosteric inhibitors that target the non-catalytic domain of a kinase.[28] Examples of such inhibitors are pleckstrin homology (PH) domain-dependent AKT inhibitors (see below) and the ABL inhibitor GNF.[32] Such inhibitors tend to have the highest degree of kinase selectivity. A fourth group of inhibitors form covalent bonds to the catalytic domain by binding to rare residues in the kinase. An example of this group is the EGFR inhibitor HKI-272.[33]

These classes of inhibitors cover most of the currently known kinase inhibitors. In the following sections, we discuss efforts in developing inhibitors for three of the most commonly deranged pathways in ovarian cancer.

PI3Kinase pathway

The AKT kinase family that consists of AKT1, AKT2 and AKT3 is known to promote cell proliferation and growth and to protect cells from apoptosis.[34] Activation of AKT is dependent on the availability of phosphatidylinositol (3,4,5)-triphosphate (PtdIns (3,4,5)P or PIP3) in the cytoplasm.[35] PIP3 interaction with the PH domain of AKT leads to its translocation to the cell membrane where it becomes phosphorylated at S473, predominantly by the mammalian target of rapamycin complex 2 (mTORC2),[36] and at T308, by phosphatidylinositol-dependent kinase 1 (PDK1),[37] leading to AKT activation. In the cell, the concentration of PIP3 is dependent on the balance between the activity of two enzymes, the kinase PI3K, which is activated by G proteins and receptor tyrosine kinases, leading to an increase in PIP3,[38] and the phosphatase PTEN that removes one phosphate group from PIP3 resulting in PtdIns (4,5)P, leading to inactivation of the AKT pathway.[39] In ovarian cancers, the PI3K/AKT pathway is known to be activated in more than 70% of cases through inactivating mutations in PTEN, or amplifications and activating mutations in PI3K and AKT, respectively.[17] Activation of AKT leads to its translocation to the cytoplasm and the nucleus where it phosphorylates several key substrates, leading to promotion of survival. Most notably, it:

1. phosphorylates and inactivates the pro-apoptotic protein BAD[40,41]
2. phosphorylates the pro-apoptotic transcription factor FOXO1, leading to its translocation out of the nucleus and into the cytoplasm[42]
3. induces the anti-apoptotic protein survivin

4. phosphorylates the ubiquitin ligase MDM2, leading to its translocation to the nucleus where MDM2 binds to the pro-apoptotic protein p53, resulting in p53 degradation.[43]

In addition, activated AKT leads to enhanced cell growth predominantly by indirect activation of mTORC1, a critical regulator of translation initiation, through phosphorylation and inactivation of the mTORC1 inhibitor tuberous sclerosis complex 2 (TSC2).[44,45] Activated AKT has also been shown to drive cell proliferation by the phosphorylation and inhibition of p27 and p21, leading to their cytoplasmic localisation and degradation.

Targeting the PI3K/AKT pathway has been performed by inhibitors of the mTOR pathway. However, there is evidence to suggest that partial inhibition of the mTOR pathway may lead to paradoxical activation of the PI3K/AKT pathway.[46] Therefore, agents that inhibit both PI3K and mTOR have been developed, such as XL765 (Exelixis/Sanofi-aventis) and NVP-BEZ235 (Novartis), which are currently in phase I trials.[47] First-generation PI3K inhibitors such as the irreversible covalent inhibitor wortmannin and LY294002, are non-specific, highly toxic and characterised by poor solubility.[48,49] Current pan-PI3K inhibitors are in early clinical trials and include either modifications of wortmannin and LY294002 such as PWT-458 (Pfizer) and SF1126 (Semafore Pharmaceuticals), respectively, or are chemically distinct such as GDC-0941 (Exelixis/Sanofi-aventis) and XL147 (Exelixis/Sanofi-aventis).[47] It is important to note that most of these inhibitors have, so far, demonstrated disease stabilisation rather than tumour regression. This may be due to activation of alternative survival pathways. Indeed, recent work has shown significant synergy between inhibitors of PI3K and MEK/ERK pathways in tumours bearing activating KRAS or PI3K mutations.[50,51] This strategy may be effectively utilised in type I ovarian cancers with activating KRAS mutations or type II ovarian cancers with PI3K activating mutations.

Several AKT inhibitors have also been developed. One such inhibitor, perifosine (Keryx Biopharmaceuticals), targets the PH domain of AKT, preventing its localisation to the cell membrane,[52] and is currently in phase II clinical trials. However, perifosine is not specific to AKT as it also inhibits the JNK pathway, and response rates to its use as a single agent have been limited.[52]

Another effective way of targeting the PH domain of AKT is through the use of phosphatidylinositol ether lipid (PIEL) analogues. PIEL analogues mimic the products of PI3K and compete with them for the PH domain, resulting in inhibition of membrane localisation or activation of AKT.[53]

Triciribine phosphate is a nucleotide analogue that inhibits the phosphorylation of all three isoforms of AKT. The exact mechanisms of this inhibition are unknown. *In vitro* studies have shown that triciribine preferentially inhibits proliferation of cancer cells with high activity of AKT.[54] In spite of its promising activity in pre-clinical trials, minimal efficacy was observed in Phase I/II trials when used as a single agent[55] and testing its use in combination therapies is planned.

A further approach that is currently in pre-clinical evaluation is the development of isotype-specific AKT inhibitors. A naphthyridinone derivative has been shown to inhibit AKT1 and AKT2 but not AKT3, resulting in improving efficacy and only transient insulin resistance.[56]

IL-6/JAK/STAT3 pathway

As in many other cancers, interleukin 6 (IL-6) is overexpressed in more than 50% of ovarian cancers, possibly as a consequence of mutations of the IL-6 transcription repressor p53.[57] IL-6 binds to its receptor IL6R (composed of ILRα and gp130), leading to its tetramerisation/hexamerisation, which in turn leads to activation of JAK1/JAK2/TYK2 kinases.[58–60] Activated JAK1/JAK2/TYK2 leads to tyrosine phosphorylation of the cytoplasmic domain of the IL6R, leading to recruitment of, predominantly, signal transducer and activator of transcription 3 (STAT3) via its SH2 domain and its subsequent phosphorylation by JAK1/JAK2/TYK2. Once phosphorylated, STAT3 dissociates from the receptor and forms active dimers. Unlike many other signalling pathways that relay signals from the membrane through the cytoplasm to the nucleus, STATs offer a direct route of signalling from the membrane to the nucleus. STAT3 activation leads to the transcription of prosurvival proteins such as the anti-apoptotic protein BCL-XL, the cell cycle promotor cyclin D1 and the oncogene c-Myc, as well as angiogenic factors.[61] In addition to activation of STAT3 by IL-6, RAS is also activated and this leads to hyperphosphorylation of the MAPK pathway, leading to activation of the transcription factor NF-IL6.[62] Activation of NF-IL6 leads to increased expression and transactivation of the multidrug resistance gene *MDR1*.[63]

Several strategies have been employed for targeting STAT3 signalling that can be broadly divided into rationalised inhibitor design and screening. Peptides, peptidomimetics and small-molecule derivatives have been developed to interrupt STAT3 dimerisation by targeting the SH2 domain or by inhibiting the interaction between STAT3 dimers and DNA.[64,65] In addition, high-throughput cell-based screening has identified quinolines as possible inhibitors of STAT3 phosphorylation.[66] Despite intense research aimed at discovering potent STAT3 inhibitors that could be tested in clinical trials, such agents still do not exist.

NF-κB pathway

The nuclear factor κB (NF-κB) pathway is highly activated in more than 50% of ovarian cancers.[17] NF-κB is a transcription factor that is kept in the cytoplasm of most cells by the action of the inhibitor of κB (IκB) that binds to NF-κB and masks the nuclear localisation signal.[67] Activation of NF-κB is achieved through the inhibitor of κB kinase (IKK) family that consists of IKKα and IKKβ and the regulatory protein IKKγ. These kinases are often activated by tumour necrosis factor α (TNF-α), which binds to its receptor TNFR leading to the recruitment of the receptor interacting protein kinase 1 (RIP1) and recruitment of IKK and its phosphorylation by RIP1, mitogen-activated protein kinase kinase kinase 3 (MEKK3) or TGFβ activated kinase 1 (TAK1).[68–70] Once activated, IKK phosphorylates IκB, leading to its dissociation from NF-κB and its degradation, unmasking the nuclear localisation signal of NF-κB, leading to its translocation to the nucleus where it promotes transcription. The activation and nuclear translocation of NF-κB to the nucleus results in promotion of survival by induction of transcription of anti-apoptotic genes such as *BCLXL* and *XIAP*[71] and the induction of transcription of the oxygen free radical scavenger enzyme manganese superoxide dismutase (MnSOD).[72] In addition, NF-κB also transactivates the expression of cyclin D1 and c-Myc, leading to increased proliferation.[73] However, it should also be noted that NF-κB can function as a pro-apoptotic protein by transactivation of *PUMA* and *BAX* and as an inhibitor of proliferation by induction of the expression of p21.[67] The mechanism leading to constitutive activation of NF-κB has remained unclear. One possible hypothesis is that the inflammatory and hypoxic environment surrounding ovarian cancer cells may lead to the secretion of TNF, establishing a positive feedback loop of activation for NF-κB.[67]

Several approaches have been used for targeting the NF-κB pathway, including:

- inhibitors of IKK[74]
- inhibition of proteosomal degradation of IκB by bortezomib[75]
- masking the nuclear localisation signal of NF-κB by complementary peptides[76]
- anti-inflammatory drugs or, more specifically, interfering with NF-κB signalling through direct binding of the adenoviral E1A[77] or small interfering RNA (siRNA) against IKK proteins.

In addition, the natural product curcumin has been shown to downregulate NF-κB and other kinases, chemokines, surface receptor proteins and cyclins, leading to effective antiproliferative activity in a variety of cancer cells.[78,79]

Targeting kinases to improve response to existing chemotherapy

In spite of the proven efficacy of paclitaxel and carboplatin in treating ovarian cancers, they only elicit a response in 70% and 42% of all patients, respectively.[4] Improving response to standard chemotherapies is likely to have a significant effect on survival outcome. Enhancing the bioavailability of existing drugs is an effective and proven way to improve chemotherapy response. For example, the incorporation of doxorubicin into PEGylated liposomes (PLD) has resulted in a significant improvement in the pharmacokinetic properties of the drug. Several studies have shown that PLD is an effective chemotherapeutic option either alone or in combination with carboplatin for the treatment of recurrent platinum-sensitive ovarian cancer.[7,8] Similarly, the incorporation of paclitaxel into albumin-based nanoparticles has been shown to improve bioavailability and reduce adverse effects exerted by current Cremophor®-based preparations.[80] In addition to improving bioavailability, targeted therapies are being investigated to enhance the activity of such drugs.

Paclitaxel targets microtubules, inducing microtubule stabilisation, mitotic arrest and induction of apoptosis. Several strategies using targeted therapies have been employed to overcome paclitaxel resistance. A widely employed approach is to target survival mechanisms in cancer cells to render such cells more susceptible to chemotherapy. For example, AKT or PI3K inhibition is thought to potentiate the activity of paclitaxel by abolishing the anti-apoptotic effect of constitutively active AKT. Similarly, inhibition of the NF-κB pathway using IKK inhibitors or E1A protein transduction significantly enhances paclitaxel response.

Another strategy that is currently in clinical trials is the use of inhibitors for the tyrosine kinase SRC that have been shown to potentiate paclitaxel activity. SRC is overexpressed in more than 50% of ovarian cancers.[17] SRC is a non-receptor tyrosine kinase that is characterised by the presence of an SH4 domain that is responsible for membrane binding, an SH2 domain that recognises and interacts with phosphorylated tyrosine residues, an SH3 domain that interacts with proline-rich proteins, an SH1 catalytic domain, and a C-terminal negative regulatory region.[81] Phosphorylation of the tyrosine 530 at the C-terminal domain induces binding to the SH2 domain, which inhibits the catalytic domain and prevents it from interacting with target proteins.[82] *SRC* is an oncogene that is known to be involved in regulating a variety of intracellular processes such as adhesion, migration, cell growth and survival. Regulation of adhesion is largely dependent on the interaction with focal adhesion kinase (FAK) and the inhibition of the GTPase RhoA and suppression of integrins attached to the extracellular matrix.[83] Regulation of cell survival is thought to be via binding and activation of PI3K, an interaction that requires FAK.[84] SRC also has the ability to activate RAS, resulting in enhanced cellular growth and proliferation.[85] How inhibition of SRC leads to sensitisation to paclitaxel or carboplatin remains unclear. *In vitro*, the mechanism is thought to involve increased caspase 3 cleavage in a caspase 9-independent fashion.[86] In addition, the SRC inhibitor dasatinib sensitises cancer cells to paclitaxel through a mechanism that is dependent on $p27^{Kip1}$ and via decreasing Bcl-2 and CDC2, and enhancing apoptosis.[87] Interestingly, inhibition of SRC leads to re-sensitisation of the cancer cell line CaOV3TaxR, known for overexpression of the multidrug resistance gene *MDR1*, to the activity of paclitaxel without changing the expression or function of *MDR1*. In this *in vitro* system, SRC inhibition may lead to a decrease in the minimum paclitaxel dose required for stabilisation of microtubules.[88] SRC inhibition also results in paclitaxel sensitisation in orthotopic models of ovarian cancer *in vivo*, and inhibition of angiogenesis has been shown to play an important role in this sensitisation,[89] possibly through an effect on angiogenesis. The SaPProC trial is a phase II trial that is currently evaluating the use of the combined SRC and ABL inhibitor saracatinib (AZD0530) in combination with paclitaxel for the treatment of platinum-resistant ovarian cancer.

Targeting kinases with novel biological functions

In addition to the progress made in targeting kinases with established biological significance in ovarian cancer, the functional significance of many other kinases is increasingly being recognised. High-throughput kinome-wide knockdown screens using siRNA identify many novel potential targets that are now in need of clinical translation.[90,91] The discovery of siRNA-mediated regulation of gene expression has provided a powerful method for studying gene function for the rapid discovery of novel targets for therapy.[91,92] These molecules are processed in the cytoplasm by the RNAse III enzyme family Dicer, leading to the critical phosphorylation of the 5′ ends of the siRNA and revealing a two to three nucleotide overhang at the 3′ end.[93] Dicer processing leads to the incorporation of the siRNA into a multiprotein RNA-inducing silencing complex (RISC), resulting in unwinding of the double-stranded siRNA and allowing the anti-sense strand to complement the mRNA strand and the RISC proteins to cleave the mRNA.[94] An alternative approach utilises the processing of the pre-miRNA molecules to yield miRNA (microRNA) through the activity of the enzymes Drosha and Dicer. Downregulation of Dicer or Drosha has been shown to correlate with outcome in women with ovarian cancer.[95] The use of synthetic siRNA technology for targeted depletion of individual genes has made it possible to conduct functional screens of the entire genomes to:

- study gene function[96]
- identify genes essential for survival[97]
- identify genes that, upon depletion, induce synthetic lethality with known mutations[98]
- discover synergistic interactions with chemotherapies.[99]

While these screens have provided important insights into novel pathways as targets for therapy, they have also posed great challenges for studying the relevance of such targets to cancer and in identifying clinically suitable methods for inhibiting interesting targets. For example, a whole-genome screen conducted to identify novel enhancers of paclitaxel response identified more than 80 targets that significantly enhanced paclitaxel response.[100] While many of these targets were mechanistically plausible and were validated, the patterns of their expression and activity in various cancers have not been previously identified, making it difficult to suggest which subgroups of patients are most likely to benefit from such a targeted approach. A siRNA screen designed to identify kinases involved in the regulation of mitosis and paclitaxel response identified six potential targets.[99] Mining published expression microarray data sets revealed that the expression of only one of these targets, salt-inducible kinase 2 (SIK2), correlated with poor survival in women with ovarian cancer. Thus, integrating functional siRNA screens with expression genomics data may provide a powerful tool for the identification of the most promising targets for therapy. At a mechanistic level, depletion of SIK2 resulted in delayed mitotic progression and paclitaxel sensitisation *in vitro* and *in vivo*. SIK2 localises at the centrosome and phosphorylates the centrosome linker protein C-NAP1, leading to its translocation to the cytoplasm and centrosome disengagement early in mitosis. Targeting SIK2 by RNA interference (RNAi) resulted in failure of centrosome separation, decreased AKT S473 phosphorylation and delayed G_1/S progression.

The emergence of promising kinases, such as SIK2, from functional screens poses a challenge for drug discovery endeavours. For example, there are currently no known specific inhibitors for SIK2. The development of such specific inhibitors would be facilitated by identifying the crystal structure of SIK2. So far, 136 catalytic domain structures have been deposited into public databases and efforts are currently under way to provide complete structural knowledge of all known kinases.[26] However, discovering inhibitors of novel kinases usually starts with identifying and synthesising analogues to inhibitors that are known to inhibit other kinases. Screening of known kinase inhibitors for their efficiency in inhibiting a novel kinase is an important first step in the development of lead kinase inhibitors that are subsequently optimised for selective targeting of the kinase of interest. Optimisation may be guided by homology models with other known kinase-ligand structures. For example, the compound PD180970,[101] which is known to target a variety of tyrosine kinases, has been modified, resulting in the discovery of the selective inhibitor of several kinases, for instance the inhibitor of polo-like kinases, BI-D1870.[102]

Beyond kinase inhibitors: nanoparticle delivery of siRNAs

As discussed earlier, RNAi as a method of gene silencing has rapidly become a powerful tool in protein function delineation and gene function discovery, and in guiding drug development. While many therapeutic targets can be adequately inhibited at the protein level by traditional approaches such as small-molecule inhibitors or antibodies, others are less conducive to this. For example, the complex three-dimensional structure of some protein targets as well as the presence of multiple phosphorylation sites limit the ability to use these conventional approaches. Compared with longer fragments, siRNA offers the potential to deliver a therapeutically 'active' agent that does not depend on the presence or functionality of host endogenous RNAi processing machinery components such as Dicer. This is of particular importance because approximately 50% of ovarian cancer cell lines and human ovarian cancers lack Dicer expression.[95] Thus, development of siRNA technology could provide a tool to overcome the shortcomings of some current therapeutic approaches. Indeed, a report published in 2010 confirmed the feasibility of siRNA-mediated silencing of gene targets as a therapeutic tool in patients.[103]

One of the challenges surrounding the use of siRNA for systemic therapy relates to the need for efficient and biocompatible delivery vehicles. The half-life of naked siRNA *in vivo* is fairly short (about 10 minutes) owing to rapid degradation by serum RNases and prompt clearance by the kidneys.[104] In addition, siRNAs must surmount tissue barriers to reach target cells, which must be efficiently penetrated.[105] To overcome these obstacles, siRNAs have been incorporated into non-viral lipids or protein carriers including, cholesterol, liposomes, cyclodextrin nanoparticles, fusogenic peptides, aptamers, biodegradable polylactide copolymers, and polymers.[106]

Liposomes, in general, have been shown to be safe in a number of clinical trials using a wide variety of anti-cancer and antimicrobial drugs. Liposomal charge, size and lipid composition can directly impact their safety, distribution and uptake by cells and tissues. We have focused on the use of a neutral nanoliposome, 1,2-dioleoyl-sn-glycero-3-phosphatidylcholine (DOPC), for *in vivo* delivery of siRNA because of the safety and efficacy against multiple targets in a variety of animal models.[99,107] Landen and colleagues[107] have successfully silenced EphA2 receptor tyrosine kinase expression using siRNA incorporated into the DOPC nanoliposomes in orthotopic mouse models of ovarian cancer. EphA2 belongs to the Eph family of protein tyrosine kinase receptors and is localised to sites of cell–cell adhesion in adult human epithelial cells.[108] EphA2 targeting using siRNA significantly reduced tumour burden in mice bearing human ovarian cancer by up to 50%. This effect was dramatically potentiated by the addition of paclitaxel, resulting in a 90% reduction in tumour size. This approach has been highly effective against multiple other targets and is being developed for clinical use.[99]

Another promising avenue for cancer therapy involves targeting tumour angiogenesis. While vascular endothelial growth factor (VEGF)-targeted therapies are showing encouraging clinical responses, additional targets are needed to make further improvements. In search of such targets, we carried out genomic profiling studies of endothelial cells from epithelial ovarian cancer and from their normal counterparts.[109] These studies showed that Zeste homologue 2 (EZH2) was overexpressed in endothelial cells from epithelial ovarian cancer and that this correlated with poor outcome.[110] EZH2 was found to promote angiogenesis by methylation and inhibition of the anti-angiogenic factor VASH1. Liposomal delivery of EZH2 siRNA resulted in reactivation of VASH1, inhibition of angiogenesis and decreased ovarian cancer tumour growth in xenograft models.[110] For delivery of siRNA into the tumour endothelium, we sought to develop additional nanoparticles that would allow siRNA delivery into both tumour and tumour-associated endothelial cells. Chitosan is desirable for biological applications owing to properties such as low immunogenicity and low toxicity. These properties make the use of chitosan for systemic *in vivo* siRNA delivery highly attractive.[111] Chitosan nanoparticles are highly effective for delivery of siRNA into both tumour and tumour-associated endothelial cells.[110] Moreover, these nanoparticles offer opportunities for attaching targeting moieties such as peptides for highly selective delivery of siRNA into the tumour vasculature.[112] Such an approach may add a powerful tool to the armamentarium for targeting angiogenesis-promoting genes.

References

1. Ferlay J, Shin HR, Bray F, Forman D, Mathers C, Parkin DM. *GLOBOCAN 2008, Cancer Incidence and Mortality Worldwide: IARC CancerBase No. 10*. Lyon: International Agency for Research on Cancer; 2010 [globocan.iarc.fr].
2. Cancer Research UK. Ovarian cancer – UK mortality statistics [info.cancerresearchuk.org/cancerstats/types/ovary/mortality].
3. National Cancer Institute. Surveillance Epidemiology and End Results (SEER) [seer.cancer.gov].

4. Muggia FM, Braly PS, Brady MF, Sutton G, Niemann TH, Lentz SL, *et al.* Phase III randomized study of cisplatin versus paclitaxel versus cisplatin and paclitaxel in patients with suboptimal stage III or IV ovarian cancer: a Gynecologic Oncology Group study. *J Clin Oncol* 2000;18:106–15.
5. Murgia V, Sorio R, Griso C, Caffo O, Arcuri C, Ferro A, *et al.* Multicenter phase 2 study of combined gemcitabine and epirubicin as second-line treatment for patients with advanced ovarian cancer. *Int J Gynecol Cancer* 2010;20:953–7.
6. Pujade-Lauraine E, Wagner U, Aavall-Lundqvist E, Gebski V, Heywood M, Vasey PA, *et al.* Pegylated liposomal doxorubicin and carboplatin compared with paclitaxel and carboplatin for patients with platinum-sensitive ovarian cancer in late relapse. *J Clin Oncol* 2010;28:3323–9.
7. ten Bokkel Huinink W, Lane SR, Ross GA. Long-term survival in a phase III, randomised study of topotecan versus paclitaxel in advanced epithelial ovarian carcinoma. *Ann Oncol* 2004;15:100–3.
8. Gordon AN, Fleagle JT, Guthrie D, Parkin DE, Gore ME, Lacave AJ. Recurrent epithelial ovarian carcinoma: a randomized phase III study of pegylated liposomal doxorubicin versus topotecan. *J Clin Oncol* 2001;19:3312–22.
9. du Bois A, Herrstedt J, Hardy-Bessard AC, Muller HH, Harter P, Kristensen G, *et al.* Phase III trial of carboplatin plus paclitaxel with or without gemcitabine in first-line treatment of epithelial ovarian cancer. *J Clin Oncol* 2010;28:4162–9.
10. Bolis G, Scarfone G, Raspagliesi F, Mangili G, Danese S, Scollo P, *et al.* Paclitaxel/carboplatin versus topotecan/paclitaxel/carboplatin in patients with FIGO suboptimally resected stage III–IV epithelial ovarian cancer a multicenter, randomized study. *Eur J Cancer* 2010;46:2905–12.
11. Pfisterer J, Weber B, Reuss A, Kimmig R, du Bois A, Wagner U, *et al.* Randomized phase III trial of topotecan following carboplatin and paclitaxel in first-line treatment of advanced ovarian cancer: a Gynecologic Cancer Intergroup trial of the AGO-OVAR and GINECO. *J Natl Cancer Inst* 2006;98:1036–45.
12. Fong PC, Yap TA, Boss DS, Carden CP, Mergui-Roelvink M, Gourley C, *et al.* Poly(ADP)-ribose polymerase inhibition: frequent durable responses in *BRCA* carrier ovarian cancer correlating with platinum-free interval. *J Clin Oncol* 2010;28:2512–9.
13. Harrison ML, Jameson C, Gore ME. Mucinous ovarian cancer. *Int J Gynecol Cancer* 2008;18209–14.
14. Mizuno M, Kikkawa F, Shibata K, Kajiyama H, Ino K, Kawai M, *et al.* Long-term follow-up and prognostic factor analysis in clear cell adenocarcinoma of the ovary. *J Surg Oncol* 2006;94138–43.
15. Tothill RW, Tinker AV, George J, Brown R, Fox SB, Lade S, *et al.* Novel molecular subtypes of serous and endometrioid ovarian cancer linked to clinical outcome. *Clin Cancer Res* 2008;14:5198–208.
16. Crum CP. Intercepting pelvic cancer in the distal fallopian tube: theories and realities. *Mol Oncol* 2009;3:165–70.
17. Bast RC Jr, Hennessy B, Mills GB. The biology of ovarian cancer: new opportunities for translation. *Nat Rev Cancer* 2009;9:415–28.
18. Singer G, Oldt R 3rd, Cohen Y, Wang BG, Sidransky D, Kurman RJ, *et al.* Mutations in BRAF and KRAS characterize the development of low-grade ovarian serous carcinoma. *J Natl Cancer Inst* 2003;95:484–6.
19. Gemignani ML, Schlaerth AC, Bogomolniy F, Barakat RR, Lin O, Soslow R, *et al.* Role of *KRAS* and *BRAF* gene mutations in mucinous ovarian carcinoma. *Gynecol Oncol* 2003;90:378–81.
20. Shih Ie M, Kurman RJ. Ovarian tumorigenesis: a proposed model based on morphological and molecular genetic analysis. *Am J Pathol* 2004;164:1511–18.
21. Schubbert S, Shannon K, Bollag G. Hyperactive Ras in developmental disorders and cancer. *Nat Rev Cancer* 2007;7:295–308.
22. Trahey M, McCormick F. A cytoplasmic protein stimulates normal N-ras p21 GTPase, but does not affect oncogenic mutants. *Science* 1987;238:542–5.
23. Dinulescu DM, Ince TA, Quade BJ, Shafer SA, Crowley D, Jacks T. Role of K-ras and Pten in the development of mouse models of endometriosis and endometrioid ovarian cancer. *Nat Med* 2005;11:63–70.
24. Johnson L, Mercer K, Greenbaum D, Bronson RT, Crowley D, Tuveson DA, *et al.* Somatic activation of the *K-ras* oncogene causes early onset lung cancer in mice. *Nature* 2001;410:1111–16.
25. Ahmed AA, Etemadmoghadam D, Temple J, Lynch AG, Riad M, Sharma R, *et al.* Driver mutations in *TP53* are ubiquitous in high grade serous carcinoma of the ovary. *J Pathol* 2010;221:49–56.

26. Fedorov O, Sundstrom M, Marsden B, Knapp S. Insights for the development of specific kinase inhibitors by targeted structural genomics. *Drug Discov Today* 2007;12:365–72.
27. Eswaran J, Knapp S. Insights into protein kinase regulation and inhibition by large scale structural comparison. *Biochim Biophys Acta* 2010;1804:429–32.
28. Zhang J, Yang PL, Gray NS. Targeting cancer with small molecule kinase inhibitors. *Nat Rev Cancer* 2009;9:28–39.
29. Liu Y, Gray NS. Rational design of inhibitors that bind to inactive kinase conformations. *Nat Chem Biol* 2006;2:358–64.
30. Schindler T, Bornmann W, Pellicena P, Miller WT, Clarkson B, Kuriyan J. Structural mechanism for STI-571 inhibition of abelson tyrosine kinase. *Science* 2000;289:1938–42.
31. Fernandez A, Sanguino A, Peng Z, Ozturk E, Chen J, Crespo A, *et al.* An anticancer C-Kit kinase inhibitor is reengineered to make it more active and less cardiotoxic. *J Clin Invest* 2007;117:4044–54.
32. Zhang J, Adrián FJ, Jahnke W, Cowan-Jacob SW, Li AG, Iacob RE, *et al.* Targeting Bcr-Abl by combining allosteric with ATP-binding-site inhibitors. *Nature* 2010;463:501–6.
33. Rabindran SK, Discafani CM, Rosfjord EC, Baxter M, Floyd MB, Golas J, *et al.* Antitumor activity of HKI-272, an orally active, irreversible inhibitor of the HER-2 tyrosine kinase. *Cancer Res* 2004;64:3958–65.
34. Manning BD, Cantley LC. AKT/PKB signaling: navigating downstream. *Cell* 2007;129:1261–74.
35. Vivanco I, Sawyers CL. The phosphatidylinositol 3-Kinase AKT pathway in human cancer. *Nat Rev Cancer* 2002;2:489–501.
36. Sarbassov DD, Guertin DA, Ali SM, Sabatini DM. Phosphorylation and regulation of Akt/PKB by the rictor-mTOR complex. *Science* 2005;307:1098–101.
37. Alessi DR, Deak M, Casamayor A, Caudwell FB, Morrice N, Norman DG, *et al.* 3-Phosphoinositide-dependent protein kinase-1 (PDK1): structural and functional homology with the Drosophila DSTPK61 kinase. *Curr Biol* 1997;7:776–89.
38. Liu P, Cheng H, Roberts TM, Zhao JJ. Targeting the phosphoinositide 3-kinase pathway in cancer. *Nat Rev Drug Discov* 2009;8:627–44.
39. Cully M, You H, Levine AJ, Mak TW. Beyond *PTEN* mutations: the PI3K pathway as an integrator of multiple inputs during tumorigenesis. *Nat Rev Cancer* 2006;6:184–92.
40. Datta SR, Katsov A, Hu L, Petros A, Fesik SW, Yaffe MB, *et al.* 14-3-3 proteins and survival kinases cooperate to inactivate BAD by BH3 domain phosphorylation. *Mol Cell* 2000;6:41–51.
41. Datta SR, Dudek H, Tao X, Masters S, Fu H, Gotoh Y, *et al.* Akt phosphorylation of BAD couples survival signals to the cell-intrinsic death machinery. *Cell* 1997;91:231–41.
42. Tran H, Brunet A, Griffith EC, Greenberg ME. The many forks in FOXO's road. *Sci STKE* 2003;2003(172):RE5.
43. Mayo LD, Donner DB. A phosphatidylinositol 3-kinase/Akt pathway promotes translocation of Mdm2 from the cytoplasm to the nucleus. *Proc Natl Acad Sci U S A* 2001;98:11598–603.
44. Tee AR, Anjum R, Blenis J. Inactivation of the tuberous sclerosis complex-1 and -2 gene products occurs by phosphoinositide 3-kinase/Akt-dependent and -independent phosphorylation of tuberin. *J Biol Chem* 2003;278:37288–96.
45. Inoki K, Li Y, Zhu T, Wu J, Guan KL. TSC2 is phosphorylated and inhibited by Akt and suppresses mTOR signalling. *Nat Cell Biol* 2002;4:648–57.
46. Wang X, Hawk N, Yue P, Kauh J, Ramalingam SS, Fu H, *et al.* Overcoming mTOR inhibition-induced paradoxical activation of survival signaling pathways enhances mTOR inhibitors' anticancer efficacy. *Cancer Biol Ther* 2008;7:1952–8.
47. Cleary JM, Shapiro GI. Development of phosphoinositide-3 kinase pathway inhibitors for advanced cancer. *Curr Oncol Rep* 2010;12:87–94.
48. Garlich JR, De P, Dey N, Su JD, Peng X, Miller A, *et al.* A vascular targeted pan phosphoinositide 3-kinase inhibitor prodrug, SF1126, with antitumor and antiangiogenic activity. *Cancer Res* 2008;68:206–15.
49. Marone R, Cmiljanovic V, Giese B, Wymann MP. Targeting phosphoinositide 3-kinase: moving towards therapy. *Biochim Biophys Acta* 2008;1784:159–85.
50. Faber AC, Li D, Song Y, Liang MC, Yeap BY, Bronson RT, *et al.* Differential induction of apoptosis in HER2 and EGFR addicted cancers following PI3K inhibition. *Proc Natl Acad Sci U S A* 2009;106:19503–8.

51. Engelman JA, Chen L, Tan X, Crosby K, Guimaraes AR, Upadhyay R, *et al.* Effective use of PI3K and MEK inhibitors to treat mutant Kras G12D and PIK3CA H1047R murine lung cancers. *Nat Med* 2008;14:1351–6.
52. Gills JJ, Dennis PA. Perifosine: update on a novel Akt inhibitor. *Curr Oncol Rep* 2009;11:102–10.
53. Gills JJ, Castillo SS, Zhang C, Petukhov PA, Memmott RM, Hollingshead M, *et al.* Phosphatidylinositol ether lipid analogues that inhibit AKT also independently activate the stress kinase, p38alpha, through MKK3/6-independent and -dependent mechanisms. *J Biol Chem* 2007;282:27020–9.
54. Yang L, Dan HC, Sun M, Liu Q, Sun XM, Feldman RI, *et al.* Akt/protein kinase B signaling inhibitor-2, a selective small molecule inhibitor of Akt signaling with antitumor activity in cancer cells overexpressing Akt. *Cancer Res* 2004;64:4394–9.
55. Hoffman K, Holmes FA, Fraschini G, Esparza L, Frye D, Raber MN, *et al.* Phase I–II study: triciribine (tricyclic nucleoside phosphate) for metastatic breast cancer. *Cancer Chemother Pharmacol* 1996;37:254–8.
56. Cherrin C, Haskell K, Howell B, Jones R, Leander K, Robinson R, *et al.* An allosteric Akt inhibitor effectively blocks Akt signaling and tumor growth with only transient effects on glucose and insulin levels *in vivo*. *Cancer Biol Ther* 2010;9:493–503.
57. Wang L, Rayanade RJ, Garcia D, Patel K, Pan H, Sehgal PB. Modulation of interleukin-6-induced plasma protein secretion in hepatoma cells by p53 species. *J Biol Chem* 1995;270:23159–65.
58. Heinrich PC, Behrmann I, Muller-Newen G, Schaper F, Graeve L. Interleukin-6-type cytokine signalling through the gp130/Jak/STAT pathway. *Biochem J* 1998;334(Pt 2):297–314.
59. Stahl N, Farruggella TJ, Boulton TG, Zhong Z, Darnell JE Jr, Yancopoulos GD. Choice of STATs and other substrates specified by modular tyrosine-based motifs in cytokine receptors. *Science* 1995;267:1349–53.
60. Stahl N, Boulton TG, Farruggella T, Ip NY, Davis S, Witthuhn BA, *et al.* Association and activation of Jak-Tyk kinases by CNTF-LIF-OSM-IL-6 beta receptor components. *Science* 1994;263:92–5.
61. Bromberg J. Stat proteins and oncogenesis. *J Clin Invest* 2002;109:1139–42.
62. Nakajima T, Kinoshita S, Sasagawa T, Sasaki K, Naruto M, Kishimoto T, *et al.* Phosphorylation at threonine-235 by a ras-dependent mitogen-activated protein kinase cascade is essential for transcription factor NF-IL6. *Proc Natl Acad Sci U S A* 1993;90:2207–11.
63. Chen GK, Sale S, Tan T, Ermoian RP, Sikic BI. CCAAT/enhancer-binding protein beta (nuclear factor for interleukin 6) transactivates the human *MDR1* gene by interaction with an inverted CCAAT box in human cancer cells. *Mol Pharmacol* 2004;65:906–16.
64. Mandal PK, Ren Z, Chen X, Xiong C, McMurray JS. Structure-affinity relationships of glutamine mimics incorporated into phosphopeptides targeted to the SH2 domain of signal transducer and activator of transcription 3. *J Med Chem* 2009;52:6126–41.
65. Mandal PK, Liao WS, McMurray JS. Synthesis of phosphatase-stable, cell-permeable peptidomimetic prodrugs that target the SH2 domain of Stat3. *Org Lett* 2009;11:3394–7.
66. Xu J, Cole DC, Chang CP, Ayyad R, Asselin M, Hao W, *et al.* Inhibition of the signal transducer and activator of transcription-3 (STAT3) signaling pathway by 4-oxo-1-phenyl-1,4-dihydroquinoline-3-carboxylic acid esters. *J Med Chem* 2008;51:4115–21.
67. Lin Y, Bai L, Chen W, Xu S. The NF-kappaB activation pathways, emerging molecular targets for cancer prevention and therapy. *Expert Opin Ther Targets* 2010;14:45–55.
68. Chen ZJ. Ubiquitin signalling in the NF-kappaB pathway. *Nat Cell Biol* 2005;7:758–65.
69. Yang J, Lin Y, Guo Z, Cheng J, Huang J, Deng L, *et al.* The essential role of MEKK3 in TNF-induced NF-kappaB activation. *Nat Immunol* 2001;2:620–4.
70. Devin A, Cook A, Lin Y, Rodriguez Y, Kelliher M, Liu Z. The distinct roles of TRAF2 and RIP in IKK activation by TNF-R1: TRAF2 recruits IKK to TNF-R1 while RIP mediates IKK activation. *Immunity* 2000;12:419–29.
71. Campbell KJ, Rocha S, Perkins ND. Active repression of antiapoptotic gene expression by RelA(p65) NF-kappa B. *Mol Cell* 2004;13:853–65.
72. Holley AK, Xu Y, St Clair DK, St Clair WH. RelB regulates manganese superoxide dismutase gene and resistance to ionizing radiation of prostate cancer cells. *Ann N Y Acad Sci* 2010;1201:129–36.

73. Dahlman JM, Wang J, Bakkar N, Guttridge DC. The RelA/p65 subunit of NF-kappaB specifically regulates cyclin D1 protein stability: implications for cell cycle withdrawal and skeletal myogenesis. *J Cell Biochem* 2009;106:42–51.
74. Lee DF, Hung MC. Advances in targeting IKK and IKK-related kinases for cancer therapy. *Clin Cancer Res* 2008;14:5656–62.
75. Gasparian AV, Guryanova OA, Chebotaev DV, Shishkin AA, Yemelyanov AY, Budunova IV. Targeting transcription factor NFkappaB: comparative analysis of proteasome and IKK inhibitors. *Cell Cycle* 2009;8:1559–66.
76. Mabuchi S, Ohmichi M, Nishio Y, Hayasaka T, Kimura A, Ohta T, *et al.* Inhibition of NFkappaB increases the efficacy of cisplatin in *in vitro* and *in vivo* ovarian cancer models. *J Biol Chem* 2004;279:23477–85.
77. Morimoto K, Gosselink J, Kartono A, Hogg JC, Hayashi S, Ogawa E. Adenovirus E1A regulates lung epithelial ICAM-1 expression by interacting with transcriptional regulators at its promoter. *Am J Physiol Lung Cell Mol Physiol* 2009;296:L361–71.
78. Lin YG, Kunnumakkara AB, Nair A, Merritt WM, Han LY, Armaiz-Pena GN, *et al.* Curcumin inhibits tumor growth and angiogenesis in ovarian carcinoma by targeting the nuclear factor-kappaB pathway. *Clin Cancer Res* 2007;13:3423–30.
79. Aggarwal BB, Kumar A, Bharti AC. Anticancer potential of curcumin: preclinical and clinical studies. *Anticancer Res* 2003;23:363–98.
80. Gradishar WJ, Krasnojon D, Cheporov S, Makhson AN, Manikhas GM, Clawson A, *et al.* Significantly longer progression-free survival with nab-paclitaxel compared with docetaxel as first-line therapy for metastatic breast cancer. *J Clin Oncol* 2009;27:3611–19.
81. Kim LC, Song L, Haura EB. Src kinases as therapeutic targets for cancer. *Nat Rev Clin Oncol* 2009;6:587–95.
82. Cartwright CA, Eckhart W, Simon S, Kaplan PL. Cell transformation by pp60c-src mutated in the carboxy-terminal regulatory domain. *Cell* 1987;49:83–91.
83. Arthur WT, Petch LA, Burridge K. Integrin engagement suppresses RhoA activity via a c-Src-dependent mechanism. *Curr Biol* 2000;10:719–22.
84. Siesser PM, Hanks SK. The signaling and biological implications of FAK overexpression in cancer. *Clin Cancer Res* 2006;12:3233–7.
85. Timpson P, Jones GE, Frame MC, Brunton VG. Coordination of cell polarization and migration by the Rho family GTPases requires Src tyrosine kinase activity. *Curr Biol* 2001;11:1836–46.
86. Chen T, Pengetnze Y, Taylor CC. Src inhibition enhances paclitaxel cytotoxicity in ovarian cancer cells by caspase-9-independent activation of caspase-3. *Mol Cancer Ther* 2005;4:217–24.
87. Le XF, Mao W, Zhang Q, Tian L, Ahmed AA, Claret F, *et al.* p27Kip1 protein levels predict dasatinib-induced potentiation of paclitaxel activity in human ovarian cancer cells. Proceedings of the 100th Annual Meeting of the American Association for Cancer Research, 2009. Abstract 824.
88. George JA, Chen T, Taylor CC. SRC tyrosine kinase and multidrug resistance protein-1 inhibitions act independently but cooperatively to restore paclitaxel sensitivity to paclitaxel-resistant ovarian cancer cells. *Cancer Res* 2005;65:10381–8.
89. Han LY, Landen CN, Trevino JG, Halder J, Lin YG, Kamat AA, *et al.* Antiangiogenic and antitumor effects of SRC inhibition in ovarian carcinoma. *Cancer Res* 2006;66:8633–9.
90. Boutros M, Ahringer J. The art and design of genetic screens: RNA interference. *Nat Rev Genet* 2008;9:554–66.
91. Dykxhoorn DM, Chowdhury D, Lieberman J. RNA interference and cancer: endogenous pathways and therapeutic approaches. *Adv Exp Med Biol* 2008;615:299–329.
92. Fire A, Xu S, Montgomery MK, Kostas SA, Driver SE, Mello CC. Potent and specific genetic interference by double-stranded RNA in *Caenorhabditis elegans*. *Nature* 1998;391:806–11.
93. Bernstein E, Caudy AA, Hammond SM, Hannon GJ. Role for a bidentate ribonuclease in the initiation step of RNA interference. *Nature* 2001;409:363–6.
94. Nykanen A, Haley B, Zamore PD. ATP requirements and small interfering RNA structure in the RNA interference pathway. *Cell* 2001;107:309–21.
95. Merritt WM, Lin YG, Han LY, Kamat AA, Spannuth WA, Schmandt R, *et al.* Dicer, Drosha, and outcomes in patients with ovarian cancer. *N Engl J Med* 2008;359:2641–50.

96. Smogorzewska A, Desetty R, Saito TT, Schlabach M, Lach FP, Sowa ME, *et al.* A genetic screen identifies FAN1, a Fanconi anemia-associated nuclease necessary for DNA interstrand crosslink repair. *Mol Cell* 2010;39:36–47.
97. Sheng Z, Li L, Zhu LJ, Smith TW, Demers A, Ross AH, *et al.* A genome-wide RNA interference screen reveals an essential CREB3L2-ATF5-MCL1 survival pathway in malignant glioma with therapeutic implications. *Nat Med* 2010;16:671–7.
98. Luo J, Emanuele MJ, Li D, Creighton CJ, Schlabach MR, Westbrook TF, *et al.* A genome-wide RNAi screen identifies multiple synthetic lethal interactions with the Ras oncogene. *Cell* 2009;137:835–48.
99. Ahmed AA, Lu Z, Jennings NB, Etemadmoghadam D, Capalbo L, Jacamo RO, *et al.* SIK2 is a centrosome kinase required for bipolar mitotic spindle formation that provides a potential target for therapy in ovarian cancer. *Cancer Cell* 2010;18:109–21.
100. Whitehurst AW, Bodemann BO, Cardenas J, Ferguson D, Girard L, Peyton M, *et al.* Synthetic lethal screen identification of chemosensitizer loci in cancer cells. *Nature* 2007;446:815–19.
101. Kraker AJ, Hartl BG, Amar AM, Barvian MR, Showalter HD, Moore CW. Biochemical and cellular effects of c-Src kinase-selective pyrido[2, 3-d]pyrimidine tyrosine kinase inhibitors. *Biochem Pharmacol* 2000;60:885–98.
102. Lenart P, Petronczki M, Steegmaier M, Di Fiore B, Lipp JJ, Hoffmann M, *et al.* The small-molecule inhibitor BI 2536 reveals novel insights into mitotic roles of polo-like kinase 1. *Curr Biol* 2007;17:304–15.
103. Davis ME, Zuckerman JE, Choi CH, Seligson D, Tolcher A, Alabi CA, *et al.* Evidence of RNAi in humans from systemically administered siRNA via targeted nanoparticles. *Nature* 2010;464:1067–70.
104. Huang C, Li M, Chen C, Yao Q. Small interfering RNA therapy in cancer: mechanism, potential targets, and clinical applications. *Expert Opin Ther Targets* 2008;12:637–45.
105. Lu PY, Woodle MC. Delivering small interfering RNA for novel therapeutics. *Methods Mol Biol* 2008;437:93–107.
106. Pirollo KF, Chang EH. Targeted delivery of small interfering RNA: approaching effective cancer therapies. *Cancer Res* 2008;68:1247–50.
107. Landen CN Jr, Chavez-Reyes A, Bucana C, Schmandt R, Deavers MT, Lopez-Berestein G, *et al.* Therapeutic *EphA2* gene targeting *in vivo* using neutral liposomal small interfering RNA delivery. *Cancer Res* 2005;65:6910–18.
108. Walker-Daniels J, Hess AR, Hendrix MJ, Kinch MS. Differential regulation of EphA2 in normal and malignant cells. *Am J Pathol* 2003;162:1037–42.
109. Lu C, Bonome T, Li Y, Kamat AA, Han LY, Schmandt R, *et al.* Gene alterations identified by expression profiling in tumor-associated endothelial cells from invasive ovarian carcinoma. *Cancer Res* 2007;67:1757–68.
110. Lu C, Han HD, Mangala LS, Ali-Fehmi R, Newton CS, Ozbun L, *et al.* Regulation of tumor angiogenesis by *EZH2*. *Cancer Cell* 2010;18:185–97.
111. Howard KA, Rahbek UL, Liu X, Damgaard CK, Glud SZ, Andersen MO, *et al.* RNA interference *in vitro* and *in vivo* using a novel chitosan/siRNA nanoparticle system. *Mol Ther* 2006;14:476–84.
112. Han HD, Mangala LS, Lee JW, Shahzad MM, Kim HS, Shen D, *et al.* Targeted gene silencing using RGD-labeled chitosan nanoparticles. *Clin Cancer Res* 2010;16:3910–22.

Chapter 14
Functional imaging: from tumour biology to the clinic

Nandita M deSouza, Evis Sala, Stavroula Kyriazi and Andrea Rockall

Introduction

The increasing demand for *in vivo* imaging to provide early biomarkers of disease response as well as to report on predictive and prognostic features of tumours is driving the need for a combined structural and functional approach. Morphological imaging is usually only useful in assessing response late after therapy and, while volumetric measures, for example in cervical cancer, are crucial prognostic indicators, their use in small, early-stage disease is less useful in this regard. With the advent of techniques such as dynamic contrast-enhanced (DCE) computed tomography (CT) or magnetic resonance imaging (MRI), diffusion-weighted (DW) imaging, lymph node-specific contrast agents and positron emission tomography (PET) with ^{18}F-FDG or other targeted radiotracers, there is a burgeoning field of 'functional' techniques that can be exploited for use in the clinic. This chapter describes the range of techniques available, their relationship to tumour biology and their utility in the context of patient management pathways.

Available techniques

Dynamic contrast-enhanced CT or MRI

The microvascular properties of tissue can be interrogated with DCE-CT or DCE-MRI, where rapid image acquisition before, during and after a bolus of intravenously injected contrast agent enables pharmacokinetic modelling of its passage through the circulation and into the tissue compartment. The presence of the contrast agent (iodinated in the case of CT, weakly paramagnetic in the case of MRI) increases X-ray attenuation or signal intensity, respectively; the degree of enhancement is determined by blood flow, vascular density, capillary permeability and capillary surface area in the early vascular phase and by extravascular space volume in the interstitial phase. With CT, the attenuation directly reflects contrast agent concentration; with MRI, the measured signal intensity is converted into T1 relaxation values and contrast concentration–time curves, which, after pharmacokinetic model fitting, yield quantitative parameters, such as the volume transfer coefficient (K^{trans}) between blood plasma and the extracellular extravascular leakage space (EES), the volume of EES (v_e) and the rate constant (k_{ep}). As a general observation, malignant lesions tend to enhance earlier, more rapidly and more avidly than benign lesions.

The methodology used in pharmacokinetic analysis is vital: a number of mathematical models exist. It is crucial to unify and standardise these if data are to be interpreted in large multicentre trials.

Diffusion-weighted MRI

An alternative to extrinsic contrast administration is to develop intrinsic image contrast through 'apparent diffusivity' (tissue water incoherent displacement over distances of ~1–20 μm).[1] The motion measured by this technique relates to distances travelled by protons as a result of thermally driven, random (Brownian) motion. The sensitivity of a DW sequence to motion is characterised by its b value, which reflects the amplitude, duration and spacing of the applied diffusion gradients. High b values increase the sensitivity to motion, interrogating shorter displacement distances of protons. Usually, the signal is measured without (S0) and with (Sb) DW gradients applied, allowing an apparent diffusion coefficient (ADC) to be calculated. The derived ADC values are represented in the form of a two-dimensional map.

In tissues, the random paths that extracellular water molecules may otherwise take are hindered by cell membranes. Foci of cancer may be highly cellular and in such an environment extracellular water would not be able to diffuse far before signal acquisition[2] and hence there is reduced ADC in the region of the tumour. DW-MRI thus has the potential to detect and characterise tumours because of the reduced diffusivity associated with highly cellular tumours.[2] In cancer imaging, initial data from single-centre studies show promise at all phases of the disease from early detection through staging to response assessment and identification of recurrence.

Magnetic resonance spectroscopy

Proton magnetic resonance spectroscopy (proton MRS) employs the same hardware as MRI to non-invasively explore the biochemical composition of tissue but forfeits spatial information and thus anatomical depiction. Proton MRS derives its signal from the different resonant frequencies of protons within a molecule due to magnetic diatomic interactions within the molecular structure. Resonant signals can be displayed as a function of frequency (i.e. as a spectrum) after Fourier transformation. The spectrum encompasses a series of peaks on the chemical shift axis (expressed in parts per million, ppm) unique for different metabolites. The ppm scale describes the shift in hertz from a reference frequency divided by the excitation frequency of the external magnetic field. In practice, inherent field inhomogeneities result in metabolites resonating at a range of frequencies instead of a unique value, which compromises spectral resolution. Nevertheless, typical peak patterns can be recognised for a variety of biochemical compounds, such as choline (3.2 ppm) and creatine (3.0 ppm), which have been characterised as biomarkers of cellular proliferation and energy, respectively. Disease causes changes in the concentration of normal metabolites and the appearance of aberrant metabolites, such as lactate (1.4 ppm), which indicates increased anaerobic activity. Absolute quantification *in vivo* is hampered by the absence of internal standards of concentration, so relative concentrations are frequently used to characterise tumours and assess response.

Positron emission tomography

PET/CT is a functional imaging tool that uses short-lived radionuclides attached to tracers to image metabolic processes in the body in combination with a low-dose CT for localisation purposes. The success of this combined modality is due to the fact that combined PET and CT data acquisition is highly synergistic in tumour staging and therapy monitoring applications. The integration of PET and CT provides precise lesion localisation on PET scans within the anatomical reference frame provided by CT, thereby increasing the specificity of examination.

The most commonly used radiotracer is ^{18}F-fluoro-2-deoxy-D-glucose (FDG), which is metabolised as glucose. Many malignant tumours are therefore identifiable owing to their increased glycolytic rate. However, it must be remembered that physiological uptake can be seen in the uterus, ovarian follicles and corpus luteum cysts in premenopausal women. FDG uptake can also be seen in certain benign ovarian and uterine tumours as well as in inflammatory and infectious processes.

Ovarian cancer

In ovarian cancer, functional imaging can be particularly useful for multi-site evaluation of treatment-induced changes, although it is technically challenging because of the extent and convoluted anatomy of the peritoneal cavity.

DCE-MRI

As a biomarker of tissue vascularity and perfusion, DCE imaging can aid characterisation of ovarian lesions. Semi-quantitative analysis of enhancement curves shows that early initiation and high rate and magnitude of enhancement are associated with malignancy.[3] Amplitude and maximal slope of enhancement reportedly achieved 100% sensitivity with 72% and 92% specificity, respectively, in identifying histological invasion.[4] These parameters correlated positively with vascular endothelial growth factor receptor 2 (VEGFR-2) expression but not with microvessel density, thus representing functional angiogenic properties, such as permeability, rather than structural hypervascularisation. Absolute quantitative metrics showed no significant changes in K^{trans} after commencing of platinum/taxane chemotherapy, suggesting that the detection of antivascular effects of standard cytotoxic agents may require more rigorous acquisition and analysis techniques.[5]

The feasibility of DCE-MRI in multiple metastatic sites with improved temporal resolution (1.6 s) and extended spatial coverage[6] is promising for adoption of DCE imaging into the clinical workflow of response assessment. In women with low-volume, asymptomatic relapsed disease, serological angiogenic markers VEGFR-1 and VEGFR-2 correlated negatively with fractional blood volume v_p and positively with K^{trans} from omental, peritoneal and nodal lesions, indicating a relationship between hypoxia-induced upregulation of angiogenic receptors and increased vascular permeability.[7] Although in the same study baseline DCE-MRI metrics were not prognostic of subsequent clinical progression, biochemical (CA125), morphological (whole tumour volume) and perfusional (enhancing tumour fraction) parameters at 4 weeks differed significantly in those with stable disease compared with those who progressed biochemically at 26 weeks of follow-up. This highlights the need for integrated multiparametric models to maximise predictive and prognostic power.

DW-MRI

There is considerable overlap of mean and lowest ADC values between benign and malignant ovarian tumours[8,9] because of histological heterogeneity: malignant tumours with abundance of desmoplastic stroma may present relatively high ADCs, whereas benign lesions such as fibromas may have lower ADC values owing to compact matrix organisation.[9]

Although contrast-enhanced CT and MRI have excellent per-patient sensitivity in detecting peritoneal deposits (92% and 95%, respectively),[10] their per-lesion performance deteriorates considerably in implants smaller than 1 cm (sensitivity 7–50%) and in certain anatomical areas, such as the right subdiaphragmatic space, omentum, root of mesentery and serosal surface of small bowel and bladder (sensitivity 12–43%),[11–13] because small serosal implants invaginated within peritoneal reflections are often obscured by their similar attenuation values/signal intensity to adjacent structures. DW-MRI depicts deposits on the visceral peritoneum as foci of high signal intensity against a background of suppressed signal from surrounding ascites, bowel contents and fat, leading to greater conspicuity (Figure 14.1). Its addition, gadolinium-enhanced MRI has been reported to improve the accuracy of tumour detection in 15 of 16 anatomical sites (accuracy of 84–88% compared with 52–72% for MRI alone

(a) (b) (c) (d)

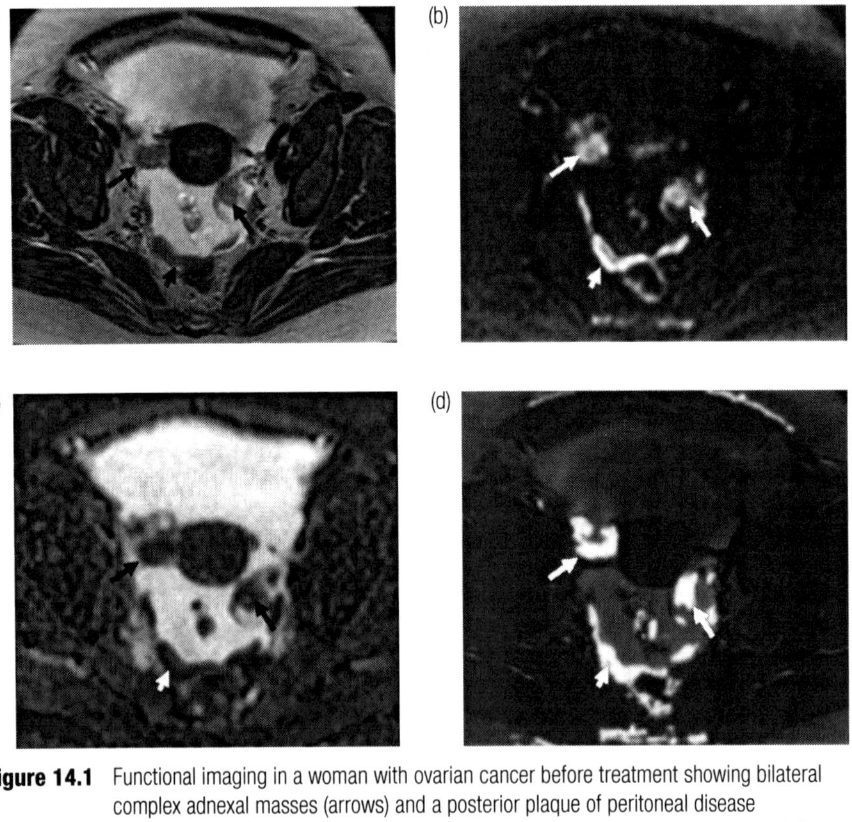

Figure 14.1 Functional imaging in a woman with ovarian cancer before treatment showing bilateral complex adnexal masses (arrows) and a posterior plaque of peritoneal disease (arrowheads): (a) axial T2-weighted; (b) dffusion-weighted (b = 1050 mm²/s); (c) ADC map (d) morphological image with functional ADC data presented as a white overlay

and 71–81% for DW-MRI alone)[14] and to achieve 90% sensitivity and 95% specificity in delineating the extent of peritoneal dissemination with satisfactory inter-observer agreement ($\kappa = 0.77$).[15] False-positive results arise from normal hypercellular tissues, such as small bowel mucosa, and non-cancerous lesions, such as tubo-ovarian abscesses, inflammatory collections, lymphoceles and proteinaceous or haemorrhagic ovarian cysts;[16] false-negative results may occur in malignant lesions of low cellularity, such as mucinous sub-types, and in predominantly cystic or calcified deposits. Preliminary results also show significantly lower ADCs in peritoneal deposits compared with primary ovarian tumours and omental cake.[17]

MRS

MRS has been validated sparsely in ovarian malignancy and almost exclusively for lesion characterisation. *Ex vivo* studies of fluid from ovarian cysts showed a significantly increased presence of lactate and alanine in combination with low glucose in malignant lesions, indicating anaerobic metabolic pathways, whereas the absence of lactate peaks was a powerful predictor of benignity.[18,19] *In vivo* studies suggested that a choline/creatine ratio greater than 3 was predictive of malignancy.[20] Although lactate peaks were significantly higher in malignant lesions, choline concentrations were not discriminatory.[21]

In metastatic epithelial ovarian cancer, choline was detected in almost all primary adnexal sites but in fewer than 50% of omental lesions.[22] The discrepancy was attributed to the poorer quality of spectral acquisitions from extra-ovarian sites because of local susceptibility artefacts and smaller voxels with lower signal to noise ratio. Moreover, large lipid peaks may interfere in the omental spectra. When choline concentration is calculated with an internal water signal as a reference, the uncertainty (estimated at 5–13%)[23] may introduce additional errors in longitudinal studies, since both water content in tissue and T2 relaxation values can be modified by effective treatment. Under current technical limitations, MRS in ovarian cancer appears to be confined to an investigatory setting.

FDG-PET/CT

FDG uptake in epithelial ovarian tumours has been shown to correlate significantly with histological grade.[24] In preoperative staging, sensitivity varies between 62% and 100%, with overall improvement in diagnostic accuracy of 5–22% compared with CT alone.[25–27] The incremental benefit of fused PET/CT in per-lesion accuracy is greater in extrapelvic sites, particularly because of its ability to characterise metastatic lymph nodes (see the lymph nodes section below) and to correctly differentiate diffuse serosal infiltration along small bowel loops from normal physiological intestinal activity, often a cause of false-negative results in standalone PET.[25,27] Nevertheless, diagnostic performance in detecting peritoneal carcinomatosis drops dramatically at an implant size threshold of 4–6 mm because of the inherent limitations in the minimum detectable level of FDG uptake and spatial resolution of the gamma camera.[28,29]

In response assessment, a metabolic response defined as a minimum 20% decrease in standardised uptake values (SUV) after the first cycle and 55% decrease after the third cycle of neoadjuvant chemotherapy was shown to predict macroscopically tumour-free surgery and median overall survival more accurately than clinical, biochemical and histopathological criteria.[30] In another study,[31] a cut-off value of 65% SUV reduction had 90% sensitivity, 82% specificity and 86% accuracy in predicting histological response.

PET/CT is the preferred modality to localise clinical and biochemical recurrence, with reported sensitivity, specificity and accuracy of 72–100%, 40–90% and 77–91%, respectively;[32–36] in comparison, the performance of contrast-enhanced CT in assessing recurrence is inferior (accuracy 43–89%), primarily because of low tumour burden at relapse and distortion of pelvic anatomy after cytoreductive surgery.[37–39] In two meta-analyses,[40,41] PET/CT had the highest pooled sensitivity and specificity (91% and 86%, respectively) compared with PET and CT alone, MRI and CA125. In four prospective studies,[42–45] PET/CT upstaged disease compared with purely anatomical imaging in 55–64% of patients by depicting additional sites, and it altered decisions on clinical management in 34–59% of cases, with 44–57% of these changes rated as high impact.

Cervical cancer

Cervical cancer shows heterogeneity relating to treatment response and to risk of metastatic spread and gene expression,[46,47] and their relationship to response and outcome is of interest.

DCE-MRI

T2-weighted MRI is used routinely to define disease extent because of excellent contrast between the intermediate signal intensity of the tumour and the low signal intensity of the cervical stroma. DCE-MRI in cervical cancer initially used for further improvements in staging[48] indicated that peritumoral enhancement overestimated disease extent[49] and parametrial involvement.[50] This prompted more complex pharmacokinetic analysis of the data in an attempt to separate tumoral from peritumoral characteristics.

Correlation of DCE-MRI parameters with histological features most closely known to affect outcome and survival (i.e. lymphovascular space involvement and lymph node status) showed no significant differences in the slope or amplitude of enhancement between aggressive and non-aggressive tumours[51] despite strong correlation with histomorphological markers of tumour angiogenesis such as microvessel density.[52] The areas of increased contrast enhancement were shown to be mainly composed of abundant cancer cell fascicles, whereas poorly perfused areas were composed of fibrous tissue with scattered cancer cells.[53]

DCE-MRI has also been explored as a predictive biomarker: poorly enhancing tumours (amplitude less than median) have significantly worse disease-specific survival and, in conjunction with volume data, have clear differences in outcome.[54] Tumour heterogeneity can be another helpful feature: a retrospective study linked the fraction of enhancing pixels within a tumour to disease-free survival.[55] Histogram analyses quoting a signal intensity value for the 5th, 10th or 20th centile of pixels to represent the level of enhancement of a particular fraction of pixels within the entire tumour[56] have shown that the signal intensity of the 10th centile of pixels (which effectively represents the poorly enhancing fraction) and tumour volume change early during radiation/chemotherapy are independent and better predictors of tumour recurrence and death than clinical prognostic factors such as stage, lymph node status and histology; the combination of clinical prognostic factors and MRI parameters can further improve early prediction of treatment failure.[56] If these data are corroborated in larger multicentre trials, they would provide a vital opportunity to alter treatment strategy.

Longitudinal studies during therapy have also shown potential for predicting treatment failure at an early time-point in treatment. In one study, persistently low perfusion pre-radiotherapy, after 20–25 Gy and 45–50 Gy indicated a high risk of treatment failure, with more favourable outcome in women with initially high perfusion or subsequent improvements of initially low perfusion,[57] while in another similar study signal intensity of the 5th centile of pixels of less than 2.05 and a residual tumour volume of more than 30 cm^3 at 2.5 weeks after commencing treatment provided the best prediction of unfavourable primary tumour control and disease-free survival.[58] Other studies have corroborated that an early onset of enhancement after radiotherapy is a better predictor of survival,[59] reflecting reoxygenation of hypoxic tumour.[60] Relative signal intensity has also been shown to correlate positively with perfusion and cell density, linking DCE parameters to a highly perfused cellular phenotype.[61]

DW-MRI

The ADC of cervical tumours is significantly lower than that of normal cervical stroma[62–64] and offers a new contrast mechanism for improved disease detection (Figure 14.2). In women with International Federation of Gynecology and Obstetrics (FIGO) stage IA and IB1 cervical cancer who are are referred following cone biopsy on which invasive disease is an unexpected finding, identifying disease within the cervix is difficult on T2-weighted imaging because it is of small volume. In these cases,

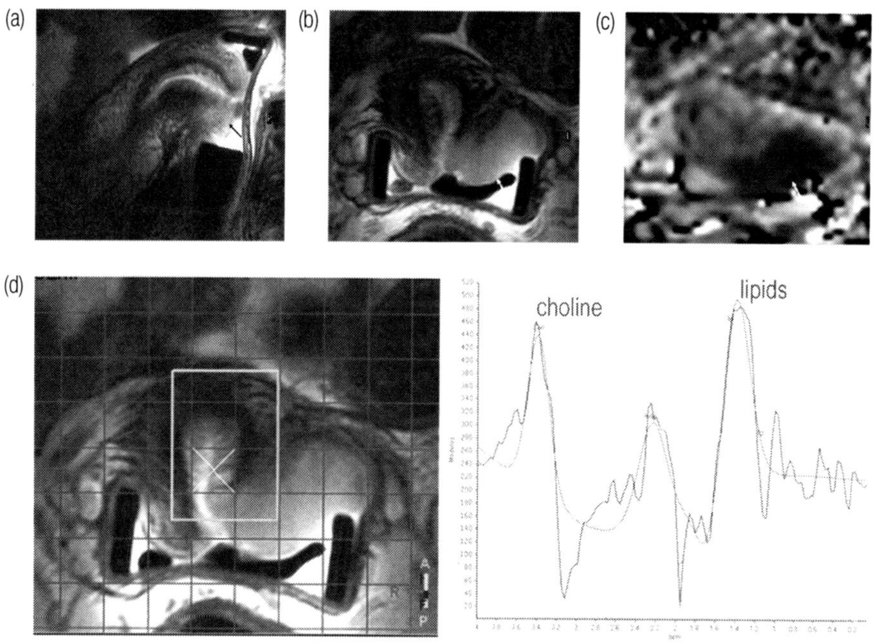

Figure 14.2 Functional imaging in a woman with cervical cancer imaged using an endovaginal coil. (a) sagittal T2-weighted; (b) coronal T2-weighted; (c) coronal ADC map; (d) two-dimensional chemical shift spectroscopy; the large left-sided tumour seen in (a) and (b) shows restricted diffusion in (c), and a high level of choline and triglycerides on the magnetic resonance spectrum in (d)

addition of DW-MRI to T2-weighted imaging improves accuracy of detection with good inter-observer agreement.[62] ADC is significantly lower in poorly differentiated compared with well or moderately differentiated tumours but is not significantly different when tumours are divided by other histological features (type, lymphovascular invasion and lymph node metastasis). However, differences between the ADCs of the well or moderately differentiated compared with the poorly differentiated tumours need quantification rather than visualisation alone for evaluation.[65]

The use of ADC in therapeutic monitoring, where extracellular water increases as tumours undergo apoptosis and necrosis, is in its infancy. Changes in ADC seen as early as 2 weeks after therapy correlate well with subsequent volumetric response.[66,67] A negative correlation was found between pretreatment ADCs and percentage size reduction after 2 months of chemoradiation, while percentage ADC change after 1 month correlated positively with percentage size reduction after 2 months of therapy.[67] As with DCE-MRI, the predictive value of ADC has been explored: in women with squamous carcinomas, the 90th centile of ADC values was lower in responders than in non-responders.[64]

MRS

Several studies have shown that tumours have elevated total choline resonances (at 3.2 ppm) compared with normal tissue, but choline is also commonly seen in normal cervical tissue.[68] Use of this biomarker for response assessment in cervical tumours has thus not proved useful.[69] MR spectra of biopsy samples from invasive cancer of the cervix also are characterised by resonances of mobile triglycerides,[70] and triglyceride-CH_2 resonances have been detected *in vivo* in 74% of cervical tumours[71] but are not detected in normal control women. The origin of these triglycerides is debated but they have been linked to the presence of necrosis[72] and apoptosis.[73]

FDG-PET/CT

In cervical tumours, FDG used in locally advanced or relapsed disease has been shown to change management in a significant percentage of patients.[74] Derived SUV_{max} has been used to distinguish prognostic groups regardless of tumour stage and volume. Preliminary reports of an association between primary tumour SUV_{max} and tumour stage, grade and volume[75] were not subsequently corroborated.[76] High SUV_{max} at presentation has also been associated with persistent abnormal FDG uptake after treatment and is associated with a reduced disease-free survival compared with low SUV_{max},[77,78] indicating that high pretreatment SUV_{max} (13.4 or higher) may identify those needing more aggressive therapy from the outset because of an increased risk of post-surgical recurrence.[77]

Tumour SUV_{max} can vary greatly across the volume of individual cervical tumours[79] and greater intratumour heterogeneity has been significantly associated with the risk of lymph node metastasis, poorer treatment response and reduced progression-free survival,[80] although the association of heterogeneity with volume was a confounding factor.

FDG-PET is useful for assessing early response to chemoradiation in locally advanced disease. Post-therapy abnormal FDG uptake has also shown potential for predicting tumour recurrence and death,[81,82] while SUV_{max} response during therapy[83] and the absence of abnormal FDG uptake on the post-therapy PET[81,84] are predictive of survival outcome.

Endometrial cancer

DCE-MRI

In endometrial cancer, DCE studies have involved a multiphase approach (rather than a continuous acquisition) where images are acquired at different time intervals after intravenous injection of contrast medium at multiple phases (usually four phases) of dynamic contrast medium enhancement. This approach allows qualitative assessment of images and does not generate semi-quantitative or quantitative parameters such as indices of perfusion and permeability.

The combination of DCE-MRI and T2-weighted images offers a 'one-stop' examination with the highest efficacy for staging.[85,86] Dynamic multiphase contrast-enhanced three-dimensional T1-weighted sequences through the uterus in the sagittal and axial (parallel to the short axis of the uterine corpus) planes are routinely used in combination with T2-weighted imaging (Figure 14.3) and significantly improve accuracy of assessment of deep myometrial invasion.[85–91] In a study published in 2009,[86] the diagnostic accuracy, specificity and negative predictive value increased from 88%, 80% and 80% to 98%, 100% and 93.7%, respectively.

Following intravenous contrast medium administration, endometrial cancer enhances early relative to the normal endometrium, allowing identification of small tumours, even those contained by the endometrium. In the later phases of enhancement (i.e the equilibrium phase), tumour appears hypointense relative to the myometrium. The equilibrium phase (2 minutes post-injection) allows better evaluation of deep myometrial invasion (FIGO stage IB) since there is maximum tumour to myometrium contrast in this phase. This is particularly important in cases where on T2-weighted images the signal intensity of the tumour is isointense to the normal myometrium. Similarly, in those cases where tumour extends into the uterine cornu it can be difficult to accurately evaluate the depth of myometrial invasion on T2-weighted images alone owing to myometrial thinning. In these cases, the addition of DCE-MRI to T2-weighted imaging can lead to significant improvement in preoperative staging accuracy.[86] Other reported pitfalls in assessing the depth of myometrial invasion in endometrial carcinoma,

(a)

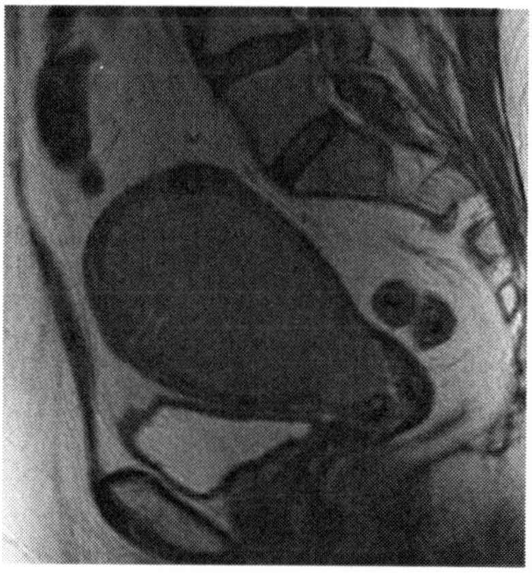

(b)

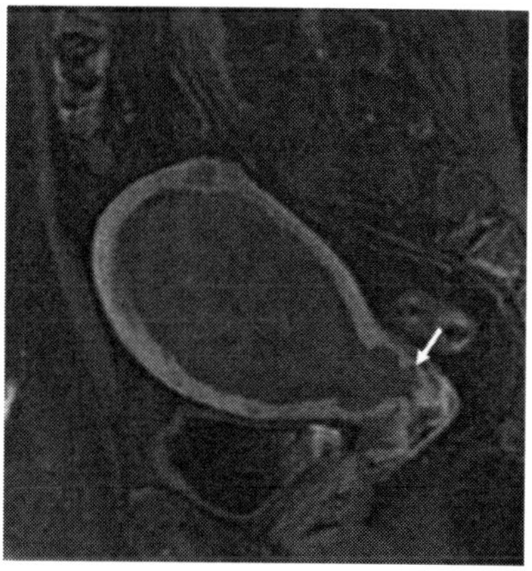

Figure 14.3 Functional imaging in endometrial cancer: (a) T2-weighted and (b) multiphase dynamic contrast-enhanced (equilibrium phase, 120 s) images demonstrate an endometrial cavity distended by presence of tumour; the invasion of cervical stroma posteriorly is much better appreciated in (b) than in (a)

such as leiomyomas, adenomyosis, loss of junctional zone definition and myometrial compression by polypoid tumour, can be minimised by the addition of DCE-MRI to T2-weighted imaging.[90–93] The tumour/myometrium interface should be assessed in at least two planes. The delayed phase (3–4 minutes) of contrast medium enhancement enables better evaluation of cervical stromal invasion as an intact enhancing cervical mucosa can reliably exclude cervical stromal invasion (FIGO stage II).

DW-MRI

DW-MRI has limited clinical utility as the diagnosis of endometrial cancer is made at endometrial biopsy and the role of MRI is to stage the disease. However, pipelle sampling has an error rate and upstaging of the tumour grade may occur in up to 15% of patients. In these cases, DW imaging may influence surgical planning by improving preoperative detection of high-grade tumours. DW-MRI can also be helpful in cases where the endometrial biopsy is technically impossible, the histopathology results are inconclusive or the MRI is performed for different clinical indications, such as evaluation of an indeterminate adnexal lesion, and the endometrial abnormality is an incidental finding. Endometrial cancer demonstrates high signal intensity on DW images and low signal intensity on ADC maps. The ADC value of endometrial cancer is significantly lower than that of endometrial polyps and of normal endometrium.[94,95] In a study published in 2008, Fujii *et al.*[94] found that ADC values can provide useful information in differentiating malignant from benign endometrial lesions with a sensitivity, specificity and accuracy of 85%, 100% and 92%, respectively. High-grade endometrial carcinomas have high cellular density and are expected to have lower ADC values than low-grade ones. However, it should be noted that there is no reliable cut-off ADC value that is diagnostic of the presence of malignancy. Also, tumour necrosis associated with poorly differentiated tumours can increase ADC values.

Although DCE-MRI is routinely used for staging endometrial cancer and is highly accurate, DW-MRI can be useful for determining the depth of myometrial invasion because it is independent of differences in tissue vascularity. This can be particularly helpful in tumours that are either iso- or hyper-intense relative to the myometrium or when the use of intravenous contrast medium is contraindicated. In a prospective study published in 2010, Rechichi *et al.*[96] suggested that the accuracy of DW-MRI in assessing myometrial invasion is comparable to that of DCE-MRI, which it could replace in preoperative evaluation. DW-MRI can also be useful in detection of drop metastases in the cervix or metastatic foci outside the uterus, such as adnexa or peritoneum.[97]

There are no published articles on the value of DW imaging in detection of tumour recurrence in endometrial cancer. This is because of difficulties in obtaining histopathological correlation in these cases where the women normally undergo further radiotherapy or chemotherapy or a combination. As with all gynaecological tumours, in our experience, DW-MRI is very useful in detecting localised tumour recurrence within the pelvis as well as detecting disseminated peritoneal recurrence. Areas of tumour recurrence appear bright on DW images and demonstrate restricted diffusion on the ADC maps.

MRS

There is no published literature on the value of MRS in endometrial cancer apart from a small pilot study[98] in which MRS was performed in 12 women with various endometrial lesions. In the three women with endometrial carcinoma, high choline and lipid signals were detected, whereas no creatine and no lactate signals were found. Lipid signals were detected only in women with endometrial carcinoma, mirroring the findings in cervical cancer.

FDG-PET/CT

The main role of PET/CT in endometrial cancer is for evaluating lymph node metastases[99] (see below) and in detecting recurrent disease, where its use reduces the frequency of equivocal interpretations.[100] However, PET/CT may play an important role in the primary staging of high-grade endometrial cancer owing to its ability to accurately detect distant metastases in the abdomen and extra-abdominal regions, thus adding relevant information that may influence patient management.[101] In 2010, Nahamura *et al.*[102] suggested that SUV_{max} of the primary tumour obtained from FDG-PET/CT may be associated with aggressive biological characteristics in endometrial cancer.

Kitajima *et al.*[103] reported that integrated FDG-PET/contrast-enhanced CT was a more accurate modality for assessing endometrial and cervical cancer recurrence and led to more appropriate subsequent clinical management than that resulting from PET alone or contrast-enhanced CT alone.

Lymph nodes

The presence of lymph node metastases has a detrimental effect on prognosis and a significant impact on management and treatment. Morphological signs of nodal involvement include visible necrosis (highly specific), a signal intensity similar to that of the primary tumour, an irregular nodal contour or visible tumour extending beyond the nodal capsule,[104–106] which are rarely seen at the time of presentation. The standard method of predicting lymph node metastases on CT and MRI is thus by applying threshold values for the short-axis diameter of a node. A threshold of 10 mm short axis is commonly considered malignant: at this value, sensitivity for detecting nodal metastases is low although specificity is over 95%, while a threshold of 8 mm increases sensitivity with a loss of specificity.[107,108] If a node is between 8 and 10 mm with a short-to-long axis ratio of more than 0.8 (that is, round in shape), this finding may further improve sensitivity.[108] Below 8 mm, the reported sensitivities of size criteria are too low to contribute to treatment planning decisions.

DCE-MRI

DCE-MRI has not been widely evaluated in assessment of pelvic nodes. A study in the mid-1990s[106] in patients with bladder cancer reported early enhancement in malignant nodes, increasing sensitivity of morphological imaging from 71% to 86%, with specificities remaining high (98% versus 95%). In breast cancer, a correlation has been reported between rapid wash-out slope of primary tumour and positive axillary dissection[109,110] and negative predictive value is high when a combination of nodal area and enhancement index is used.[111] In patients with head and neck cancer, the contrast enhancement parameters have been found to be significantly different between benign and malignant nodes.[112] These studies suggest that DCE-MRI may have role in assessment of pelvic nodes but further work is needed.

DW-MRI

Lymph nodes can be easily detected on DW-MRI as discrete, non-continuous, high signal intensity ovoid structures[113] with increased conspicuity (Figure 14.4), although correlation with T2-weighted images is advised. In one study of 18 women with gynaecological malignancy,[114] a greater number of nodes was identified on DW-MRI than on conventional T2-weighted MRI (73% compared with 40% of the 340 dissected nodes). The wide variation in quantified results in differentiating benign and malignant nodes may relate to low resolution and signal to noise ratio. In small nodes, the region of interest may only encompass a single voxel, with the risk of inaccurate data. Despite these difficulties, several studies have evaluated the measurement of ADC for detecting nodal metastases. A significant increase in sensitivity in women with an endometrial or cervical cancer using mean ADC and relative ADC between tumour and nodes was demonstrated at 3 T; the addition of nodal size to relative ADC values significantly improved sensitivity from 25% to 83%, while specificity remained high 99% (versus 98%).[115] Similar results in cervical cancer have been reported,[116] with sensitivity and specificity of ADC for differentiating metastatic from nonmetastatic lymph nodes at 87% and 80%, respectively; there has also been some success in differentiating hyperplastic from metastatic nodes.[117] Other studies have not reproduced these results and have reported an inability to distinguish benign from malignant nodes using ADC values.[114,118] Early data tentatively support a correlation between minimum nodal ADC and FDG-PET positivity.[119]

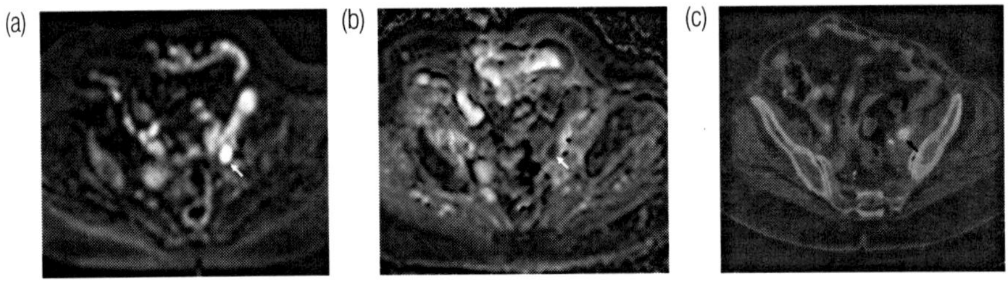

Figure 14.4 Nodal metastasis in gynaecological malignancy: (a) axial diffusion-weighted ($b = 1000\,mm^2/s$), (b) ADC map and (c) PET/CT images through the pelvis showing a nodal metastasis along the left pelvic side wall (arrows) in a woman with recurrent cervical cancer

FDG-PET/CT

There are only a few studies specifically addressing FDG uptake in nodal metastases in ovarian cancer where retroperitoneal and extra-abdominal nodal metastases may be detected[120,121] and malignant involvement in normal-sized para-aortic lymph nodes may be detectable.[27]

In endometrial cancer, reported sensitivities for detection of nodal metastases are not sufficiently high to effectively rule out nodal metastases (Table 14.1), although the high specificity may be helpful in clinical practice – an FDG positive node is highly likely to be metastatic and therefore may direct surgical or radiotherapy planning. In cervical cancer, the diagnostic accuracy is relatively high in advanced stage disease but is limited in early stage (Table 14.2). One study evaluated 60 women with early-stage disease (tumour less than 4 cm and no node larger than 10 mm on MRI) with

Table 14.1 Diagnostic performance of FDG-PET in detecting nodal metastases in endometrial cancer

Study	Women (*n*)	Sensitivity	Specificity	Comment
Kitajima *et al.* (2008)[126]	45	51% by nodal site Node 5–9 mm 66.7% Node ≥10 mm 100% 50% by patient	99% by nodal site 86.7% by patient	NPV 98.9%
Nayot *et al.* (2008)[127]	12	53%	99.6%	Pilot study
Park *et al.* (2008)[128]	53	69%	90%	No difference when compared with MRI (*P*=0.25 [sensitivity])
Horowitz *et al.* (2004)[129]	19	60%	98%	In women with grade 2 or 3 clear-cell, serous papillary or sarcomatous histology
Picchio *et al.* (2010)[101]	32	57%	100%	Greater detection of extra-nodal metastases
Signorelli *et al.* (2009)[99]	37	66.7% by nodal site 77% by patient	Nodal site 99.4% Patient-based 100%	High-risk disease (grade 2 with deep invasion and grade 3) Very high NPV for nodal metastases

FDG-PET = ^{18}F-fluoro-2-deoxy-D-glucose positron emission tomography; MRI = magnetic resonance imaging; NPV = negative predictive value

Table 14.2 Diagnostic performance of FDG-PET in detecting nodal metastases in cervical cancer (selected studies)

Study	Study design	Women (*n*)	Sensitivity	Specificity
Advanced disease				
Lin *et al.* (2003)[130]	Prospective	50	PA nodes 86%	PA nodes 87%
Choi *et al.* (2006)[131]	Prospective	22	Pelvic nodes 77%	Pelvic nodes 55%
Loft *et al.* (2007)[132]	Prospective	119	Pelvic nodes 96% PA nodes 100%	Pelvic nodes 75% PA nodes 95%
Early disease				
Chou *et al.* (2006)[122]	Prospective (no nodal enlargement on MRI)	60	10%	–
Sironi *et al.* (2006)[133]	Prospective	47	73%	97%

FDG-PET = ^{18}F-fluoro-2-deoxy-D-glucose positron emission tomography; MRI = magnetic resonance imaging; PA = para-aortic

only one of ten positive nodes being successfully identified.[122] FDG-PET has been explored as a prognostic as well as a predictive biomarker. In a retrospective study of 83 women with cervical cancer, the SUV_{max} of pelvic nodal metastases predicted treatment response, pelvic recurrence risk and disease-specific survival.[123] FDG uptake in nodes before treatment has been shown to predict prognosis and to correlate with the 3 year disease-specific survival.[124] An SUV_{max} of more than 3.3 in para-aortic nodes was associated with 5 year disease recurrence and mortality.[125]

Iron oxide magnetic resonance lymphography

Magnetic resonance lymphography (MRL) using iron oxide nanoparticles has been found to significantly increase sensitivity for detection of nodal metastases with no loss of specificity in women with endometrial or cervical cancer.[107] The combination of DW-MRI and MRL is a very exciting development reported in prostate cancer, with an important reduction in the time taken for interpretation of the images.[113] Sensitivity for the detection of nodal metastases was 92%. The false-negative cases were both of micrometastatic nodal deposits.

References

1. Charles-Edwards EM, deSouza NM. Diffusion-weighted magnetic resonance imaging and its application to cancer. *Cancer Imaging* 2006;6:135–43.
2. Naganawa S, Sato C, Kumada H, Ishigaki T, Miura S, Takizawa O. Apparent diffusion coefficient in cervical cancer of the uterus: comparison with the normal uterine cervix. *Eur Radiol* 2005;15:71–8.
3. Sohaib SA, Sahdev A, Van Trappen P, Jacobs IJ, Reznek RH. Characterization of adnexal mass lesions on MR imaging. *AJR Am J Roentgenol* 2003;180:1297–304.
4. Thomassin-Naggara I, Bazot M, Darai E, Callard P, Thomassin J, Cuenod CA. Epithelial ovarian tumors: value of dynamic contrast-enhanced MR imaging and correlation with tumor angiogenesis. *Radiology* 2008;248:148–59.
5. Lankester KJ, Taylor NJ, Stirling JJ, Boxall J, d'Arcy JA, Leach MO, *et al.* Effects of platinum/taxane based chemotherapy on acute perfusion in human pelvic tumours measured by dynamic MRI. *Br J Cancer* 2005;93:979–85.
6. Priest AN, Gill AB, Kataoka M, McLean MA, Joubert I, Graves MJ, *et al.* Dynamic contrast-enhanced MRI in ovarian cancer: Initial experience at 3 tesla in primary and metastatic disease. *Magn Reson Med* 2010;63:1044–9.
7. Mitchell CL, O'Connor JP, Jackson A, Parker GJ, Roberts C, Watson Y, *et al.* Identification of early predictive imaging biomarkers and their relationship to serological angiogenic markers in patients with ovarian cancer with residual disease following cytotoxic therapy. *Ann Oncol* 2010;21:1982–9.
8. Katayama M, Masui T, Kobayashi S, Ito T, Sakahara H, Nozaki A, *et al.* Diffusion-weighted echo planar imaging of ovarian tumors: is it useful to measure apparent diffusion coefficients? *J Comput Assist Tomogr* 2002;26:250–6.
9. Thomassin-Naggara I, Darai E, Cuenod CA, Fournier L, Toussaint I, Marsault C, *et al.* Contribution of diffusion-weighted MR imaging for predicting benignity of complex adnexal masses. *Eur Radiol* 2009;19:1544–52.
10. Tempany CM, Zou KH, Silverman SG, Brown DL, Kurtz AB, McNeil BJ. Staging of advanced ovarian cancer: comparison of imaging modalities – report from the Radiological Diagnostic Oncology Group. *Radiology* 2000;215:761–7.
11. Coakley FV, Choi PH, Gougoutas CA, Pothuri B, Venkatraman E, Chi D, *et al.* Peritoneal metastases: detection with spiral CT in patients with ovarian cancer. *Radiology* 2002;223:495–9.
12. de Bree E, Koops W, Kroger R, van Ruth S, Witkamp AJ, Zoetmulder FA. Peritoneal carcinomatosis from colorectal or appendiceal origin: correlation of preoperative CT with intraoperative findings and evaluation of interobserver agreement. *J Surg Oncol* 2004;86:64–73.
13. Jacquet P, Jelinek JS, Steves MA, Sugarbaker PH. Evaluation of computed tomography in patients with peritoneal carcinomatosis. *Cancer* 1993;72:1631–6.
14. Low RN, Sebrechts CP, Barone RM, Muller W. Diffusion-weighted MRI of peritoneal tumors: comparison with conventional MRI and surgical and histopathologic findings: a feasibility study. *AJR Am J Roentgenol* 2009;193:461–70.
15. Fujii S, Matsusue E, Kanasaki Y, Kanamori Y, Nakanishi J, Sugihara S, *et al.* Detection of peritoneal dissemination in gynecological malignancy: evaluation by diffusion-weighted MR imaging. *Eur Radiol* 2008;18:18–23.
16. Feuerlein S, Pauls S, Juchems MS, Stuber T, Hoffmann MH, Brambs HJ, *et al.* Pitfalls in abdominal diffusion-weighted imaging: how predictive is restricted water diffusion for malignancy. *AJR Am J Roentgenol* 2009;193:1070–6.

17. Sala E, Priest AN, Kataoka M, Graves MJ, McLean MA, Joubert I, *et al.* Apparent diffusion coefficient and vascular signal fraction measurements with magnetic resonance imaging: feasibility in metastatic ovarian cancer at 3 Tesla: technical development. *Eur Radiol* 2010;20:491–6.
18. Boss EA, Moolenaar SH, Massuger LF, Boonstra H, Engelke UF, de Jong JG, *et al.* High-resolution proton nuclear magnetic resonance spectroscopy of ovarian cyst fluid. *NMR Biomed* 2000;13:297–305.
19. Massuger LF, van Vierzen PB, Engelke U, Heerschap A, Wevers R. 1H-magnetic resonance spectroscopy: a new technique to discriminate benign from malignant ovarian tumors. *Cancer* 1998;82:1726–30.
20. Stanwell P, Russell P, Carter J, Pather S, Heintze S, Mountford C. Evaluation of ovarian tumors by proton magnetic resonance spectroscopy at three Tesla. *Invest Radiol* 2008;43:745–51.
21. Okada T, Harada M, Matsuzaki K, Nishitani H, Aono T. Evaluation of female intrapelvic tumors by clinical proton MR spectroscopy. *J Magn Reson Imaging* 2001;13:912–17.
22. McLean MA, Priest AN, Joubert I, Lomas DJ, Kataoka MY, Earl H, *et al.* Metabolic characterization of primary and metastatic ovarian cancer by 1H-MRS *in vivo* at 3T. *Magn Reson Med* 2009;62:855–61.
23. Bolan PJ, Meisamy S, Baker EH, Lin J, Emory T, Nelson M, *et al. In vivo* quantification of choline compounds in the breast with 1H MR spectroscopy. *Magn Reson Med* 2003;50:1134–43.
24. Kurokawa T, Yoshida Y, Kawahara K, Tsuchida T, Fujibayashi Y, Yonekura Y, *et al.* Whole-body PET with FDG is useful for following up an ovarian cancer patient with only rising CA-125 levels within the normal range. *Ann Nucl Med* 2002;16:491–3.
25. Dirisamer A, Schima W, Heinisch M, Weber M, Lehner HP, Haller J, *et al.* Detection of histologically proven peritoneal carcinomatosis with fused 18F-FDG-PET/MDCT. *Eur J Radiol* 2009;69:536–41.
26. Kitajima K, Murakami K, Yamasaki E, Kaji Y, Fukasawa I, Inaba N, *et al.* Diagnostic accuracy of integrated FDG-PET/contrast-enhanced CT in staging ovarian cancer: comparison with enhanced CT. *Eur J Nucl Med Mol Imaging* 2008;35:1912–20.
27. Yoshida Y, Kurokawa T, Kawahara K, Tsuchida T, Okazawa H, Fujibayashi Y, *et al.* Incremental benefits of FDG positron emission tomography over CT alone for the preoperative staging of ovarian cancer. *AJR Am J Roentgenol* 2004;182:227–33.
28. Nakamoto Y, Saga T, Ishimori T, Mamede M, Togashi K, Higuchi T, *et al.* Clinical value of positron emission tomography with FDG for recurrent ovarian cancer. *AJR Am J Roentgenol* 2001;176:1449–54.
29. Rose PG, Faulhaber P, Miraldi F, Abdul-Karim FW. Positive emission tomography for evaluating a complete clinical response in patients with ovarian or peritoneal carcinoma: correlation with second-look laparotomy. *Gynecol Oncol* 2001;82:17–21.
30. Avril N, Sassen S, Schmalfeldt B, Naehrig J, Rutke S, Weber WA, *et al.* Prediction of response to neoadjuvant chemotherapy by sequential F-18-fluorodeoxyglucose positron emission tomography in patients with advanced-stage ovarian cancer. *J Clin Oncol* 2005;23:7445–53.
31. Nishiyama Y, Yamamoto Y, Kanenishi K, Ohno M, Hata T, Kushida Y, *et al.* Monitoring the neoadjuvant therapy response in gynecological cancer patients using FDG PET. *Eur J Nucl Med Mol Imaging* 2008;35:287–95.
32. Fagotti A, Fanfani F, Rossitto C, Lorusso D, De Gaetano AM, Giordano A, *et al.* A treatment selection protocol for recurrent ovarian cancer patients: the role of FDG-PET/CT and staging laparoscopy. *Oncology* 2008;75:152–8.
33. Pannu HK, Cohade C, Bristow RE, Fishman EK, Wahl RL. PET-CT detection of abdominal recurrence of ovarian cancer: radiologic–surgical correlation. *Abdom Imaging* 2004;29:398–403.
34. Risum S, Hogdall C, Markova E, Berthelsen AK, Loft A, Jensen F, *et al.* Influence of 2-(18F) fluoro-2-deoxy-D-glucose positron emission tomography/computed tomography on recurrent ovarian cancer diagnosis and on selection of patients for secondary cytoreductive surgery. *Int J Gynecol Cancer* 2009;19:600–4.
35. Sironi S, Messa C, Mangili G, Zangheri B, Aletti G, Garavaglia E, *et al.* Integrated FDG PET/CT in patients with persistent ovarian cancer: correlation with histologic findings. *Radiology* 2004;233:433–40.
36. Thrall MM, DeLoia JA, Gallion H, Avril N. Clinical use of combined positron emission tomography and computed tomography (FDG-PET/CT) in recurrent ovarian cancer. *Gynecol Oncol* 2007;105:17–22.

37. Kubik-Huch RA, Dorffler W, von Schulthess GK, Marincek B, Kochli OR, Seifert B, *et al.* Value of (18F)-FDG positron emission tomography, computed tomography, and magnetic resonance imaging in diagnosing primary and recurrent ovarian carcinoma. *Eur Radiol* 2000;10:761–7.
38. Sebastian S, Lee SI, Horowitz NS, Scott JA, Fischman AJ, Simeone JF, *et al.* PET-CT vs. CT alone in ovarian cancer recurrence. *Abdom Imaging* 2008;33:112–18.
39. Topuz E, Aydiner A, Saip P, Eralp Y, Tas F, Salihoglu Y, *et al.* Correlations of serum CA125 level and computerized tomography (CT) imaging with laparotomic findings following intraperitoneal chemotherapy in patients with ovarian cancer. *Eur J Gynaecol Oncol* 2000;21:599–602.
40. Gu P, Pan LL, Wu SQ, Sun L, Huang G. CA 125, PET alone, PET-CT, CT and MRI in diagnosing recurrent ovarian carcinoma: a systematic review and meta-analysis. *Eur J Radiol* 2009;71:164–74.
41. Havrilesky LJ, Kulasingam SL, Matchar DB, Myers ER. FDG-PET for management of cervical and ovarian cancer. *Gynecol Oncol* 2005;97:183–91.
42. Fulham MJ, Carter J, Baldey A, Hicks RJ, Ramshaw JE, Gibson M. The impact of PET-CT in suspected recurrent ovarian cancer: a prospective multi-centre study as part of the Australian PET Data Collection Project. *Gynecol Oncol* 2009;112:462–8.
43. Mangili G, Picchio M, Sironi S, Vigano R, Rabaiotti E, Bornaghi D, *et al.* Integrated PET/CT as a first-line re-staging modality in patients with suspected recurrence of ovarian cancer. *Eur J Nucl Med Mol Imaging* 2007;34:658–66.
44. Simcock B, Neesham D, Quinn M, Drummond E, Milner A, Hicks RJ. The impact of PET/CT in the management of recurrent ovarian cancer. *Gynecol Oncol* 2006;103:271–6.
45. Soussan M, Wartski M, Cherel P, Fourme E, Goupil A, Le Stanc E, *et al.* Impact of FDG PET-CT imaging on the decision making in the biologic suspicion of ovarian carcinoma recurrence. *Gynecol Oncol* 2008;108:160–5.
46. Britten RA, Evans AJ, Allalunis-Turner MJ, Franko AJ, Pearcey RG. Intratumoral heterogeneity as a confounding factor in clonogenic assays for tumour radioresponsiveness. *Radiother Oncol* 1996;39:145–53.
47. Bachtiary B, Boutros PC, Pintilie M, Shi W, Bastianutto C, Li JH, *et al.* Gene expression profiling in cervical cancer: an exploration of intratumor heterogeneity. *Clin Cancer Res* 2006;12:5632–40.
48. Yamashita Y, Takahashi M, Sawada T, Miyazaki K, Okamura H. Carcinoma of the cervix: dynamic MR imaging. *Radiology* 1992;182:643–8.
49. Tsuda K, Murakami T, Kurachi H, Ogawa H, Oi H, Miyake A, *et al.* MR imaging of cervical carcinoma: comparison among T2-weighted, dynamic, and postcontrast T1-weighted images with histopathological correlation. *Abdom Imaging* 1997;22:103–7.
50. Postema S, Pattynama PM, Broker S, van der Geest RJ, van Rijswijk CS, Baptist TJ. Fast dynamic contrast-enhanced colour-coded MRI in uterine cervix carcinoma: useful for tumour staging? *Clin Radiol* 1998;53:729–34.
51. Postema S, Pattynama PM, van Rijswijk CS, Trimbos JB. Cervical carcinoma: can dynamic contrast-enhanced MR imaging help predict tumor aggressiveness? *Radiology* 1999;210:217–20.
52. Hawighorst H, Knapstein PG, Knopp MV, Vaupel P, van Kaick G. Cervical carcinoma: standard and pharmacokinetic analysis of time–intensity curves for assessment of tumor angiogenesis and patient survival. *MAGMA* 1999;8:55–62.
53. Yamashita Y, Baba T, Baba Y, Nishimura R, Ikeda S, Takahashi M, *et al.* Dynamic contrast-enhanced MR imaging of uterine cervical cancer: pharmacokinetic analysis with histopathologic correlation and its importance in predicting the outcome of radiation therapy. *Radiology* 2000;216:803–9.
54. Loncaster JA, Carrington BM, Sykes JR, Jones AP, Todd SM, Cooper R, *et al.* Prediction of radiotherapy outcome using dynamic contrast enhanced MRI of carcinoma of the cervix. *Int J Radiat Oncol Biol Phys* 2002;54:759–67.
55. Donaldson SB, Buckley DL, O'Connor JP, Davidson SE, Carrington BM, Jones AP, *et al.* Enhancing fraction measured using dynamic contrast-enhanced MRI predicts disease-free survival in patients with carcinoma of the cervix. *Br J Cancer* 2010;102:23–6.
56. Mayr NA, Yuh WT, Jajoura D, Wang JZ, Lo SS, Montebello JF, *et al.* Ultra-early predictive assay for treatment failure using functional magnetic resonance imaging and clinical prognostic parameters in cervical cancer. *Cancer* 2010;116:903–12.

57. Mayr NA, Yuh WT, Magnotta VA, Ehrhardt JC, Wheeler JA, Sorosky JI, *et al.* Tumor perfusion studies using fast magnetic resonance imaging technique in advanced cervical cancer: a new noninvasive predictive assay. *Int J Radiat Oncol Biol Phys* 1996;36:623–33.
58. Yuh WT, Mayr NA, Jarjoura D, Wu D, Grecula JC, Lo SS, *et al.* Predicting control of primary tumor and survival by DCE MRI during early therapy in cervical cancer. *Invest Radiol* 2009;44:343–50.
59. Boss EA, Massuger LF, Pop LA, Verhoef LC, Huisman HJ, Boonstra H, *et al.* Post-radiotherapy contrast enhancement changes in fast dynamic MRI of cervical carcinoma. *J Magn Reson Imaging* 2001;13:600–6.
60. Cooper RA, Carrington BM, Loncaster JA, Todd SM, Davidson SE, Logue JP, *et al.* Tumour oxygenation levels correlate with dynamic contrast-enhanced magnetic resonance imaging parameters in carcinoma of the cervix. *Radiother Oncol* 2000;57:53–9.
61. Lyng H, Vorren AO, Sundfor K, Taksdal I, Lien HH, Kaalhus O, *et al.* Assessment of tumor oxygenation in human cervical carcinoma by use of dynamic Gd-DTPA-enhanced MR imaging. *J Magn Reson Imaging* 2001;14:750–6.
62. Charles-Edwards EM, Messiou C, Morgan VA, De Silva SS, McWhinney NA, Katesmark M, *et al.* Diffusion-weighted imaging in cervical cancer with an endovaginal technique: potential value for improving tumor detection in stage Ia and Ib1 disease. *Radiology* 2008;249:541–50.
63. Liu Y, Bai R, Sun H, Liu H, Wang D. Diffusion-weighted magnetic resonance imaging of uterine cervical cancer. *J Comput Assist Tomogr* 2009;33:858–62.
64. McVeigh PZ, Syed AM, Milosevic M, Fyles A, Haider MA. Diffusion-weighted MRI in cervical cancer. *Eur Radiol* 2008;18:1058–64.
65. Payne GS, Schmidt M, Morgan VA, Giles S, Bridges J, Ind T, *et al.* Evaluation of magnetic resonance diffusion and spectroscopy measurements as predictive biomarkers in stage 1 cervical cancer. *Gynecol Oncol* 2010;116:246–52.
66. Semple SI, Harry VN, Parkin DE, Gilbert FJ. A combined pharmacokinetic and radiologic assessment of dynamic contrast-enhanced magnetic resonance imaging predicts response to chemoradiation in locally advanced cervical cancer. *Int J Radiat Oncol Biol Phys* 2009;75:611–17.
67. Liu Y, Bai R, Sun H, Liu H, Zhao X, Li Y. Diffusion-weighted imaging in predicting and monitoring the response of uterine cervical cancer to combined chemoradiation. *Clin Radiol* 2009;64:1067–74.
68. Mahon MM, deSouza NM, Dina R, Soutter WP, McIndoe GA, Williams AD, *et al.* Preinvasive and invasive cervical cancer: an *ex vivo* proton magic angle spinning magnetic resonance spectroscopy study. *NMR Biomed* 2004;17:144–53.
69. deSouza NM, Soutter WP, Rustin G, Mahon MM, Jones B, Dina R, *et al.* Use of neoadjuvant chemotherapy prior to radical hysterectomy in cervical cancer: monitoring tumour shrinkage and molecular profile on magnetic resonance and assessment of 3-year outcome. *Br J Cancer* 2004;90:2326–31.
70. Delikatny EJ, Russell P, Hunter JC, Hancock R, Atkinson KH, Haaften-Day C, *et al.* Proton MR and human cervical neoplasia: *ex vivo* spectroscopy allows distinction of invasive carcinoma of the cervix from carcinoma *in situ* and other preinvasive lesions. *Radiology* 1993;188:791–6.
71. Mahon MM, Williams AD, Soutter WP, Cox IJ, McIndoe GA, Coutts GA, *et al.* 1H magnetic resonance spectroscopy of invasive cervical cancer: an *in vivo* study with *ex vivo* corroboration. *NMR Biomed* 2004;17:1–9.
72. Kuesel AC, Sutherland GR, Halliday W, Smith IC. 1H MRS of high grade astrocytomas: mobile lipid accumulation in necrotic tissue. *NMR Biomed* 1994;7:149–55.
73. Blankenberg FG, Katsikis PD, Storrs RW, Beaulieu C, Spielman D, Chen JY, *et al.* Quantitative analysis of apoptotic cell death using proton nuclear magnetic resonance spectroscopy. *Blood* 1997;89:3778–86.
74. Bjurberg M, Kjellen E, Ohlsson T, Ridderheim M, Brun E. FDG-PET in cervical cancer: staging, re-staging and follow-up. *Acta Obstet Gynecol Scand* 2007;86:1385–91.
75. Eschmann SM, Friedel G, Paulsen F, Reimold M, Hehr T, Budach W, *et al.* Is standardised (18) F-FDG uptake value an outcome predictor in patients with stage III non-small cell lung cancer? *Eur J Nucl Med Mol Imaging* 2006;33:263–9.
76. Kidd EA, Siegel BA, Dehdashti F, Grigsby PW. The standardized uptake value for F-18 fluorodeoxyglucose is a sensitive predictive biomarker for cervical cancer treatment response and survival. *Cancer* 2007;110:1738–44.

77. Lee YY, Choi CH, Kim CJ, Kang H, Kim TJ, Lee JW, *et al.* The prognostic significance of the SUVmax (maximum standardized uptake value for F-18 fluorodeoxyglucose) of the cervical tumor in PET imaging for early cervical cancer: preliminary results. *Gynecol Oncol* 2009;115:65–8.
78. Xue F, Lin LL, Dehdashti F, Miller TR, Siegel BA, Grigsby PW. F-18 fluorodeoxyglucose uptake in primary cervical cancer as an indicator of prognosis after radiation therapy. *Gynecol Oncol* 2006;101:147–51.
79. Miller TR, Pinkus E, Dehdashti F, Grigsby PW. Improved prognostic value of 18F-FDG PET using a simple visual analysis of tumor characteristics in patients with cervical cancer. *J Nucl Med* 2003;44:192–7.
80. Kidd EA, Grigsby PW. Intratumoral metabolic heterogeneity of cervical cancer. *Clin Cancer Res* 2008;14:5236–41.
81. Grigsby PW, Siegel BA, Dehdashti F, Rader J, Zoberi I. Posttherapy [18F] fluorodeoxyglucose positron emission tomography in carcinoma of the cervix: response and outcome. *J Clin Oncol* 2004;22:2167–71.
82. Grigsby PW, Siegel BA, Dehdashti F, Mutch DG. Posttherapy surveillance monitoring of cervical cancer by FDG-PET. *Int J Radiat Oncol Biol Phys* 2003;55:907–13.
83. Lin LL, Yang Z, Mutic S, Miller TR, Grigsby PW. FDG-PET imaging for the assessment of physiologic volume response during radiotherapy in cervix cancer. *Int J Radiat Oncol Biol Phys* 2006;65:177–81.
84. Schwarz JK, Siegel BA, Dehdashti F, Grigsby PW. Association of posttherapy positron emission tomography with tumor response and survival in cervical carcinoma. *JAMA* 2007;298:2289–95.
85. Manfredi R, Mirk P, Maresca G, Margariti PA, Testa A, Zannoni GF, *et al.* Local-regional staging of endometrial carcinoma: role of MR imaging in surgical planning. *Radiology* 2004;231:372–8.
86. Sala E, Crawford R, Senior E, Shaw A, Simcock B, Vrotsou K, *et al.* Added value of dynamic contrast-enhanced magnetic resonance imaging in predicting advanced stage disease in patients with endometrial carcinoma. *Int J Gynecol Cancer* 2009;19:141–6.
87. Ito K, Matsumoto T, Nakada T, Nakanishi T, Fujita N, Yamashita H. Assessing myometrial invasion by endometrial carcinoma with dynamic MRI. *J Comput Assist Tomogr* 1994;18:77–86.
88. Nakao Y, Yokoyama M, Hara K, Koyamatsu Y, Yasunaga M, Araki Y, *et al.* MR imaging in endometrial carcinoma as a diagnostic tool for the absence of myometrial invasion. *Gynecol Oncol* 2006;102:343–7.
89. Seki H, Kimura M, Sakai K. Myometrial invasion of endometrial carcinoma: assessment with dynamic MR and contrast-enhanced T1-weighted images. *Clin Radiol* 1997;52:18–23.
90. Sironi S, Colombo E, Villa G, Taccagni G, Belloni C, Garancini P, *et al.* Myometrial invasion by endometrial carcinoma: assessment with plain and gadolinium-enhanced MR imaging. *Radiology* 1992;185:207–12.
91. Yamashita Y, Harada M, Sawada T, Takahashi M, Miyazaki K, Okamura H. Normal uterus and FIGO stage I endometrial carcinoma: dynamic gadolinium-enhanced MR imaging. *Radiology* 1993;186:495–501.
92. Hricak H, Stern JL, Fisher MR, Shapeero LG, Winkler ML, Lacey CG. Endometrial carcinoma staging by MR imaging. *Radiology* 1987;162:297–305.
93. Lien HH, Blomlie V, Trope C, Kaern J, Abeler VM. Cancer of the endometrium: value of MR imaging in determining depth of invasion into the myometrium. *AJR Am J Roentgenol* 1991;157:1221–3.
94. Fujii S, Matsusue E, Kigawa J, Sato S, Kanasaki Y, Nakanishi J, *et al.* Diagnostic accuracy of the apparent diffusion coefficient in differentiating benign from malignant uterine endometrial cavity lesions: initial results. *Eur Radiol* 2008;18:384–9.
95. Tamai K, Koyama T, Saga T, Umeoka S, Mikami Y, Fujii S, *et al.* Diffusion-weighted MR imaging of uterine endometrial cancer. *J Magn Reson Imaging* 2007;26:682–7.
96. Rechichi G, Galimberti S, Signorelli M, Perego P, Valsecchi MG, Sironi S. Myometrial invasion in endometrial cancer: diagnostic performance of diffusion-weighted MR imaging at 1.5-T. *Eur Radiol* 2010;20:754–62.
97. Shen SH, Chiou YY, Wang JH, Yen MS, Lee RC, Lai CR, *et al.* Diffusion-weighted single-shot echo-planar imaging with parallel technique in assessment of endometrial cancer. *AJR Am J Roentgenol* 2008;190:481–8.

98. Celik O, Hascalik S, Sarac K, Meydanli MM, Alkan A, Mizrak B. Magnetic resonance spectroscopy of premalignant and malignant endometrial disorders: a feasibility of *in vivo* study. *Eur J Obstet Gynecol Reprod Biol* 2005;118:241–5.

99. Signorelli M, Guerra L, Buda A, Picchio M, Mangili G, Dell'Anna T, *et al.* Role of the integrated FDG PET/CT in the surgical management of patients with high risk clinical early stage endometrial cancer: detection of pelvic nodal metastases. *Gynecol Oncol* 2009;115:231–5.

100. Kitajima K, Suzuki K, Nakamoto Y, Onishi Y, Sakamoto S, Senda M, *et al.* Low-dose non-enhanced CT versus full-dose contrast-enhanced CT in integrated PET/CT studies for the diagnosis of uterine cancer recurrence. *Eur J Nucl Med Mol Imaging* 2010;37:1490–8.

101. Picchio M, Mangili G, Samanes Gajate AM, De Marzi P, Spinapolice EG, Mapelli P, *et al.* High-grade endometrial cancer: value of [(18)F]FDG PET/CT in preoperative staging. *Nucl Med Commun* 2010;31:506–12.

102. Nakamura K, Kodama J, Okumura Y, Hongo A, Kanazawa S, Hiramatsu Y. The SUVmax of 18F-FDG PET correlates with histological grade in endometrial cancer. *Int J Gynecol Cancer* 2010;20:110–15.

103. Kitajima K, Murakami K, Yamasaki E, Domeki Y, Kaji Y, Morita S, *et al.* Performance of integrated FDG-PET/contrast-enhanced CT in the diagnosis of recurrent uterine cancer: comparison with PET and enhanced CT. *Eur J Nucl Med Mol Imaging* 2009;36:362–72.

104. Brown G, Richards CJ, Bourne MW, Newcombe RG, Radcliffe AG, Dallimore NS, *et al.* Morphologic predictors of lymph node status in rectal cancer with use of high-spatial-resolution MR imaging with histopathologic comparison. *Radiology* 2003;227:371–7.

105. Yang WT, Lam WW, Yu MY, Cheung TH, Metreweli C. Comparison of dynamic helical CT and dynamic MR imaging in the evaluation of pelvic lymph nodes in cervical carcinoma. *AJR Am J Roentgenol* 2000;175:759–66.

106. Barentsz JO, Jager GJ, van Vierzen PB, Witjes JA, Strijk SP, Peters H, *et al.* Staging urinary bladder cancer after transurethral biopsy: value of fast dynamic contrast-enhanced MR imaging. *Radiology* 1996;201:185–93.

107. Rockall AG, Sohaib SA, Harisinghani MG, Babar SA, Singh N, Jeyarajah AR, *et al.* Diagnostic performance of nanoparticle-enhanced magnetic resonance imaging in the diagnosis of lymph node metastases in patients with endometrial and cervical cancer. *J Clin Oncol* 2005;23:2813–21.

108. Jager GJ, Barentsz JO, Oosterhof GO, Witjes JA, Ruijs SJ. Pelvic adenopathy in prostatic and urinary bladder carcinoma: MR imaging with a three-dimensional TI-weighted magnetization-prepared-rapid gradient-echo sequence. *AJR Am J Roentgenol* 1996;167:1503–7.

109. Bahri S, Chen JH, Yu HJ, Kuzucan A, Nalcioglu O, Su MY. Can dynamic contrast-enhanced MRI (DCE-MRI) predict tumor recurrence and lymph node status in patients with breast cancer? *Ann Oncol* 2008;19:822–4.

110. Tuncbilek N, Karakas HM, Okten OO. Dynamic magnetic resonance imaging in determining histopathological prognostic factors of invasive breast cancers. *Eur J Radiol* 2005;53:199–205.

111. Murray AD, Staff RT, Redpath TW, Gilbert FJ, Ah-See AK, Brookes JA, *et al.* Dynamic contrast enhanced MRI of the axilla in women with breast cancer: comparison with pathology of excised nodes. *Br J Radiol* 2002;75:220–8.

112. Noworolski SM, Fischbein NJ, Kaplan MJ, Lu Y, Nelson SJ, Carvajal L, *et al.* Challenges in dynamic contrast-enhanced MRI imaging of cervical lymph nodes to detect metastatic disease. *J Magn Reson Imaging* 2003;17:455–62.

113. Thoeny HC, Triantafyllou M, Birkhaeuser FD, Froehlich JM, Tshering DW, Binser T, *et al.* Combined ultrasmall superparamagnetic particles of iron oxide-enhanced and diffusion-weighted magnetic resonance imaging reliably detect pelvic lymph node metastases in normal-sized nodes of bladder and prostate cancer patients. *Eur Urol* 2009;55:761–9.

114. Nakai G, Matsuki M, Inada Y, Tatsugami F, Tanikake M, Narabayashi I, *et al.* Detection and evaluation of pelvic lymph nodes in patients with gynecologic malignancies using body diffusion-weighted magnetic resonance imaging. *J Comput Assist Tomogr* 2008;32:764–8.

115. Lin G, Ho KC, Wang JJ, Ng KK, Wai YY, Chen YT, *et al.* Detection of lymph node metastasis in cervical and uterine cancers by diffusion-weighted magnetic resonance imaging at 3T. *J Magn Reson Imaging* 2008;28:128–35.

116. Kim JK, Kim KA, Park BW, Kim N, Cho KS. Feasibility of diffusion-weighted imaging in the differentiation of metastatic from nonmetastatic lymph nodes: early experience. *J Magn Reson Imaging* 2008;28:714–19.
117. Chen YB, Liao J, Xie R, Chen GL, Chen G. Discrimination of metastatic from hyperplastic pelvic lymph nodes in patients with cervical cancer by diffusion-weighted magnetic resonance imaging. *Abdom Imaging* 2011;36:102–9.
118. Roy C, Bierry G, Matau A, Bazille G, Pasquali R. Value of diffusion-weighted imaging to detect small malignant pelvic lymph nodes at 3 T. *Eur Radiol* 2010;20:1803–11.
119. Choi EK, Kim JK, Choi HJ, Park SH, Park BW, Kim N, *et al*. Node-by-node correlation between MR and PET/CT in patients with uterine cervical cancer: diffusion-weighted imaging versus size-based criteria on T2WI. *Eur Radiol* 2009;19:2024–32.
120. Drieskens O, Stroobants S, Gysen M, Vandenbosch G, Mortelmans L, Vergote I. Positron emission tomography with FDG in the detection of peritoneal and retroperitoneal metastases of ovarian cancer. *Gynecol Obstet Invest* 2003;55:130–4.
121. Fanti S, Nanni C, Castellucci P, Farsad M, Rampin L, Gross MD, *et al*. Supra-clavicular lymph node metastatic spread in patients with ovarian cancer disclosed at 18F-FDG-PET/CT: an unusual finding. *Cancer Imaging* 2006;6:20–3.
122. Chou HH, Chang TC, Yen TC, Ng KK, Hsueh S, Ma SY, *et al*. Low value of [18F]-fluoro-2-deoxy-D-glucose positron emission tomography in primary staging of early-stage cervical cancer before radical hysterectomy. *J Clin Oncol* 2006; 4:123–8.
123. Kidd EA, Siegel BA, Dehdashti F, Grigsby PW. Pelvic lymph node F-18 fluorodeoxyglucose uptake as a prognostic biomarker in newly diagnosed patients with locally advanced cervical cancer. *Cancer* 2010;116:1469–75.
124. Singh AK, Grigsby PW, Dehdashti F, Herzog TJ, Siegel BA. FDG-PET lymph node staging and survival of patients with FIGO stage IIIb cervical carcinoma. *Int J Radiat Oncol Biol Phys* 2003;56:489–93.
125. Yen TC, See LC, Lai CH, Tsai CS, Chao A, Hsueh S, *et al*. Standardized uptake value in para-aortic lymph nodes is a significant prognostic factor in patients with primary advanced squamous cervical cancer. *Eur J Nucl Med Mol Imaging* 2008;35:493–501.
126. Kitajima K, Murakami K, Yamasaki E, Fukasawa I, Inaba N, Kaji Y, *et al*. Accuracy of 18F-FDG PET/CT in detecting pelvic and paraaortic lymph node metastasis in patients with endometrial cancer. *AJR Am J Roentgenol* 2008;190:1652–8.
127. Nayot D, Kwon JS, Carey MS, Driedger A. Does preoperative positron emission tomography with computed tomography predict nodal status in endometrial cancer? A pilot study. *Curr Oncol* 2008;15:123–5.
128. Park JY, Kim EN, Kim DY, Suh DS, Kim JH, Kim YM, *et al*. Comparison of the validity of magnetic resonance imaging and positron emission tomography/computed tomography in the preoperative evaluation of patients with uterine corpus cancer. *Gynecol Oncol* 2008;108:486–92.
129. Horowitz NS, Dehdashti F, Herzog TJ, Rader JS, Powell MA, Gibb RK, *et al*. Prospective evaluation of FDG-PET for detecting pelvic and para-aortic lymph node metastasis in uterine corpus cancer. *Gynecol Oncol* 2004;95:546–51.
130. Lin WC, Hung YC, Yeh LS, Kao CH, Yen RF, Shen YY. Usefulness of (18)F-fluorodeoxyglucose positron emission tomography to detect para-aortic lymph nodal metastasis in advanced cervical cancer with negative computed tomography findings. *Gynecol Oncol* 2003;89:73–6.
131. Choi HJ, Roh JW, Seo SS, Lee S, Kim JY, Kim SK, *et al*. Comparison of the accuracy of magnetic resonance imaging and positron emission tomography/computed tomography in the presurgical detection of lymph node metastases in patients with uterine cervical carcinoma: a prospective study. *Cancer* 2006;106:914–22.
132. Loft A, Berthelsen AK, Roed H, Ottosen C, Lundvall L, Knudsen J, *et al*. The diagnostic value of PET/CT scanning in patients with cervical cancer: a prospective study. *Gynecol Oncol* 2007;106:29–34.
133. Sironi S, Buda A, Picchio M, Perego P, Moreni R, Pellegrino A, *et al*. Lymph node metastasis in patients with clinical early-stage cervical cancer: detection with integrated FDG PET/CT. *Radiology* 2006;238:272–9.

Section 4

What questions are being asked by current clinical trials?

15

Chapter 15

Current clinical trials in ovarian cancer

Christina Fotopoulou, Angus McIndoe, Jalid Sehouli and Hani Gabra

Epithelial ovarian cancer (EOC) is the most common cause of death among women who develop gynaecological cancer and the fifth most common cause of cancer-related death in females in western countries.[1,2] The latest data show that one in 43 women will develop EOC during their lifetime. Women with a mutated *BRCA1* or *BRCA2* gene are at increased risk, ranging between 25% and 60% depending on the specific mutation.[3]

Owing to its unusual tumour biology and clinical behaviour, the disease presents late, typically with extensive locoregional dissemination throughout the peritoneal cavity with surprisingly rare incidence of truly visceral metastatic disease, although nodal involvement is not uncommon and of unclear significance.[4]

This unusual natural history has led to unique therapeutic strategies that reflect the importance of locoregional control to survival for this disease.

Primary cytoreduction: quality criteria

Surgery aimed at maximal tumour reduction, ideally without any macroscopic tumour residual disease, followed by adjuvant systemic chemotherapy typically with paclitaxel and carboplatin, constitutes the current gold standard in the primary management of the disease.[5,6] Nevertheless, median progression-free survival (PFS) ranges only between 16 and 22 months, and median overall survival (OS) is rather limited, at 3–5 years.[4–6] There is thus a great need for future strategies to improve the OS.

The rate of optimal residual disease (less than 1 cm), particularly the rate of complete macroscopic tumour resection, is broadly considered to be an appropriate evaluation tool for assessing surgical quality in advanced EOC.[7] Validated data show that, in the primary presentation of the disease, for each 10% increase in cytoreduction there is a direct correlation to a 5.5% increase in median survival.[8] However, no reliable parameters have as yet become established for routine clinical use to allow prediction of complete or at least optimal tumour resection in individual women with advanced EOC, and optimal tumour debulking rates range widely between 12% and 76 % according to institution or trial.[9,10] The wide variety of surgical outcome in terms of optimal and total macroscopic resection rates and morbidity are, however, not only dependent on the stage of the disease and the extensive tumour dissemination patterns associated with this. Increasingly, investigators are calling for objective validation of surgical skills quality, which is one of the most important determinants of the likelihood of optimal primary resection, especially in advanced stages of the disease.[11–13] Increasing surgical effort, continual education and practice, and growing expertise are associated with improved rates of primary cytoreduction.[7,8,11–14]

This issue is being considered in the current German Arbeitsgemeinschaft Gynaekologische Onkologie Studiengruppe Ovarialkarzinom (AGO-OVAR) OP.3 LION trial that is assessing the value of systematic lymphadenectomy in primary EOC and its impact on patients' survival. In this study, only centres that have proven high surgical quality with appropriate validated experience in the management of EOC are able to participate. Women up to age 75 years with International Federation of Gynecology and Obstetrics (FIGO) stages IIB–IV primary EOC and with an overall good performance index (that is, ECOG [Eastern Cooperative Oncology Group] 0/1) are being intraoperatively randomised in systematic pelvic and para-aortic lymphadenectomy versus none where their debulking achieves a result with no residual extra- or intra-abdominal disease in the absence of bulky lymph nodes. By March 2011, 1165 women had been recruited and 393 of them had been randomised. Women with non-epithelial histology at fresh frozen section, intraoperative bulky nodes and/or with tumour residuals were excluded from randomisation. The primary endpoint of the study is to assess the impact of systematic lymphadenectomy in primary advanced EOC on OS. Secondary endpoints are the impact on PFS, operative morbidity and quality of life. The defined follow-up time is set to a maximum of 6 years, while the estimated duration of the study is programmed for 9.5 years or until 247 deaths occur. The estimated number of overall randomised patients needed to reach statistically significant results is defined as 640. Since current data regarding the true value of systematic lymph node dissection in the absence of bulky nodes versus resection of merely enlarged nodes are clearly controversial and international guidelines and personal experiences in this area vary widely,[15–18] the results of the LION study are keenly awaited so that new standards in the surgical treatment of advanced ovarian cancer can be established.

Value of the neoadjuvant approach in primary advanced ovarian cancer

The value of the neoadjuvant approach in the primary treatment of advanced EOC is currently one of the most debated issues in gynaecological oncology worldwide.[19] Various studies have shown that interval debulking surgery (IDS) after three cycles of neoadjuvant chemotherapy (NAC) appears to be associated with both reduced operative morbidity and higher complete tumour resection rates, or even prolonged survival, compared with primary tumour debulking.[9,19–21] Nevertheless, equally numerous practice-based analyses yield contradictory results showing no clear benefit from the neoadjuvant approach over primary cytoreduction,[22–24] rendering the potential benefit of IDS post NAC strongly controversial. Certain investigators argue that NAC as a primary treatment strategy for advanced EOC should be reserved for cases with comorbidities, especially in elderly patients where an initial attempt at radical cytoreduction appears to be too hazardous.[25]

In 2010, Vergote *et al.*[9] presented the results of the large European Organisation for Research and Treatment of Cancer–Gynecological Cancer Group (EORTC-GCG)/ National Cancer Institute Canada–Clinical Trial Group (NCIC-CTG) prospective multicentre randomised study evaluating NAC in advanced EOC. Of the 670 randomly assigned women with extensive stage IIIC or IV disease, 632 (94.3%) were eligible and started treatment. At primary debulking surgery, the majority of women

(74.5%) had peritoneal lesions larger than 5 cm in diameter and 61.6% had lesions larger than 10 cm. Postoperative rates of adverse effects and mortality tended to be higher after primary debulking than after IDS. Complete resection of all macroscopic disease (at primary or interval surgery) was the strongest independent variable in predicting OS. Complete tumour resection rates at IDS post NAC were significantly higher compared with primary debulking surgery. Nevertheless, importantly, the significantly enhanced resection rates associated with NAC-IDS did not translate to significantly better OS or PFS, a very curious result given the apparent prognostic importance of optimal/total clearance rates described above.

Higher tumour resection rates in the NAC-IDS setting have also been confirmed in various other single-centre studies from Canada and Europe.[26,27] NAC-IDS patients therefore appear to be significantly more likely to be optimally debulked compared with those undergoing primary debulking surgery. In the EORTC/NCIC-CTG trial, however, surgical quality and survival varied very widely among the participating centres, so it is important that wholesale adoption of NAC-IDS as used in this trial should only be integrated into clinical routine with caution and understanding of the population and practice issues within this trial.

A 2009 meta-analysis of the Cochrane Central Register of Controlled Trials[28] showed that there is currently no conclusive evidence at to whether IDS improves the survival rate in women with advanced ovarian cancer.

The morphological changes of ovarian cancer after NAC also have to be addressed. Many reports clearly indicate that both macroscopic and microscopic appearances of the tumour are influenced by chemotherapy. Histological features such as the presence of pronounced stromal changes, necrosis and regressive alterations are seen, and accurate tumour typing and grading is obviously significantly affected.[29–31] In some cases, it may even be difficult to confirm the presence of residual tumour, while for definite confirmation additional multiple histological sections and immunohistochemistry are required. All these chemotherapy-induced alterations may render the tumour undetectable or hardly traceable, not only for the pathologist at a microscopic level but also for the surgeon at the time of IDS.[29–32]

The currently recruiting CHORUS trial sponsored by the Royal College of Obstetricians and Gynaecologists also addresses the issue of the neoadjuvant approach in advanced EOC. In this pilot multicentre study, women are randomised to either undergo radical surgery with subsequent adjuvant platinum-based chemotherapy or to receive three courses of platinum-based chemotherapy and then undergo radical tumour debulking within 3 weeks of NAC. Within 6 weeks of surgery, patients then commence an additional three courses of chemotherapy. The women will be followed up at 9 months after randomisation. The primary outcome measures are OS, PFS and quality of life as assessed by the Questionnaire Core 30 Items (QLQ-C30) and the QLQ-Ovarian Cancer (QLQ-OV28).

Surgical cytoreduction at recurrence

The value of tumour debulking surgery for recurrent EOC remains highly controversial. While many proponents of cytoreduction at relapse advocate that complete tumour resection may result in higher survival rates, opponents of this radical approach argue instead that high complication rates, longer hospitalisation times and a clear indication for systemic treatment in pretreated patients weigh against this approach.[33–37]

Many authors have attempted to define a preoperative algorithm that would identify optimal candidates for secondary cytoreduction based on well-defined selection criteria. The disease-free interval, the number of recurrence sites, the patient's performance status, the surgical outcome of the primary surgery and the current amount of ascites have been variously discussed as possible predictive factors of clinical outcome in surgery at recurrence.[37,38] However, no well-established, prospective data yet exist that could set universal standards to inform operability. In the retrospective AGO DESKTOP I trial,[38] women appeared to benefit from surgery in recurrent EOC only when total macroscopic clearance was achieved. Good performance status, complete resection at primary surgery and absence of ascites were identified as independent predictors for complete debulking, leading to the so-called 'AGO score'. An exploratory analysis of the DESKTOP I results to evaluate the role of peritoneal carcinomatosis present in recurrent EOC clearly showed that, even though peritoneal carcinomatosis was a negative predictor for complete resection in recurrent disease, it appeared to have no negative impact on survival if total macroscopic clearance could be achieved. The authors concluded that improving surgical skills might increase the patient proportion that could benefit from surgery for recurrent disease.[39]

Further confirmation and validation of the AGO score occurred within the prospective multicentre DESKTOP II trial,[40] in which it was confirmed as a useful and reliable tool to predict complete tumour resection in more than two-thirds of patients with platinum-sensitive relapsed EOC. Participating centres prospectively enrolled women with platinum-sensitive first or second relapse. The AGO score was then applied to all patients but each centre was free to decide the therapeutic management. A total of 516 women were screened within 19 months; of these, 261 (51%) were classified as score positive, and 129 women with a positive score and first relapse received a secondary tumour debulking. The rate of complete resection was 76%, thus confirming the validity of this score regarding positive prediction of complete resectability in more than two-thirds of patients.

The multicentre randomised DESKTOP III (AGO-OVAR OP.4) trial commenced in June 2010 to prospectively evaluate the impact of recurrent EOC surgery in platinum-sensitive women with a positive AGO score (tumour-free initial surgery, good performance status and ascites less than 500 ml). As at March 2011, ten women had been recruited and randomised, with the intention being to to recruit 385 women. This important study is expected to finally settle the question as to whether surgery at relapse is associated with a benefit in survival and quality of life.

Venturing beyond secondary cytoreduction, the largest series evaluating tertiary cytoreduction in 135 women with recurrent disease demonstrated that, even in a tertiary setting, nearly 40% complete tumour resection rates are feasible in highly specialised gynaecological oncology centres. In this series, the presence of peritoneal carcinomatosis was reported to have an almost three-fold worse prognosis than in those without peritoneal carcinomatosis,[39] and no significant impact on survival could be identified in tertiary cytoreduction, regardless of the diameter of postoperative residual tumour. Furthermore, previously defined negative predictors of survival such as advanced FIGO stage and the presence of ascites could not be shown to retain prognostic significance in the tertiary setting.[41] In an analysis assessing the survival benefit of quaternary surgery published in 2010 by Shih et al,[42] there remained a significant relationship between postoperative residual disease that was identified at the time of surgery for third relapse. These authors, however, failed to demonstrate any significant impact of platinum sensitivity on disease-specific survival.

Systemic therapy

First-line chemotherapy: dose-dense regimens

The currently established management of advanced primary EOC consisting of maximal effort surgery and platinum-based combination chemotherapy is associated with a more than 70% recurrence rate within the first 2 years after initial diagnosis.[5,14] Thus, first-line studies are warranted to improve survival and reduce recurrence risk. During the past decade, in attempting to improve on the gold standard of paclitaxel–carboplatin chemotherapy, various large collaborative trials that have included more than 10 000 women have investigated the substitution of docetaxel for paclitaxel (demonstrating equivalence),[43] the addition of one-third cytotoxic agent such as gemcitabine, liposomal doxorubicin, epirubicin or topotecan (without improvement in PFS or OS),[44,45] and consolidation treatment with an additional six cycles of 3-weekly paclitaxel versus no consolidation (without improvement in PFS or OS).[46]

Dose-dense administration of cytotoxic agents in a weekly schedule is another potential strategy to enhance anti-tumour activity and prolong survival.[47] In particular, preclinical studies have suggested that duration of exposure rather than dose of paclitaxel is an important determinant of response.[48] Dose density refers to increasing dose frequency while maintaining the same dose per cycle, with the overall dose typically remaining the same. Dose intensity is therefore increased and overall treatment time is shorter.[49]

In 2009, the Japanese Gynecologic Oncology Group (JGOG) reported results from their JGOG3016 phase III trial that identified a clear PFS and OS benefit from weekly administration of paclitaxel combined with 3-weekly carboplatin compared with standard paclitaxel–carboplatin 3-weekly in women with newly diagnosed epithelial ovarian, fallopian tube or primary peritoneal carcinoma.[47] Six hundred and thirty-seven women were enrolled in this open-label randomised controlled trial at 85 centres in Japan. Median PFS was longer in the dose-dense treatment group (28.0 months; 95% CI 22.3–35.4 months) than in the conventional treatment group (17.2 months; 95% CI 15.7–21.1 months, HR 0.71; 95% CI 0.58–0.88; P=0.0015). OS at 3 years was also significantly higher in the dose-dense regimen group (72.1%) than in the conventional treatment group (65.1%; HR 0.75; 95% CI 0.57–0.98; P=0.03). Withdrawal due to toxicity was higher in the dose-dense regimen group than in the conventional regimen group (113 women versus 69 women). The most common adverse event was neutropenia (dose-dense regimen 92% versus 88% in the conventional arm). The frequency of grade 3/4 anaemia was also higher in the dose-dense treatment group (69% versus 44%; P<0.0001). The frequencies of other toxic effects were similar between groups.[47] If confirmed, the impressive results of this study, in particular in improving the median PFS, will result in a step change in the first-line treatment of advanced EOC.

Building on the results of the JGOG3016 trial, the ICON8 international three-stage randomised trial of dose-fractionated chemotherapy compared with standard 3-weekly chemotherapy is designed to evaluate the dose-dense schedule in the first-line setting of patients after primary surgery or delayed primary surgery. Patients will be prospectively stratified according to whether they receive immediate or delayed primary surgery. It is estimated that 30–40% of UK women with stage IIIC/IV disease will undergo delayed primary tumour debulking. This study is a UK- and academic investigator-led trial with no pharmaceutical industry support. It is planned that 1485 women will be recruited over 3 years and assigned to one of three arms:

1. standard carboplatin (AUC = 5) every 3 weeks and paclitaxel 175 mg/m^2 every 3 weeks
2. carboplatin (AUC = 5) every 3 weeks and paclitaxel 80 mg/m^2 weekly (JGOG3016 schedule)
3. carboplatin (AUC = 2) weekly and paclitaxel 80 mg/m^2 weekly.

The principle for Arm 3 is that the weekly fractionation of carboplatin improves tolerability and thus the ability to deliver weekly chemotherapy, it is hoped without decreasing efficacy. This trial will commence in mid-2011.

Another dose-dense trial that is currently recruiting is the MITO-7 trial from the MITO (Multicenter Italian Trials in Ovarian Cancer and Gynecologic Malignancies) group in collaboration with the MaNGO (Mario Negri Gynecologic Oncology) group. The purpose of this phase III trial is to study efficacy and the effects on quality of life in women with EOC treated with a weekly schedule of carboplatin and paclitaxel chemotherapy compared with those treated with the standard 3-weekly schedule of the same chemotherapy. The primary outcome measures are quality of life and PFS. The estimated study completion date is December 2012.

Intraperitoneal chemotherapy and biotherapy in first-line and relapsed settings

EOC is a disease mainly restricted to the peritoneal cavity, with locoregional peritoneal disease affecting parietal and visceral peritoneum and typically causing ascites. Even in advanced stages, visceral metastases are often absent, with disease limited to pleural or peritoneal space. Based on this, a hypothesis was developed around locoregional therapy of peritoneal carcinomatosis suggesting that EOC might be treated by direct infusion of the anti-cancer agents into the site of origin – the peritoneal cavity itself.

There have been many randomised trials comparing intraperitoneal (IP) with intravenous (IV) chemotherapy. The common factor is that all included platinum, and most added a second drug. Meta-analysis[50–52] of these trials shows a significant reduction in hazards of 0.78 with a confidence interval of 0.69–0.89 and an improvement in median OS of about 12 months over an expected median survival for this optimally debulked group of 4 years for patients receiving IV chemotherapy.

One of the most prominent of these trials, by the Gynecologic Oncology Group (GOG) and known as GOG 172,[53,54] showed the largest difference ever in a randomised ovarian cancer trial at its time of publication with median OS of 67 months for IP chemotherapy versus 49 months in the IV control arm, the improvement being 17.4 months with a hazard ratio of 0.71. The test regimen was IV paclitaxel on day 1, IP cisplatin on day 2 and IP paclitaxel on day 8 in a 21 day cycle for six cycles randomised against standard IV chemotherapy. However, IP chemotherapy was associated with enhanced toxicities, including neuropathy, gastrointestinal toxicity and myelotoxicity. A further criticism of this trial was the imbalance of dosing between the arms, with higher cisplatin IP dose (compared with IV dose) and an additional IP paclitaxel dose on day 8. For these reasons, among others, the GOG 172 regimen did not become widely adopted. However, there are now two new IP trials that may help to clarify this area of therapy.

The continuing Japanese JGOG3019 phase II/III trial is an elegant and rational trial that builds on the recent JGOG dose-dense weekly therapy data and evaluates, in a dose- and schedule-balanced trial, the efficacy and safety of the route of administration of carboplatin (IP versus IV). All patients receive paclitaxel 80 mg/m^2 IV weekly and are randomised to either IP or IV carboplatin (AUC = 6) 3-weekly over six to eight cycles. Women with EOC at advanced FIGO stages II–IV are included. The primary endpoint is PFS, with secondary endpoints of OS, toxicity and quality of life, with planned recruitment of 746 patients.

The UK/Canadian NCIC-CTG PETROC/OV21 study is another balanced trial of IP versus IV in women who have undergone delayed primary surgery after three to four cycles of neoadjuvant 3-weekly paclitaxel–carboplatin IV chemotherapy. Initially, the trial will assess the feasibility of either cisplatin or carboplatin as IP agents in combination with paclitaxel on days 1 and 8, subsequently randomisng the 'winner' against standard carboplatin–paclitaxel. The endpoints of the study will be PFS and OS.

These two studies will define the magnitude of the benefit of route change for platinum therapy. The questions that arise regarding IP therapy are whether such a treatment improves outcome/survival and whether the perceived benefits of IP treatment are mainly about dose intensity rather than a dose-dense schedule.

In the relapse setting, in women with malignant ascites due to EOC, the trifunctional antibody catumaxomab has demonstrated the ability to destroy EpCAM-positive tumour cells in the peritoneal cavity and to control the malignant ascites in recurrent disease. Catumaxomab (bifunctional anti-EPCAM/anti-CD3 monoclonal antibody) enhances the anti-tumour activity by redirecting T cells and Fc-gamma receptor I/III-positive accessory cells to the tumour.[55–57]

In the first phase II trial,[58] catumaxomab was administered directly into the peritoneal cavity via intraperitoneal port catheters during primary cytoreductive surgery and postoperatively before standard systemic chemotherapy with paclitaxel and platinum. The women received one intraoperative (10 μg) followed by four subsequent IP doses (10, 20, 50 and 150 μg) of catumaxomab over 3 hours on days 7, 10, 13 and 16, respectively. The study was conducted to investigate the tolerability and feasibility of such a treatment. Of the 58 screened patients, 41 were evaluable for the safety analysis. All 41 experienced at least one treatment-related adverse event, with a total of 871 events. The most common adverse events were pyrexia, nausea, abdominal pain and vomiting due to cytokine release. The complications decreased continuously down to zero up to the fourth and fifth infusion. The observed postoperative complication rate was 51.2%, including anastomosis insufficiencies (three women), infections (eight women) and pleural effusions (ten women). The authors concluded that the intraoperative treatment approach with a highly immunogenic agent is feasible but its potential role with regard to postoperative complications, especially for anastomosis insufficiencies, needs to be further investigated. Survival data are expected to be presented in 2011.

Two further trials with the immunogenic agent catumaxomab are continuing: the CASIMAS study and the SECIMAS study. CASIMAS is a randomised phase IIIb study investigating the premedication of prednisolone in patients treated with IP catumaxomab for EpCAM-positive malignant ascites. A total of 208 patients are being allocated to two treatment groups in a 1 : 1 ratio. The study closed recruiting at the beginning of 2011.

SECIMAS is a phase II single-arm open-label study investigating the safety of a second cycle of catumaxomab in patients with malignant ascites requiring their first therapeutic puncture after treatment in the CASIMAS study. The trial is still recruiting.

The incorporation of targeted therapies into first-line and and post-first-line maintenance therapy

Anti-angiogenic therapy represents a huge effort in translational research, with high expectations from investigators and patients alike. The first angiogenesis inhibitor to enter phase III trials, bevacizumab, was evaluated in combination with established cytotoxic schedules in the GOG-218 trial.[59] The questions that were addressed in this trial were whether anti-angiogenic therapy is potent in combination with conventional chemotherapy, what the optimal dose and duration of therapy are, and whether or not bevacizumab's benefit may principally be in the maintenance phase for selected patients. Many unusual claims have been made about the benefits of bevacizumab, although most observers regard the benefits as somewhat modest despite the publicity and cost associated with this drug.

The first case history of single-agent activity of bevacizumab was reported in 2005,[60] and 2 years later the first phase II trial showed single-agent activity,[61] which was confirmed in a subsequent phase II trial of combination therapy that was published in 2008.[62] The first randomised phase III trial, GOG-218, was reported at the annual meeting of the American Society of Clinical Oncology (ASCO 2010) by Burger *et al.*[59] The Eastern Cooperative Oncology Group (ECOG), the North Central Cancer Treatment Group (NCCTG), the National Surgical Adjuvant Breast and Bowel Project (NSABP) and the Southwest Oncology Group (SWOG) also participated in this large multicentre trial that recruited 1800 women with optimal or suboptimal stage III–IV operated EOC. The trial compared conventional paclitaxel and carboplatin against the combination with concurrent bevacizumab plus bevacizumab in maintenance over an additional 15 months. The trial met its primary objective of increasing PFS in first-line treatment of advanced EOC by 3.8 months in the maintenance versus conventional arm. The PFS benefit between conventional and merely concurrent arms was not statistically significant, indicating that the value of bevacizumab is principally in a maintenance setting. No significant differences in OS were noted.

An equivalent European Medical Research Council (MRC)/National Cancer Research Institute (NCRI) study, the ICON7 trial,[63] with the participation of NCIC-CTG, AGO-OVAR, the French Group d'Investigateurs Nationaux pour l'Etude des Cancers Ovariens (GINECO), the Spanish Grupo Espanol de Investigacion en Cancer de Ovario (GEICO), EORTC, the Australia New Zealand Gynaecological Oncology Group (ANZGOG) and the Nordic Society of Gynaecological Oncology (NSGO), randomised 1528 women with primary epithelial ovarian, fallopian tube or peritoneal cancer to receive conventional paclitaxel and carboplatin or concurrent bevacizumab which was continued as maintenance treatment for an additional 18 cycles. The addition of concurrent and maintenance bevacizumab (7.5 mg/kg 3-weekly for 12 months) to standard chemotherapy statistically significantly improved PFS by a median of 1.5 months. Bevacizumab treatment was well tolerated and there were no new safety concerns. The quality of life analyses are continuing and longer term PFS, mature OS and translational research results are expected in 2012. The authors concluded that carboplatin and paclitaxel in combination with bevacizumab with subsequent single-agent bevacizumab at 15 mg/kg for a total of 15 months should be considered a standard treatment option for advanced EOC.

Nevertheless, mature OS and quality of life data will be necessary before introducing bevacizumab into clinical practice. If the 3.8 month median PFS gain (from the GOG-218 trial) is upheld, this will bring a cost of $229,187/year of PFS gained.

Pazopanib is a potent and selective multitargeted receptor tyrosine kinase inhibitor of VEGFR-1, VEGFR-2, VEGFR-3, PDGFR-α/β and c-Kit that blocks tumour growth and inhibits angiogenesis. The multicentre randomised AGO-OVAR16 trial is studying the effect of pazopanib as a consolidation treatment for 1 year after completion of conventional carboplatin and paclitaxel chemotherapy. The trial is still recruiting and numerous study groups are participating – AGO-Austria, ANZGOG, the Belgian Gynaecological Oncology Group (BGOG), GEICO, GINECO, the All-Ireland Co-operative Oncology Research Group (ICORG), JGOG, the Korean Gynecologic Oncology Group (KGOG), MaNGO, MITO, NSGO, California Consortium, the New York Gynecologic Oncology Group (NYGOG) and SWOG. To date, 752 of the planned 900 patients have been randomised.

The triple kinase inhibitor BIBF 1120 (which inhibits VEGF receptors, FGF receptors and PDGF receptors, thereby inhibiting angiogenesis) is being tested in a phase III randomised trial sponsored by Boehringer Ingelheim and supported by the AGO. The trial is evaluating whether BIBF 1120 in combination with paclitaxel and carboplatin is more effective than placebo in combination with paclitaxel and carboplatin in first-line treatment of women with advanced EOC. Safety information about BIBF 1120/paclitaxel/carboplatin will be obtained.

A further consolidation regimen with a targeted therapy is being assessed in the EORTC trial 55041. This randomised open-label phase III trial is active although no longer recruiting, and evaluates erlotinib compared with observation alone as maintenance therapy for patients with no evidence of disease progression after conventional first-line chemotherapy for ovarian, peritoneal or fallopian tube cancer. Erlotinib is a tyrosine kinase inhibitor that acts on the epidermal growth factor receptor (EGFR). In collaboration with AGO-Austria, ANZGOG, GINECO, MRC/NCIC and MaNGO, the trial recruited 835 patients to receive erlotinib consolidation for 2 years or no therapy.

The multicentre placebo-controlled phase II TRIO 014 trial of the Cancer International Research Group is investigating the value of adding AMG 479 (a fully human monoclonal antibody against IGF-1R) to paclitaxel and carboplatin first-line chemotherapy in women with optimally debulked (smaller than 1 cm) FIGO stage III and IV (positive pleural cytology only) ovarian epithelial (including fallopian tube and primary peritoneal) carcinoma.

Ovarian cancer sub-types with rare histology

Each sub-type of ovarian carcinoma is known to have different biological behaviour and varying responses to chemotherapy. Newer molecular studies support the notion that the various sub-types represent histopathologically, genetically and biologically distinct diseases exhibiting a large degree of molecular heterogeneity and are thus associated with different response and survival rates. Even though there is clear evidence that women with non-serous ovarian cancer sub-types, especially mucinous and clear cell, have worse overall outcome, the histological sub-type does not currently influence treatment.[64] In the recurrent situation, the question of the development of intrinsic platinum resistance arises. Some authors have considered in isolated cases the application of regimens such as FOLFOX (folinic acid, 5-fluorouracil and oxaliplatin) in mucinous EOC sub-types or even favour the use of anti-angiogenic agents such as bevacizumab, both of which are treatment regimens used in colorectal cancers.[65]

The multicentre intergroup randomised factorial mEOC/GOG 241 trial compares the combination of oxaliplatin, capecitabine and bevacizumab with conventional carboplatin and paclitaxel in women with previously untreated mucinous EOC. The trial will enrol primary patients with advanced mucinous EOC (FIGO stages II–IV) or chemo-naïve patients with recurrent mucinous disease after initial FIGO stage I disease. In total, 332 women are planned to be recruited, 83 in each of four arms:

1. carboplatin and paclitaxel 3-weekly for six cycles
2. oxaliplatin and capecitabine 3-weekly for six cycles
3. carboplatin and paclitaxel 3-weekly for six cycles with bevacizumab 15 mg/kg 3-weekly for five or six cycles
4. oxaliplatin and capecitabine 3-weekly for six cycles with bevacizumab 15 mg/kg 3-weekly for five or six cycles.

Patients in arms 3 and 4 will receive bevacizumab 15 mg/kg 3-weekly for 12 cycles as maintenance therapy. Clinical assessment will be performed by computed tomography (CT) scans for the entire follow-up period up to a maximum of 5 years.

A further histology-based study is the Japanese JGOG3017 trial for women with a histological diagnosis of clear-cell carcinoma. GINECO, GOG, KGOG, MITO and the Scottish Gynaecological Cancer Trials Group (SGCTG) are also participating in this trial. This randomised phase III trial compares the efficacy and safety of standard-arm paclitaxel plus carboplatin versus the experimental arm of irinotecan plus cisplatin in clear-cell carcinoma of the ovary. The primary endpoint is PFS and secondary endpoints are OS, response assessment and adverse effects. The trial plans to recruit 652 women and that is now nearly complete.

Studies beyond first line

Despite the initial high response rates to first-line platinum-based therapies, the majority of women with EOC will experience relapse and die of the disease.[66] Several therapeutic options are available and the decision as to which therapy to commence is dependent on the platinum-free interval (PFI).[67,68] The PFI is a predictor of response not only to second-line treatment with platinum-based chemotherapy but also to other active agents including the taxanes, topoisomerase I inhibitors and anthracyclines.[66,69] In platinum-sensitive patients (that is, those with PFI longer than 6 months), a platinum rechallenge in combination regimens should be undertaken. The probability of response increases with the PFI, from less than 10% for PFI shorter than 6 months to more than 60% for PFI longer than 12 months.[67]

Platinum-sensitive EOC relapse (PFI longer than 6 months)

In 2010, the results of the large multicentre phase III CALYPSO trial demonstrated the superiority in terms of PFS and better therapeutic index of the combination of PEGylated liposomal doxorubicin (PLD) with carboplatin over standard carboplatin and paclitaxel in women with platinum-sensitive late relapse recurrent EOC.[70] The median PFS for the experimental arm was statistically superior to that for the conventional arm (n=976; HR 0.821; 95% CI 0.72–0.94; P=0.005; median PFS 11.3 versus 9.4 months). The OS data remain immature but will be reported in due course.

At ASCO 2010, the preliminary safety results from the phase III HECTOR trial of topotecan plus carboplatin versus standard therapy with paclitaxel plus carboplatin or gemcitabine plus carboplatin or carboplatin plus PLD were presented.[71] This Nord-Ostdeutsche Gesellschaft für Gynäkologische Onkologie (NOGGO)/AGO/AGO-Austria and GEICO-Gynecologic Cancer Intergroup (GCIG) trial completed recruiting in December 2009 but final results are not available yet. This preliminary analysis was an evaluation of the safety profile of the experimental arm and the standard therapy control arm. The data from the first 200 of the 550 randomised patients were analysed. Haematological toxicity contributed to 41% of cycle delays in the control arm and 36% in the topotecan plus carboplatin arm. Neutropenia and infection rates were similar in both arms. Granulocyte colony-stimulating factor (G-CSF) was administered more frequently to patients in the control arm (26%) than in the topotecan plus carboplatin arm (21%). Grade 2 or higher non-haematological toxicity was not more frequent in the control arm. There were more severe adverse events in the control arm (66%) than in the topotecan plus carboplatin arm (55%).

The ICON6 phase III study will assess the safety and efficacy of cediranib in concurrent and maintenance design in women with platinum-sensitive relapsed EOC. Cediranib, also known as AZD2171, is a potent inhibitor of VEGFR tyrosine kinases (VEGFR-1, VEGFR-2 and VEGFR-3). The first stage is about trial safety; in the second stage of the trial, the primary endpoint will be PFS and in the third stage OS.

A further trial for platinum-sensitive recurrent EOC is the interventional phase II ECHO trial. This study is continuing but not recruiting any more participants. The purpose of this study is to compare PFS in women with advanced EOC treated with zibotentan (ZD4054), an endothelin pathway blocker, in combination with carboplatin plus paclitaxel versus placebo in combination with carboplatin plus paclitaxel.

Based on the property of EOC cells demonstrating overexpression of the α-folate receptor in more than 90% of ovarian cancers, the humanised monoclonal antibody against α-folate receptor farletuzumab may constitute an important upregulated target for therapy to reverse platinum resistance. It inhibits the receptor and its downstream signalling and it also activates antibody-dependent cell-mediated cytotoxicity (ADCC) and the cell-division cycle causing receptor internalisation. Compared with historical progression and historical PFI, farletuzumab increased the overall response rate (70% compared with historical response rate of less than 30%), and CA125 normalised in 89% of patients receiving combination treatment (carboplatin/paclitaxel/farletuzumab).[72]

The phase III MORAb-003-004 study that is currently recruiting will test the efficacy and safety of farletuzumab in women with platinum-sensitive EOC in first relapse. Carboplatin and taxane will be combined with MORAb-003 (farletuzumab) 1.25 mg/kg or 2.5 mg/kg and compared with carboplatin and taxane with placebo. The primary outcome measure will be PFS as measured by RECIST and secondary outcome measures will be OS, CA125 PFS, GCIG PFS, length of first versus second remission, tumour response, serological response (CA125), quality of life and resource utilisation.

In an attempt to replace platinum in the treatment of women with relapsed EOC, the open-label multicentre randomised phase III OVA-301 study compared the combination of PLD and trabectedin with PLD alone in women with advanced relapsed EOC (PFI longer than 6 months). The study, now closed, still requires an updated interim analysis of OS (cut-off, 31 May 2009) but results were presented in 2010 showing that, when combined with PLD, trabectedin improves PFS and overall response rate compared with PLD alone, with acceptable tolerance, in the second-line treatment of recurrent EOC. Median PFS in the trabectedin/PLD arm was 7.3 months versus 5.8 months in the PLD arm (HR 0.79; 95% CI 0.65–0.96; $P=0.0190$). When evaluating efficacy for the partially platinum-sensitive subset of patients (PFI of 6–12 months), the median PFS was 9.2 months versus 7.5 months (HR 0.73; 95% CI 0.56–0.95; $P=0.0170$). The overall response rate was 27.6% versus 18.8% ($P=0.0080$); for platinum-sensitive patients, it was 35.3% versus 22.6%

($P = 0.0042$) and thus highly statistically significant. The overall response rate, PFS and OS among platinum-resistant patients were not statistically different.[73]

Intermediate platinum response in EOC relapse (PFI 6–12 months)

Women with an intermediate response to platinum (that is, PFI between 6 and 12 months) represent a therapeutic challenge. There have been various trials addressing this particular subset of patients. The Italian MaNGO study group leads the OVATYON trial evaluating PLD 30 mg/m^2 1 hour IV plus carboplatin (AUC = 5) 30–60 minutes IV on day 1 4-weekly, with treatment allowed up to six cycles or to progression versus PLD 30 mg/m^2 1 hour IV plus trabectedin 1.1 mg/m^2 3 hours IV on day 1 3-weekly, with up to six cycles or to progression, in women with EOC relapse with a PFI of 6–12 months. The women will be stratified according to their ECOG status, the measurable disease and PFI. The trial has commenced and it may take some time to achieve the recruitment target of 588 women.

A further study is the phase III MITO-8 trial that aims to test the hypothesis that artificial prolongation of the PFI with a non-platinum treatment will improve the effectiveness of overall therapy in women with EOC progression occurring 6–12 months after first-line treatment with a platinum derivative. The study groups MaNGO and AGO-OVAR are also participating and 46 of the overall estimated 253 women have been already recruited. In the experimental arm patients are treated with PLD followed at subsequent progression by carboplatin and paclitaxel, while in the conventional arm patients receive carboplatin and paclitaxel followed at subsequent progression by PLD.

Platinum-resistant/refractory EOC relapse (PFI shorter than 6 months)

Women with platinum-resistant/refractory EOC relapse are a difficult group in which to demonstrate benefit. In 2009, Sharma *et al.*[66] reported their experience of extended weekly carboplatin and paclitaxel in this population. Twenty women with platinum-resistant/refractory ovarian cancer received carboplatin (AUC = 3) and paclitaxel 70 mg/m^2 weekly for 3 out of 4 weeks. The RECIST response rate was 60% by radiological criteria and 76% by CA125 assessment and this was therefore a highly active regimen in this platinum-resistant situation. Despite the dose-dense regimen in these heavily pretreated patients, no grade 3/4 thombocytopenia occurred. The dynamics of response to dose-dense therapy were as rapid as with first-line therapy within the same patient. The authors stated that this dose-dense regimen is routinely extended to at least 18 weekly cycles over 6 months and that it forms a highly active and tolerable cytotoxic scaffold to which molecular-targeted therapies can be added in platinum-resistant ovarian cancer.

As with primary disease, in the recurrent situation targeted therapies are being incorporated into conventional cytotoxic regimens to enhance response. Various anti-angiogenics and small molecules such as sorafenib, bevacizumab, cediranib, zibotentan (ZD4054) and farletuzumab (MORAb-003) are being evaluated.

The phase II multicentre German TRIAS 2009 efficacy and safety study of sorafenib with topotecan in women with platinum-resistant recurrent ovarian cancer is currently recruiting. Sorafenib is a multitargeted tyrosine kinase inhibitor of VEGFR, PDGFR and Raf. The trial has a randomised double-blind placebo-controlled design.

Another large multicentre study for the platinum-resistant setting is the AURELIA phase III study. This randomised open-label two-arm study is evaluating the efficacy and safety of bevacizumab added to chemotherapy versus chemotherapy alone in women with epithelial ovarian, fallopian tube or primary peritoneal cancer with disease progression within 6 months of platinum therapy. Three cytotoxic agents will be used as monotherapy or in combination with bevacizumab: paclitaxel (weekly), topotecan (weekly) or PLD (4-weekly). The trial is led by GINECO, with AGO-OVAR, GEICO, MITO and NSGO as collaborators, and is currently still recruiting patients.

Conclusion

The proliferation of clinical trials in ovarian cancer reflects the focus and determination of investigators internationally and many promising hypotheses are being explored within these international collaborative efforts. While the cure rates for ovarian cancer have not improved substantially over the past 20 years, the median PFS and OS have steadily increased. It is to be hoped that these approaches will yield agents and approaches that result in a step change in improved survival.

References

1. Jemal A, Siegel R, Ward E, Murray T, Xu J, Smigal C, *et al*. Cancer statistics, 2006. *Cancer J Clin* 2006;56:106–30.
2. WrongDiagnosis.com. Prevalence and Incidence of Ovarian Cancer [www.wrongdiagnosis.com/o/ovarian_cancer/prevalence.htm].
3. Young RC. Gynecologic malignancies. In: Jameson JN, Kasper DL, Harrison TR, Braunwald E, Fauci AS, Hauser SL, *et al*, editors. Harrison's Principles of Internal Medicine. 16th ed. New York: McGraw-Hill Medical Publishing Division; 2005. p. 83–92.
4. Sehouli J, Senyuva F, Fotopoulou C, Neumann U, Denkert C, Werner L, Gülten OO. Intra-abdominal tumor dissemination pattern and surgical outcome in 214 patients with primary ovarian cancer. *J Surg Oncol* 2009;99:424–7.
5. du Bois A, Reuss A, Pujade-Lauraine E, Harter P, Ray-Coquard I, Pfisterer J. Role of surgical outcome as prognostic factor in advanced epithelial ovarian cancer: a combined exploratory analysis of 3 prospectively randomized phase 3 multicenter trials: by the Arbeitsgemeinschaft Gynaekologische Onkologie Studiengruppe Ovarialkarzinom (AGO-OVAR) and the Groupe d'Investigateurs Nationaux Pour les Etudes des Cancers de l'Ovaire (GINECO). *Cancer* 2009;115:1234–44.
6. Bristow RE, Berek JS. Surgery for ovarian cancer: how to improve survival. *Lancet* 2006;367:1558–60.
7. Aletti GD, Dowdy SC, Gostout BS, Jones MB, Stanhope RC, Wilson TO, *et al*. Quality improvement in the surgical approach to advanced ovarian cancer: the Mayo Clinic experience. *J Am Coll Surg* 2009;208:614–20.
8. Aletti GD, Gostout BS, Podratz KC, Cliby WA. Ovarian cancer surgical resectability: relative impact of disease, patient status, and surgeon. *Gynecol Oncol* 2006;100:33–7.
9. Vergote I, Tropé CG, Amant F, Kristensen GB, Ehlen T, Johnson N, *et al*; European Organization for Research and Treatment of Cancer–Gynaecological Cancer Group; NCIC Clinical Trials Group. Neoadjuvant chemotherapy or primary surgery in stage IIIC or IV ovarian cancer. *N Engl J Med* 2010;363:943–53.
10. Fotopoulou C, Richter R, Braicu EI, Schmidt SC, Lichtenegger W, Sehouli J. Can complete tumor resection be predicted in advanced primary epithelial ovarian cancer? A systematic evaluation of 360 consecutive patients. *Eur J Surg Oncol* 2010;36:1202–10.
11. Vernooij F, Heintz P, Witteveen E, van der Graaf Y. The outcomes of ovarian cancer treatment are better when provided by gynecologic oncologists and in specialized hospitals: a systematic review. *Gynecol Oncol* 2007;105:801–12.

12. Eisenkop SM, Spirtos NM, Montag TW, Nalick RH, Wang HJ. The impact of subspecialty training on the management of advanced ovarian cancer. *Gynecol Oncol* 1992;47:203–9.
13. Paulsen T, Kjaerheim K, Kaern J, Tretli S, Tropé C. Improved short-term survival for advanced ovarian, tubal, and peritoneal cancer patients operated at teaching hospitals. *Int J Gynecol Cancer* 2006;16 Suppl 1:11–17.
14. Colombo PE, Mourregot A, Fabbro M, Gutowski M, Saint-Aubert B, Quenet F, *et al.* Aggressive surgical strategies in advanced ovarian cancer: a monocentric study of 203 stage IIIC and IV patients. *Eur J Surg Oncol* 2009;35:135–43.
15. Angioli R, Plotti F, Palaia I, Calcagno M, Montera R, Cafà EV, *et al.* Update on lymphadenectomy in early and advanced ovarian cancer. *Curr Opin Obstet Gynecol* 2008;20:34–9.
16. Panici PB, Maggioni A, Hacker N, Landoni F, Ackermann S, Campagnutta E, *et al.* Systematic aortic and pelvic lymphadenectomy versus resection of bulky nodes only in optimally debulked advanced ovarian cancer: a randomized clinical trial. *J Natl Cancer Inst* 2005;97:560–6.
17. Maggioni A, Benedetti Panici P, Dell'Anna T, Landoni F, Lissoni A, Pellegrino A, *et al.* Randomised study of systematic lymphadenectomy in patients with epithelial ovarian cancer macroscopically confined to the pelvis. *Br J Cancer* 2006;95:699–704.
18. Benedetti Panici P, Perniola G, Angioli R, Zullo MA, Manci N, Palaia I, *et al.* Bulky lymph node resection in patients with recurrent epithelial ovarian cancer: impact of surgery. *Int J Gynecol Cancer* 2007;17:1245–51.
19. Onda T, Yoshikawa H, Yasugi T, Matsumoto K, Taketani Y. The optimal debulking after neoadjuvant chemotherapy in ovarian cancer: proposal based on interval look during upfront surgery setting treatment. *Jpn J Clin Oncol* 2010;40:36–41.
20. Bristow RE, Eisenhauer EL, Santillan A, Chi DS. Delaying the primary surgical effort for advanced ovarian cancer: a systematic review of neoadjuvant chemotherapy and interval cytoreduction. *Gynecol Oncol* 2007;104:480–90.
21. van der Burg ME, van Lent M, Buyse M, Kobierska A, Colombo N, Favalli G, *et al.* The effect of debulking surgery after induction chemotherapy on the prognosis in advanced epithelial ovarian cancer. Gynecological Cancer Cooperative Group of the European Organization for Research and Treatment of Cancer. *N Engl J Med* 1995;332:629–34.
22. Rose PG, Nerenstone S, Brady MF, Clarke-Pearson D, Olt G, Rubin SC, *et al*; Gynecologic Oncology Group. Secondary surgical cytoreduction for advanced ovarian carcinoma. *N Engl J Med* 2004;351:2489–97.
23. Scholz HS, Tasdemir H, Hunlich T, Turnwald W, Both A, Egger H. Multivisceral cytoreductive surgery in FIGO stages IIIC and IV epithelial ovarian cancer: results and 5-year follow-up. *Gynecol Oncol* 2007;106:591–5.
24. Sehouli J, Savvatis K, Braicu EI, Schmidt SC, Lichtenegger W, Fotopoulou C. Primary versus interval debulking surgery in advanced ovarian cancer: results from a systematic single-center analysis. *Int J Gynecol Cancer* 2010;20:1331–40.
25. Steer CB. Chemotherapy for ovarian cancer in the older adult. *Curr Treat Options Oncol* 2009;10:159–70.
26. Baekelandt M. The potential role of neoadjuvant chemotherapy in advanced ovarian cancer. *Int J Gynecol Cancer* 2003;13 Suppl 2:163–8.
27. Steed H, Oza AM, Murphy J, Laframboise S, Lockwood G, DE Petrillo D, *et al.* A retrospective analysis of neoadjuvant platinum-based chemotherapy versus up-front surgery in advanced ovarian cancer. *Int J Gynecol Cancer* 2006;16 Suppl 1:47–53.
28. Tangjitgamol S, Manusirivithaya S, Laopaiboon M, Lumbiganon P. Interval debulking surgery for advanced epithelial ovarian cancer. *Cochrane Database Syst Rev* 2009;(2):CD006014.
29. Chew I, Soslow RA, Park KJ. Morphologic changes in ovarian carcinoma after neoadjuvant chemotherapy: report of a case showing extensive clear cell changes mimicking clear cell carcinoma. *Int J Gynecol Pathol* 2009;28:442–6.
30. Sassen S, Schmalfeldt B, Avril N, Kuhn W, Busch R, Höfler H, *et al.* Histopathologic assessment of tumor regression after neoadjuvant chemotherapy in advanced-stage ovarian cancer. *Hum Pathol* 2007;38:926–34.
31. McCluggage WG, Lyness RW, Atkinson RJ, Dobbs SP, Harley I, McClelland HR, *et al.* Morphological effects of chemotherapy on ovarian carcinoma. *J Clin Pathol* 2002;55:27–31.

32. Ferron JG, Uzan C, Rey A, Gouy S, Pautier P, Lhommé C, *et al.* Histological response is not a prognostic factor after neoadjuvant chemotherapy in advanced-stage ovarian cancer with no residual disease. *Eur J Obstet Gynecol Reprod Biol* 2009;147:101–5.
33. Schorge JO, Wingo SN, Bhore R, Heffernan TP, Lea JS. Secondary cytoreductive surgery for recurrent platinum-sensitive ovarian cancer. *Int J Gynaecol Obstet* 2010;108:123–7.
34. Zang RY, Zhang ZY, Li ZT, Chen J, Tang MQ, Liu Q, *et al.* Effect of cytoreductive surgery on survival of patients with recurrent epithelial ovarian cancer. *J Surg Oncol* 2000;75:24–30.
35. Zang RY, Li ZT, Tang J, Cheng X, Cai SM, Zhang ZY, *et al.* Secondary cytoreductive surgery for patients with relapsed epithelial ovarian carcinoma: who benefits? *Cancer* 2004;100:1152–61.
36. Chi DS, McCaughty K, Diaz JP, Huh J, Schwabenbauer S, Hummer AJ, *et al.* Guidelines and selection criteria for secondary cytoreductive surgery in patients with recurrent, platinum-sensitive epithelial ovarian carcinoma. *Cancer* 2006;106:1933–9.
37. Bae J, Lim MC, Choi JH, Song YJ, Lee KS, Kang S, *et al.* Prognostic factors of secondary cytoreductive surgery for patients with recurrent epithelial ovarian cancer. *J Gynecol Oncol* 2009;20:101–6.
38. Harter P, du Bois A, Hahmann M, Hasenburg A, Burges A, Loibl S, *et al*; Arbeitsgemeinschaft Gynaekologische Onkologie Ovarian Committee; AGO Ovarian Cancer Study Group. Surgery in recurrent ovarian cancer: the Arbeitsgemeinschaft Gynaekologische Onkologie (AGO) DESKTOP OVAR trial. *Ann Surg Oncol* 2006;13:1702–10.
39. Harter P, Hahmann M, Lueck HJ, Poelcher M, Wimberger P, Ortmann O, *et al.* Surgery for recurrent ovarian cancer: role of peritoneal carcinomatosis: exploratory analysis of the DESKTOP I Trial about risk factors, surgical implications, and prognostic value of peritoneal carcinomatosis. *Ann Surg Oncol* 2009;16:1324–30.
40. Harter P, Sehouli J, Reuss A, Hasenburg A, Scambia G, Cibula D, *et al.* Prospective validation study of a predictive score for operability of recurrent ovarian cancer. The Multicenter Intergroup study DESKTOP II. A project of the of AGO KOMMISSION OVAR, AGO Study group, NOGGO, AGO AUSTRIA and MITO. *Int J Gynecol Cancer* 2011;21:289–95.
41. Fotopoulou C, Richter R, Braicu IE, Schmidt SC, Neuhaus P, Lichtenegger W, *et al.* Clinical outcome of tertiary surgical cytoreduction in patients with recurrent epithelial ovarian cancer. *Ann Surg Oncol* 2011;18:49–57.
42. Shih KK, Chi DS, Barakat RR, Leitao MM Jr. Beyond tertiary cytoreduction in patients with recurrent epithelial ovarian, fallopian tube, or primary peritoneal cancer. *Gynecol Oncol* 2010;116:364–9.
43. Vasey PA, Jayson GC, Gordon A, Gabra H, Coleman R, Atkinson R, *et al*; Scottish Gynaecological Cancer Trials Group. Phase III randomized trial of docetaxel-carboplatin versus paclitaxel-carboplatin as first-line chemotherapy for ovarian carcinoma. *J Natl Cancer Inst* 2004;96:1682–91.
44. Bookman MA, Brady MF, McGuire WP, Harper PG, Alberts DS, Friedlander M, *et al.* Evaluation of new platinum-based treatment regimens in advanced-stage ovarian cancer: a phase III trial of the Gynecologic Cancer Intergroup. *J Clin Oncol* 2009;27:1419–25.
45. Bookman MA. Dose-dense chemotherapy in advanced ovarian cancer. *Lancet* 2009;374:1303–4.
46. Pecorelli S, Favalli G, Gadducci A, Katsaros D, Panici PB, Carpi A, *et al*; After 6 Italian Cooperative Group. Phase III trial of observation versus six courses of paclitaxel in patients with advanced epithelial ovarian cancer in complete response after six courses of paclitaxel/platinum-based chemotherapy: final results of the After-6 protocol 1. *J Clin Oncol* 2009;27:4642–8.
47. Katsumata N, Yasuda M, Takahashi F, Isonishi S, Jobo T, Aoki D, *et al*; Japanese Gynecologic Oncology Group. Dose-dense paclitaxel once a week in combination with carboplatin every 3 weeks for advanced ovarian cancer: a phase 3, open-label, randomised controlled trial. *Lancet* 2009;374:1331–8.
48. Lopes NM, Adams EG, Pitts TW, Bhuyan BK. Cell kill kinetics and cell cycle effects of taxol on human and hamster ovarian cell lines. *Cancer Chemother Pharmacol* 1993;32:235–42.
49. Simon R, Norton L. The Norton–Simon hypothesis: designing more effective and less toxic chemotherapeutic regimens. *Nat Clin Pract Oncol* 2006;3:406–7.

50. Dovern E, de Hingh IH, Verwaal VJ, van Driel WJ, Nienhuijs SW. Hyperthermic intraperitoneal chemotherapy added to the treatment of ovarian cancer. A review of achieved results and complications. *Eur J Gynaecol Oncol* 2010;31:256–61.
51. Markman M. Clinical efficacy supporting the role of intraperitoneal drug delivery in the primary chemotherapeutic management of small-volume residual advanced ovarian cancer. *Semin Oncol* 2006;33(6 Suppl 12):S3–7.
52. Armstrong DK, Brady MF. Intraperitoneal therapy for ovarian cancer: a treatment ready for prime time. *J Clin Oncol* 2006;24:4531–3.
53. Wenzel LB, Huang HQ, Armstrong DK, Walker JL, Cella D; Gynecologic Oncology Group. Health-related quality of life during and after intraperitoneal versus intravenous chemotherapy for optimally debulked ovarian cancer: a Gynecologic Oncology Group Study. *J Clin Oncol* 2007;25:437–43.
54. Armstrong DK, Bundy B, Wenzel L, Huang HQ, Baergen R, Lele S, *et al*; Gynecologic Oncology Group. Intraperitoneal cisplatin and paclitaxel in ovarian cancer. *N Engl J Med* 2006;354:34–43.
55. Woopen H, Sehouli J. Current and future options in the treatment of malignant ascites in ovarian cancer. *Anticancer Res* 2009;29:3353–9.
56. Ströhlein MA, Siegel R, Jäger M, Lindhofer H, Jauch KW, Heiss MM. Induction of anti-tumour immunity by trifunctional antibodies in patients with peritoneal carcinomatosis. *J Exp Clin Cancer Res* 2009;28:18.
57. Burges A, Wimberger P, Kümper C, Gorbounova V, Sommer H, Schmalfeldt B, *et al*. Effective relief of malignant ascites in patients with advanced ovarian cancer by a trifunctional anti-EpCAM x anti-CD3 antibody: a phase I/II study. *Clin Cancer Res* 2007;13:3899–905.
58. Chekerov R, Reinthaller A, Reimer D, Reimer T, Angleitner-Boubenizek L, Halfen M, *et al*. Intraoperative immunotherapy with the trifunctional antibody catumaxomab in patients with ovarian cancer: Results from a phase II study. *J Clin Oncol* 2010;28(suppl):15s, abstract 5039.
59. Burger RA, Brady MF, Bookman MA, Walker JL, Homesley HD, Fowler J, *et al*. Phase III trial of bevacizumab (BEV) in the primary treatment of advanced epithelial ovarian cancer (EOC), primary peritoneal cancer (PPC), or fallopian tube cancer (FTC): A Gynecologic Oncology Group study. *J Clin Oncol* 2010;28(18s):abstr LBA1.
60. Monk BJ, Choi DC, Pugmire G, Burger RA. Activity of bevacizumab (rhuMAB VEGF) in advanced refractory epithelial ovarian cancer. *Gynecol Oncol* 2005;96:902–5.
61. Burger RA, Sill MW, Monk BJ, Greer BE, Sorosky JI. Phase II trial of bevacizumab in persistent or recurrent epithelial ovarian cancer or primary peritoneal cancer: a Gynecologic Oncology Group study. *J Clin Oncol* 2007;25:5165–71.
62. Garcia AA, Hirte H, Fleming G, Yang D, Tsao-Wei DD, Roman L, *et al*. Phase II clinical trial of bevacizumab and low-dose metronomic oral cyclophosphamide in recurrent ovarian cancer: a trial of the California, Chicago, and Princess Margaret Hospital phase II consortia. *J Clin Oncol* 2008;26:76–82.
63. Pfisterer J, Perren T, Swart AM, Ledermann J, Selle F, Kristensen G, *et al*. ICON7: A randomised controlled trial of bevacizumab in women with newly diagnosed epithelial ovarian, primary peritoneal or fallopian tube cancer. 13th Biennial Meeting of the International Gynecologic Cancer Society (IGCS 2010), 25–26 October 2010, Prague, Czech Republic. Abstract 2010_805.
64. Bamias A, Psaltopoulou T, Sotiropoulou M, Haidopoulos D, Lianos E, Bournakis E, *et al*. Mucinous but not clear cell histology is associated with inferior survival in patients with advanced stage ovarian carcinoma treated with platinum-paclitaxel chemotherapy. *Cancer* 2010;116:1462–8.
65. Sholi A, Martino MA, Pirigyi M, Rosenblum NG, Markman M, Peterson CS, *et al*. Mucinous adenocarcinoma of the ovary. *Semin Oncol* 2010;37:314–20.
66. Sharma R, Graham J, Mitchell H, Brooks A, Blagden S, Gabra H. Extended weekly dose-dense paclitaxel/carboplatin is feasible and active in heavily pretreated platinum-resistant recurrent ovarian cancer. *Br J Cancer* 2009;100:707–12.
67. Markman M, Rothman R, Hakes T, Reichman B, Hoskins W, Rubin S, *et al*. Second-line platinum therapy in patients with ovarian cancer previously treated with cisplatin. *J Clin Oncol* 1991;9:389–93.

68. van der Burg ME, Hoff AM, van Lent M, Rodenburg CJ, van Putten WL, Stoter G. Carboplatin and cyclophosphamide salvage therapy for ovarian cancer patients relapsing after cisplatin combination chemotherapy. *Eur J Cancer* 1991;27:248–50.
69. Eisenhauer EA, ten Bokkel Huinink WW, Swenerton KD, Gianni L, Myles J, van der Burg ME, *et al.* European-Canadian randomized trial of paclitaxel in relapsed ovarian cancer: high-dose versus low-dose and long versus short infusion. *J Clin Oncol* 1994;12:2654–66.
70. Pujade-Lauraine E, Wagner U, Aavall-Lundqvist E, Gebski V, Heywood M, Vasey PA, *et al.* Pegylated liposomal doxorubicin and carboplatin compared with paclitaxel and carboplatin for patients with platinum-sensitive ovarian cancer in late relapse. *J Clin Oncol* 2010;28:3323–9.
71. Meier W, Lichtenegger W, Marth C, Gonzalez-Martin AJ, Harter P, Tome O, *et al.* Topotecan plus carboplatin versus standard therapy with paclitaxel plus carboplatin (PC) or gemcitabin plus carboplatin (GC) or carboplatin plus pegylated doxorubicin (PLDC): a planned 200-pt interim safety analysis of the NOGGO-AGO-Germany-AGO Austria and GEICO-GCIG Intergroup Study (HECTOR). *J Clin Oncol* 2010;28 Suppl:15s, abstract 5071.
72. Konner JA, Bell-McGuinn KM, Sabbatini P, Hensley ML, Tew WP, Pandit-Taskar N, *et al.* Farletuzumab, a humanized monoclonal antibody against folate receptor alpha, in epithelial ovarian cancer: a phase I study. *Clin Cancer Res* 2010;16:5288–95.
73. Monk BJ, Herzog TJ, Kaye SB, Krasner CN, Vermorken JB, Muggia FM, *et al.* Trabectedin plus pegylated liposomal doxorubicin in recurrent ovarian cancer. *J Clin Oncol* 2010;28:3107–14.

Chapter 16

Clinical trials in cervical cancer

Karen Tipples and Melanie Powell

Introduction

The introduction in 1987 of a national cervical screening programme in the UK led, in little more than a decade, to a halving in the incidence of cervical cancer from 16 per 100 000 to 8 per 100 000 by the year 2000.[1,2] Despite similar success in other developed countries, cervical cancer remains a major international problem. It is the second most common female cancer worldwide, with almost 500 000 new cases diagnosed annually and 250 000 deaths each year.

The standard of care for early-stage disease (International Federation of Gynecology and Obstetrics [FIGO] stage IA, IB1) remains surgery. For more advanced disease chemoradiotherapy is preferred. Despite recent improvements in survival, due in the main to the introduction of chemoradiotherapy, the overall pelvic relapse rate remains significant, with the disease recurring in the pelvis in over a quarter of women. This highlights the need for continued effort to improve outcome in this disease. Five year survival rates are around 90%, 75%, 50% and 20% for FIGO stages I, IB2/II, III and IV, respectively.[3,4]

The challenges in treating cervical cancer are centred on improvements in survival and local control and minimising treatment-related morbidity. This chapter focuses on the evidence for current practice and highlights future research issues.

The role of surgery

Surgery remains the treatment of choice in early-stage disease. The most widely quoted data to support this come from an article published in 1997.[5] This study randomly assigned 327 women with stage IB or IIA disease to either radical hysterectomy or radical radiotherapy. Concomitant chemotherapy was not given as this study predates the US National Cancer Institute alert of 1999 that recommended concurrent cisplatin chemoradiation. Overall survival (OS) and disease-free survival were equivalent but it is noteworthy that two-thirds of women in the surgical arm also received radiotherapy for what were considered to be adverse pathological features. Toxicity in the surgical group at 28% was more than double that seen in the radiotherapy arm.

It is probably more reasonable to conclude from this one randomised study that surgery plus radiotherapy is equivalent to radiotherapy and that the combination of the two treatments has higher morbidity than radiotherapy alone. It has been postulated that chemoradiation is likely to be superior to surgery in terms of survival. This will, however, never be evaluated in a randomised controlled trial. With the simplicity of a single procedure and the added advantage of preservation of ovarian function in younger women, surgery remains the gold standard treament for early disease.

For stage IB2 tumours, the incidence of microscopic lymph node metastasis is about 30%. If a surgical approach is chosen, there is a high probability of requiring additional pelvic chemoradiotherapy and, with the increased morbidity of combined treatment, surgery is not recommended for tumours of stage IB2.[6]

Typically, surgery involves a radical hysterectomy with pelvic lymph node dissection. A review of the Surveillance, Epidemiology and End Results (SEER) data of almost 13 000 patients from 1988 to 1998 supports the role of lymphadenectomy, with an improvement in OS for each stage after lymph node dissection and also with the number of nodes removed.[7]

With the increasing focus on reducing treatment-associated problems, there is a move towards less radical surgery for early-stage low-risk cervical cancer. An international collaborative study led by Australia and the USA for women with stage IA2 and IB1 cervical cancer that compares laparoscopic with abdominal radical hysterectomy is now recruiting and has an endpoint of disease-free survival.[8] Consideration is now also being given to evaluating the role of simple rather than radical hysterectomy in selected low-risk stage IA2 and IB1 cervical cancers by a randomised controlled clinical trial.

The role of neoadjuvant chemotherapy before surgery is much discussed, particularly by the surgical community. Six randomised controlled studies that included 1072 women have now been evaluated as part of a Cochrane review.[9] In all of these studies, the women were randomised to receive a cisplatin-based chemotherapy regimen before surgery or to surgery alone. Although additional chemotherapy conferred a statistical improvement in progression-free survival (PFS), there was no benefit in OS. Three of the the six studies were stopped early – one because the OS in the neoadjuvant chemotherapy arm was inferior to the surgical arm,[10] one because there was a statistically significant benefit to the chemotherapy arm[11] and one because of the widespread use of additional radiotherapy.[12] Although the use of radiotherapy was balanced between the treatment groups, there was considerable variation among trials, which may partly explain the differing results among the studies. In one study,[11] every woman received radiotherapy; in the others, the proportion varied between 36% and 61%.

There was no consensus over chemotherapy regimens other than that all contained cisplatin. Data from the Italian SNAP-02 trial that used three cycles of TIP (paclitaxel, ifosfamide and cisplatin) before surgery in stages IB–IV cervical cancer showed encouraging results, with 43% of women achieving an optimal response.[13] However, with high toxicity (76% grade 3 or 4 neutropenia), this combination has been rejected outside of Italy.

Overall, based on the currently available data, there is no consistent benefit for preoperative chemotherapy and it is not advocated outside of a clinical study.

The continuing European Organisation for Research and Treatment of Cancer (EORTC) 55994 trial is a randomised phase III study that compares neoadjuvant chemotherapy followed by surgery with concomitant chemoradiotherapy in stage IB2, IIA or IIB cervical cancer. This trial, which has now been open for 9 years, has been very slow to recruit its target of 686 patients but should help to answer the question as to the benefit of chemotherapy before sugery.[14]

Fertility-conservation surgery

Where the woman wishes to preserve fertility, radical trachelectomy may be an alternative to radical hysterectomy, provided the tumour size is no greater than

2 cm and lymphovascular space invasion is not present. In this situation, radical trachelectomy does not appear to increase the rate of recurrence[15,16] and many women are able subsequently to conceive spontaneously and deliver near term.[17]

While new techniques should be evaluated as part of a clinical trial, it would now be almost impossible to ask young women, in whom fertility is usually a major issue, to accept randomisation between trachelectomy and hysterectomy.

The role of concurrent chemoradiotherapy

For women with FIGO stage IB2 disease and higher, chemoradiotherapy is the treatment of choice. This followed an unprecedented alert issued by the National Cancer Institute after the simultaneous publication of five studies recommending that cervical cancer be treated with concurrent chemoradiotherapy rather than radiotherapy alone.

Two subsequent meta-analyses of randomised trials confirmed improved OS and local control rates when concurrent cisplatin-containing chemotherapy was added to radiotherapy in the treatment of cervical cancer. The Cochrane Collaborative meta-analysis[18] included data from 19 trials (comprising 4580 patients), 12 of which used platinum-based chemotherapy. The meta-analysis showed a highly significant survival benefit with concurrent chemoradiation (HR 0.71; $P<0.00001$), which represented a 12% absolute benefit in survival. The addition of chemotherapy was, however, shown to increase acute haematological and gastrointestinal toxicity.

A Canadian study[19] that was based on eight randomised trials exclusively examined platinum-based chemoradiation and estimated the survival benefit as 11%.

These reviews highlighted important issues that could have led to an overestimate of the benefit. For instance, many studies used different radiotherapy treatment in their standard arm and many trials had a different definition of outcome. To overcome these issues, a new analysis using individual patient data was carried out and published in 2010.[20] This latest meta-analysis of thirteen studies with 3128 women confirmed the benefit of additional chemotherapy, with an absolute benefit in survival of 6% and in disease-free survival of 8%. It is interesting that the advantage of chemotherapy was not as great as had initially been thought and it is of note that non-platinum-containing regimens, in particular those containing 5-fluorouracil and/or mitomycin, showed similar benefit. This suggests that for women who are unable to receive platinum, such as those with renal impairment, there are alternative effective drugs.

Neoadjuvant and adjuvant treatment

Neoadjuvant chemotherapy and radiotherapy

The issue of neoadjuvant chemotherapy before radiotherapy for cervical cancer remains controversial. Theoretical benefits of neoadjuvant chemotherapy include the eradication of micrometastases and reduction in tumour size before definitive treatment. A Cochrane meta-analysis published in 2004 by Tierney[21] evaluated 2074 women from 18 studies that compared neoadjuvant chemotherapy before radiotherapy with radiotherapy alone. Combining all of the trials together showed no evidence of benefit for neoadjuvant chemotherapy but there was a high level of statistical heterogeneity. Results were then reanalysed according to how chemotherapy was delivered and this showed a trend towards a survival advantage for more intense chemotherapy given either in cycles of less than 14 days or using cisplatin doses of greater than 25 mg/m^2. Giving cisplatin at lower doses or over longer intervals appeared to be detrimental to outcome.

Interest in neoadjuvant chemotherapy before chemoradiotherapy has now been rekindled using dose-dense regimens. One such regimen is the combination of carboplatin and paclitaxel given weekly for 6 weeks before standard cisplatin chemoradiotherapy which has shown a high response rate and good tolerability.[22] Phase III randomised controlled trials are being considered to evaluate this approach.

Adjuvant chemotherapy and radiotherapy

An alternative and widely used approach in other tumour sites is to consider additional chemotherapy following definitive treatment, with the aim of improving survival. This has so far been less successful in cervical cancer. There have been encouraging results from an international study of 515 women with stage IIB–IVA carcinoma of the cervix randomised to either concurrent gemcitabine plus cisplatin and radiation followed by adjuvant gemcitabine and cisplatin or standard concurrent cisplatin chemoradiotherapy.[23] PFS at 3 years was 74% in the experimental arm compared with 65% in the control group ($P=0.029$). OS was also significantly improved. However, with grade 3/4 toxicity in the experimental group being almost double that seen in the control group (87% versus 46%) and two treatment-related deaths, this novel regimen is unlikely to be widely used without modification and further evaluation.

There is currently a randomised phase III trial of tri-modality treatment, comparing concurrent chemotherapy and radiotherapy with versus without adjuvant chemotherapy with high-risk early-stage cervical carcinoma after radical hysterectomy. This US trial is recruiting 400 patients and adjuvant chemotherapy will be in the form of 3-weekly carboplatin/paclitaxel given for four cycles.[24]

After surgery for early cervical cancer, certain histopathological features increase the risk of recurrence and reduce PFS. These include positive pelvic lymph nodes, lymphovascular space invasion, parametrial involvement, positive margins and tumour size of more than 4 cm. With one or more of these features, the 5 year survival drops to between 50% and 70%.[25] It is well recognised that combining surgery and radiotherapy increases the acute and late morbidities associated with both modalities. A 2009 Cochrane review considered the role of adjuvant radiotherapy following surgery in early cervical cancer.[26] Only two trials (397 women) fulfilled the criteria for evaluation. They showed that, while adjuvant radiotherapy reduced the risk of local recurrence by between 40% and 90%, it did not confer a statistically significant survival benefit. This highlights the importance of carefully selecting the initial primary treatment for an individual patient and to consider the risks and benefits for each patient before considering the role of adjuvant radiotherapy.

The current RTOG 0724 phase III trial is set to answer the question as to whether adjuvant chemotherapy (four cycles of carboplatin and paclitaxel) following standard postoperative chemoradiotherapy is of benefit in high-risk patients with positive surgical margins, parametrial involvement or involved nodes.[27] With a projected 400 patients to be recruited, this question will take some time to answer.

Improving radiotherapy treatment

Improving the outcome from radiotherapy is important from two key perspectives. Firstly, morbidity of treatment, particularly in long-term survivors, is now recognised as an issue needing to be addressed. Secondly, since almost one-third of patients relapse in the pelvis, enhancing the effectiveness of radiotherapy is critical. Improving the outcome from radiotherapy might be achieved by improving delivery of treatment, increasing dose to tumour or the addition of radiosensitisers.

Intensity-modulated radiotherapy

The integration of computed tomography (CT) imaging into the radiotherapy planning process has allowed the dose of radiation to match or conform to the outline of the target. This shaping of the radiation fields is known as conformal radiotherapy and would now be considered best practice when treating the pelvis. Intensity-modulated radiotherapy (IMRT) is an extension of this principle. By varying the intensity of the radiation beam, it allows more accurate shaping, even around concavities. The dose distribution with IMRT fits even more precisely to the target volume, producing a concave shape both at the posterior aspect of the target volume, reducing dose to the rectum, and also anteriorly, curving around the lateral lymph node target volume while sparing more of the central bladder and bowel.

The data using IMRT are encouraging. Mundt *et al.*[28] have published the progress of their initial cohort of women treated with IMRT at the University of Chicago. Acute toxicity in the first 40 women (70% postoperative, 30% primary radiotherapy) was compared retrospectively with that in the preceding 35 patients treated with conventional radiotherapy. Grade 2 gastrointestinal symptoms were reduced from 91% to 60% and grade 2 genitourinary morbidity reduced from 20% to 10% with IMRT. After further follow-up, late gastrointestinal toxicity was reduced from 50% to 11%.[29]

IMRT also allows allocation of different dose targets to discrete areas within the target volume, as well as enabling delivery of a boost to all sites of bulk disease. This may improve the therapeutic ratio by delivering a higher total dose to all of the macroscopic disease while maintaining standard doses to the areas of potential microscopic spread. This principle is currently being evaluated in the UK in a phase II study.[30]

Current trials in early-stage cervical cancer

Much current research in early-stage cervical cancer is focused on developing new drugs to either complement or replace cisplatin-based chemoradiotherapy regimens. Sorafenib has not been previously combined with conventional chemoradiotherapy to treat cervical cancer. A phase I/II trial in Canada will add sorafenib at least a week before starting chemoradiotherapy and then throughout treatment in women with both early-stage and locally advanced cervical cancers.[31] A further study is exploring the anti-tumour activity of cetuximab before chemoradiotherapy and the safety and tolerability of cetuximab with concurrent chemoradiation.[32]

The fully human agonist monoclonal antibody mapatumumab binds to the tumour necrosis factor-related apoptosis-inducing ligand receptor 1 (TRAIL-R1; DR4) and induces cytotoxicity in multiple tumour cell lines *in vitro* and *in vivo*. In multiple phase I and phase II studies, mapatumumab appeared to be safe both as single agent and in combination with chemotherapy, including cisplatin, and in cervical cancer cell lines induced apoptosis in 51% of the cells, increasing to 83% in combination with irradiation.[33] A Dutch phase I/II study is currently evaluating the safety, tolerability and efficacy of mapatumumab in combination with cisplatin and radiotherapy in women with locally advanced cervical cancer.[34]

Management of recurrent disease

The prognosis for women who develop recurrent disease remains poor - of the order of 6 months to 2 years.[1] It is possible to identify subgroups with local relapse for whom the prognosis is better and who may be cured with salvage surgery or radical chemoradiotherapy. However, for those relapsing outside the pelvis, treatment is usually palliative chemotherapy or best supportive care.

Since radiotherapy is offered to women with more advanced cancer, most cases of recurrence occur in those who have been irradiated. For these women, provided relapsed disease is confined to the central pelvis, the only potentially curative option is pelvic exenteration. However, this procedure carries with it a high morbidity and mortality, with fewer than 50% of patients surviving 5 years.[35]

There have been no randomised trials comparing chemotherapy with best supportive care in advanced cervical carcinoma. Cisplatin has been used for nearly three decades to treat recurrent and metastatic cancer and remains the mainstay of treatment. However, the high mortality rate, low response rate to available treatments and short survival mandates investigation into more effective therapies.[36]

Grendys *et al*,[37] in the GOG-0179 randomised phase III trial, demonstrated for the first time a survival advantage for combination chemotherapy over single-agent cisplatin in advanced cervical cancer. Cisplatin was compared with cisplatin plus topotecan and with a methotroxate, vinblastine, doxorubicin and cisplatin (MVAC) arm. The MVAC arm was closed owing to four treatment-related deaths among 63 patients and was not included in the final analysis. Of the remaining women, 146 received cisplatin and 147 received cisplatin plus topotecan. This trial demonstrated improved OS and PFS when compared with single-agent therapy, with median OS of 9.4 and 6.5 months, respectively ($P = 0.017$), and PFS of 4.6 and 2.9 months, respectively ($P = 0.014$).

The Gynecologic Oncology Group (GOG) instituted a multi-arm trial in 2003 with four different platinum-based intravenous doublets containing topotecan, paclitaxel, vinorelbine or gemcitabine.[38] None of the experimental regimens was found to be superior to the control arm of cisplatin plus paclitaxel. Response rates were 29.1% for the control, 25.9% for cisplatin plus vinorelbine, 22.3% for cisplatin plus gemcitabine and 23.4% for cisplatin plus topotecan. Unfortunately, the toxicity data from the four arms will not be revealed until the survival data are mature, which makes it difficult, given the similar response rates, to conclude whether one arm is superior on the basis of toxicity.

As expected, more women in this trial had received prior cisplatin therapy in conjunction with radiation therapy than in previous trials. As cisplatin-based chemoradiation has now been readily adopted as the standard of care for locally advanced disease, it follows that, for those women in whom disease ultimately recurs, palliative therapy with cisplatin-based regimens may be less effective owing to prior platinum exposure with resulting acquired drug resistance. Indeed, in successive trials the response to platinum-based chemotherapy at relapse is demonstrably inferior in those who have received prior platinum therapy. There is a clear need for alternatives to standard cisplatin-based salvage therapy for this population. Potential options include the inclusion of non-cross-resistant platinum analogues, reversal of platinum resistance and use of non-platinum chemotherapy doublets.

Symonds *et al.*[39] have reported results of a Scottish phase II trial of docetaxel (75 mg/m^2 on day 1) plus gemcitabine (1000 mg/m^2 on days 1 and 8) as second-line chemotherapy in cervical cancer. Twenty-three out of 24 women had had prior chemoradiotherapy.

The principal toxicity was neutropenia (grade 3 in eight women and grade 4 in eight women), with four women experiencing grade 3 febrile neutropenia. Among 18 women evaluable for response, there was one complete response, four partial responses, six with stable disease and seven with progressive disease.

Tiersten *et al.*[40] investigated paclitaxel plus topotecan in 15 women with recurrent or metastatic cervical carcinoma. The women were treated with paclitaxel 175 mg/m^2 on day 1 and topotecan 1 mg/m^2 on days 1–5 of a 21 day cycle with growth factor support. Among 13 evaluable patients, there were seven (54%) responses (one complete response and six partial responses) and three women (23%) experienced stable disease. The PFS and OS were 3.8 and 8.6 months, respectively. Grade 3/4 toxicities included anaemia (47%), leucopenia (27%), thrombocytopenia (13%), neurotoxicity (13%) and diarrhoea (13%).

Bevacizumab, an anti-angiogenic agent, is also under investigation in the GOG-0240 phase III multicentre four-arm study. This is comparing the OS of women with stage IVB, recurrent, or persistent carcinoma of the cervix treated with paclitaxel in combination with cisplatin or topotecan with or without bevacizumab.[41] The study will enrol 450 women and will prospectively evaluate independent prognostic factors (for example, prior radiosensitiser and time interval from diagnosis to recurrence) identified by Moore *et al.*[42] in a post-hoc analysis of three GOG protocols.

CIRCCa (cediranib in recurrent cervical cancer) is a continuing randomised double-blind phase II trial of carboplatin–paclitaxel plus cediranib versus carboplatin–paclitaxel plus placebo in metastatic/recurrent cervical cancer.[43] Cediranib is an inhibitor of all three vascular endothelial growth factor receptor (VEGFR-1, -2 and -3) tyrosine kinases, thereby blocking VEGF signalling and angiogenesis.

Conclusion

Cervical cancer remains a significant worldwide problem. Over the past decade, the improvement in outcome seen with the introduction of chemoradiotherapy in 1999 has not been improved upon. The challenge in the coming decade is not only to look for ways to improve local control and survival but also to improve quality of life by minimising morbidity of treatment.

References

1. Cancer Research UK. Cervical cancer – UK incidence statistics [info.cancerresearchuk.org/cancerstats/types/cervix/incidence/].
2. Quinn MJ, Babb P, Jones J, Allen E. Effect of screening on incidence of and mortality from cervix cancer in England: evaluation based on routinely collected statistics. *Br Med J* 1999;318:904–8.
3. Baalbergen A, Helmerhorst TJ, Burger CW. Prognostic factors that predict survival after relapse of cervical cancer. *CME J Gynecol Oncol* 2001;6:391–7.
4. Office for National Statistics. Mortality statistics: Deaths registered in England and Wales [www.statistics.gov.uk].
5. Landoni F, Maneo A, Colombo A, Placa F, Milani R, Perego P, *et al.* Randomised study of radical surgery versus radiotherapy for stage Ib–IIa cervical cancer. *Lancet* 1997;350:535–40.
6. Piver MS, Chung WS. Prognostic significance of cervical lesion size and pelvic node metastases in cervical carcinoma. *Obstet Gynecol* 1975;46:507–10.
7. Rossi PJ, Horowitz IR, Johnstone PA, Jani AB. Lymphadenectomy for patients with cervical cancer: is it of value? *J Surg Oncol* 2009;100:404–6.
8. National Cancer Institute. PDQ Clinical Trials Database: Laparoscopic Approach to Cervical Cancer [www.cancer.gov/search/ResultsClinicalTrials.aspx?protocolsearchid=8504756].

9. Rydzewska L, Tierney J, Vale CL, Symonds PR. Neoadjuvant chemotherapy plus surgery versus surgery for cervical cancer. *Cochrane Database Syst Rev* 2010;(1):CD007406.

10. Katsumata N, Yoshikawa H, Hirakawa T, Saito T, Kuzuya K, Fujii T, *et al.* Phase III randomized trial of neoadjuvant chemotherapy (NAC) followed by radical hysterectomy (RH) versus RH for bulky stage I/II cervical cancer (JCOG 0102). *Proc Am Soc Clin Oncol* 2006;24(18s):abstr 5013.

11. Sardi JE, Giaroli A, Sananes C, Ferreira M, Soderini A, Bermudez A, *et al.* Long-term follow-up of the first randomized trial using neoadjuvant chemotherapy in stage Ib squamous carcinoma of the cervix: the final results. *Gynecol Oncol* 1997;67:61–9.

12. Eddy GL, Bundy BN, Creasman WT, Spirtos NM, Mannel RS, Hannigan E, *et al.* Treatment of ("bulky") stage IB cervical cancer with or without neoadjuvant vincristine and cisplatin prior to radical hysterectomy and pelvic/para-aortic lymphadenectomy: a phase III trial of the Gynecologic Oncology Group. *Gynecol Oncol* 2007;106:362–9.

13. Lissoni AA, Colombo N, Pellegrino A, Parma G, Zola P, Katsaros D, *et al.* A phase II, randomized trial of neo-adjuvant chemotherapy comparing a three-drug combination of paclitaxel, ifosfamide, and cisplatin (TIP) versus paclitaxel and cisplatin (TP) followed by radical surgery in patients with locally advanced squamous cell cervical carcinoma: the Snap-02 Italian Collaborative Study. *Ann Oncol* 2009;20:660–5.

14. National Cancer Institute. PDQ Clinical Trials Database: Phase III Randomized Study of Neoadjuvant Cisplatin-based Chemotherapy Followed by Radical Hysterectomy versus Standard Therapy with Concurrent Radiotherapy and Cisplatin-based Chemotherapy in Patients with Stage IB2, IIA, or IIB Cervical Cancer [www.cancer.gov/clinicaltrials/search/view?cdrid=69375&version=HealthProfessional&protocolsearchid=8966809].

15. Koliopoulos G, Sotiriadis A, Kyrgiou M, Martin-Hirsch P, Makrydimas G, Paraskevaidis E. Conservative surgical methods for FIGO stage IA2 squamous cervical carcinoma and their role in preserving women's fertility. *Gynecol Oncol* 2004;93:469–73.

16. Covens A, Shaw P, Murphy J, DePetrillo D, Lickrish G, Laframboise S, *et al.* Is radical trachelectomy a safe alternative to radical hysterectomy for patients with stage IA–B carcinoma of the cervix? *Cancer* 1999;86:2273–9.

17. Plante M, Renaud MC, Hoskins IA, Roy M. Vaginal radical trachelectomy: a valuable fertility-preserving option in the management of early-stage cervical cancer. A series of 50 pregnancies. *Gynecol Oncol* 2005;98:3–10.

18. Green J, Kirwan J, Tierney J, Vale C, Symonds P, Fresco L, *et al.* Concomitant chemotherapy and radiation therapy for cancer of the uterine cervix. *Cochrane Database System Rev* 2005;(3):CD002225.

19. Lukka H, Hirte H, Fyles A, Thomas G, Elit L, Johnston M, *et al.* Concurrent cisplatin-based chemotherapy plus radiotherapy for cervical cancer: a meta-analysis. *Clin Oncol* 2002;14:203–12.

20. Chemoradiotherapy for Cervical Cancer Meta-analysis Collaboration (CCCMAC). Reducing uncertainties about the effects of chemoradiotherapy for cervical cancer: individual patient data meta-analysis. *Cochrane Database Syst Rev* 2010;(1):CD008285.

21. Tierney J. Neoadjuvant chemotherapy for cervical cancer meta-analysis collaboration (NACCCMA). *Cochrane Database Syst Rev* 2004;(1):CD001774.

22. McCormack M, Ledermann JA, Hall-Craggs MA, Symonds RP, Warwick V, Simonds H, *et al.* A phase II study of weekly neoadjuvant chemotherapy followed by radical chemoradiation for locally advanced cervical cancer. *J Clin Oncol* 2009;27(15s):abstr 5586.

23. Dueñas-González, A, Zarba JJ, Alcedo JC, Pattarunataporn P, Beslija S, Patel F, *et al.* A phase III study comparing concurrent gemcitabine (Gem) plus cisplatin (Cis) and radiation followed by adjuvant Gem plus Cis versus concurrent Cis and radiation in patients with stage IIB to IVA carcinoma of the cervix *J Clin Oncol* 2009;27(18s):abstr CRA5507.

24 National Cancer Institute. PDQ Clinical Trials Database: Phase III Randomized Study of Concurrent Chemotherapy and Pelvic Radiotherapy with versus without Adjuvant Chemotherapy in Patients with High-Risk Early-Stage Cervical Carcinoma after Radical Hysterectomy [www.cancer.gov/search/ViewClinicalTrials.aspx?cdrid=654709&version=HealthProfessional&protocolsearchid=8073290].

25. Peters WA 3rd, Liu PY, Barrett RJ 2nd, Stock RJ, Monk BJ, Berek JS, *et al.* Concurrent chemotherapy and pelvic radiation therapy compared with pelvic radiation alone as adjuvant

therapy after radical surgery in high-risk early -stage cancer of the cervix. *J Clin Oncol* 2000;18:1606–13.

26. Rogers L, Siu SS, Luesley D, Bryant A, Dickinson HO. Adjuvant radiotherapy and chemoradiation after surgery for cervical cancer. *Cochrane Database Syst Rev* 2009;(4):CD007583.
27. Radiation Therapy Oncology Group. RTOG 0724 Protocol Information: Phase III Randomized Study of Concurrent Chemotherapy and Pelvic Radiation Therapy with or without Adjuvant Chemotherapy in High-Risk Patients with Early-Stage Cervical Carcinoma following Radical Hysterectomy [www.rtog.org/ClinicalTrials/ProtocolTable/StudyDetails.aspx?study=0724].
28. Mundt AJ, Lujan AE, Rotmensch J, Waggoner SE, Yamada SD, Fleming G, *et al.* Intensity-modulated whole pelvic radiotherapy in women with gynaecologic malignancies. *Int J Radiat Oncol Biol Phys* 2002;52:1330–7.
29. Mundt AJ, Mell LK, Roeske JC. Preliminary analysis of chronic gastrointestinal toxicity in gynecology patients treated with intensity-modulated whole pelvic radiation therapy. *Int J Radiat Oncol Biol Phys* 2003;56:1354–60.
30. ClinicalTrials.gov. Cisplatin and Radiation Therapy in Treating Patients With Locally Advanced Cervical Cancer (DEPICT: A Phase I/II, Multi-Center Dose Escalation Study of Simultaneous Boost Intensity-Modulated Radiotherapy for Locally Advanced Cervical Cancer) [clinicaltrials.gov/ct2/show/NCT01230996?term=NCT01230996&rank=1].
31. National Cancer Institute. PDQ Clinical Trials Database: A Phase I/II Study of Cisplatin and Radiation in Combination with Sorafenib in Cervical Cancer [www.cancer.gov/search/ViewClinicalTrials.aspx?cdrid=563765&version=HealthProfessional&protocolsearchid=8081330].
32. National Cancer Institute. PDQ Clinical Trials Database: Phase II Randomized Study of Pelvic Irradiation and Cisplatin with versus without Cetuximab in Patients with Stage IB2, II, or IIIB Cervical Cancer [www.cancer.gov/search/ViewClinicalTrials.aspx?cdrid=651250&version=HealthProfessional&protocolsearchid=8081332].
33. Leong S, Cohen RB, Gustafon DL, Langer CJ, Camidge DR, Padavic K, *et al.* Mapatumumab, an antibody targeting TRAIL-R1, in combination with paclitaxel and carboplatin in patients with advanced solid malignancies: results of a phase I and pharmacokinetic study. *J Clin Oncol* 2009;27:4413–21.
34. National Cancer Institute. PDQ Clinical Trials Database: Mapatumumab, Cisplatin and Radiotherapy for Advanced Cervical Cancer [www.cancer.gov/search/ViewClinicalTrials.aspx?cdrid=681011&version=HealthProfessional&protocolsearchid=8081338].
35. Chang HK, Lo KY, Chiang HS. Complications of urinary diversion after pelvic exenteration for gynecological malignancy. *Int Urogynecol J* 2000;11:358–60.
36. Robati M, Holtz D, Dunton CJ. A review of topotecan in combination chemotherapy for advanced cervical cancer. *Ther Clin Risk Manag* 2008;4:213–18.
37. Grendys EC Jr, Long HJ, Bundy BN, Benda J, McMeekin DS, Sorosky JI, *et al.* Randomized phase III trial of cisplatin vs cisplatin plus topotecan vs the combination of methotrexate, vinblastine, doxorubicin, and cisplatin (MVAC) in stage IVB, recurrent or persistent carcinoma of the uterine cervix: a Gynecologic Oncology Group study. *Int J Gynecol Cancer* 2004;14:12.
38. Monk BJ, Sill MW, McMeekin DS, Cohn DE, Ramondetta LM, Boardman CH, *et al.* Phase III trial of four cisplatin containing doublet combinations in stage IVB, recurrent, or persistent cervical carcinoma: a Gynecologic Oncology Group study. *J Clin Oncol* 2009;27:4649–55.
39. Symonds R, Davidson S, Chan S, Reed N, McMahon T, Paul J. SCOTCERV: a phase II trial of docetaxel and gemcitabine as second-line chemotherapy in cervical cancer. *J Clin Oncol* 2007;25(18s):abstr 5548.
40. Tiersten AD, Selleck MJ, Hershman DL, Smith D, Resnik EE, Troxel AB, *et al.* Phase II study of topotecan and paclitaxel for recurrent, persistent, or metastatic cervical carcinoma. *Gynecol Oncol* 2004;92:635–8.
41. National Cancer Institute. PDQ Clinical Trials Database: Phase III Randomized Study of Paclitaxel in Combination with Cisplatin or Topotecan Hydrochloride with versus without Bevacizumab in Patients with Stage IVB, Recurrent, or Persistent Carcinoma of the Cervix [www.cancer.gov/search/ViewClinicalTrials.aspx?cdrid=628746&version=HealthProfessional&protocolsearchid–8081374].

42. Moore DH, Tian C, Monk BJ, Long HJ, Omura GA, Bloss JD. Prognostic factors for response to cisplatin-based chemotherapy in advanced cervical carcinoma: a Gynecologic Oncology Group study. *Gynecol Oncol* 2010;116:44–9.

43. International Standard Randomised Controlled Trial Number Register: CIRCCa (Cediranib In Recurrent Cervical Cancer): a trial of carboplatin-paclitaxel plus cediranib versus carboplatin-paclitaxel plus placebo in metastatic/recurrent cervical cancer [www.isrctn.org/ISRCTN23516549].

Chapter 17
Clinical trials in vulval cancer

Tito Lopes

Introduction

Vulval cancer is rare and constitutes approximately 3% of gynaecological cancers worldwide. It is estimated that approximately 27 000 women are diagnosed with vulval cancer each year and the rates range from less than 0.3 per 100 000 women in parts of Asia to more than 1.5 per 100 000 in North America and Europe.[1] This variation is thought to be due to differing prevalence of human papillomavirus (HPV) infection and other factors such as smoking.

In the UK, vulval cancer accounts for fewer than 1% of all cancers (excluding non-melanoma skin cancer) and 6% of gynaecological cancers. In 2007, there were 1120 new cases diagnosed, giving an incidence of 2.4 (European standardised rate per 100 000 population). In 2008, the mortality rate was 0.7 per 100 000 population, with 400 deaths. It has been estimated that the lifetime risk of developing vulval cancer is one in 316 women in the UK.[2]

The incidence of vulval cancer has increased since the mid-1990s owing to the increased incidence in younger women, which has doubled over the past 30 years. The proportion of cases diagnosed in women under the age of 50 years increased from 6% in 1975 to 13% in 2005.[2] A similar trend has been seen in other countries[3,4] and has been linked to the increase in HPV-induced vulval intraepithelial neoplasia (VIN).

The disease has two aetiologies. The first, associated with high-risk HPV infection, usually occurs in young women and is related to VIN and to basaloid carcinoma. In contrast, keratinising carcinomas are associated with lichen sclerosis and are HPV independent. This difference in aetiology is crucial when looking at prevention and non-surgical treatment strategies for VIN.

Other risk factors for vulval cancer include herpes simplex and HIV infection, cancers at other anogenital sites, systemic lupus erythematosus, smoking, and immunosuppression such as in women who have had a renal transplant.

Squamous cell carcinomas account for about 90% of cases, with melanomas, adenocarcinomas, verrucous carcinomas and basal cell carcinomas accounting for the remainder.

The majority of women present with an enlarging vulval mass or ulcer occasionally associated with bleeding or an offensive discharge. There may be a long history of vulval irritation and soreness and there may be long-standing VIN or lichen sclerosus.

International Federation of Gynecology and Obstetrics (FIGO) staging in vulval cancer has been surgically staged since 1988, with the final diagnosis dependent on the histopathological evaluation of the primary tumour and the lymph nodes. The most recent revision of the staging was in 2009,[5] with major changes to stages IB, II, III and IVA.

There are no screening tests for the prevention of vulval cancer but the introduction of vaccination programmes using the HPV vaccines Cervarix® (GlaxoSmithKline) or Gardasil® (Sanofi Pasteur) is likely to prevent HPV 16- and HPV 18-induced VIN and vulval cancer in those vaccinated.

The mainstay of treatment for invasive disease is surgery with wide excision of the primary tumour, and with inguinofemoral/groin lymph node dissection except in FIGO stage IA disease and basal cell cancers where the risk of metastases is rare. Sentinel lymph node sampling is increasingly used for tumours smaller than 4 cm in diameter.

Adjuvant radiotherapy is administered to the groin and pelvis when inguinal nodes are involved and may also be used when excision margins are deemed inadequate. Radical radiotherapy with or without chemotherapy is used as primary treatment in cases of advanced disease when surgery is not an option. Neoadjuvant chemoradiation has also been used for large primary tumours to reduce tumour size and avoid extensive surgery.

In the UK, overall 5 year survival is 58% and is dependent on stage and lymph node involvement.

Clinical trials in vulval cancer can be divided into two categories – trials in women with vulval cancer and, more recently, trials on the prevention of vulval cancer by preventing or treating HPV-related VIN. Large-scale randomised clinical trials are rare in vulval cancer because of the rarity of the condition.

Trials in vulval cancer

There are currently no active trials in vulval cancer being run by the Gynecologic Oncology Group (GOG) in the USA or by the European Organisation for Research and Treatment of Cancer (EORTC). The only active UK Clinical Research Network (UKCRN) trial in the UK is the Groningen International Study on Sentinel Nodes in Vulval Cancer (GROINSS-V) II, which is a prospective observational study.

In recent years, clinical studies and trials have concentrated primarily on two aspects of clinical practice:

- avoiding or reducing morbidity from inguinal lymphadenectomy
- the non-surgical treatment of advanced local or distant disease and recurrent disease with radiotherapy and/or chemotherapy.

Groin lymphadenectomy is associated with significant morbidity. Short-term morbidity includes wound infection and breakdown, leaking of lymph fluid and lymphocyst formation. The most significant long-term complication is lymphoedema, and in a small series from Gateshead we found that 81% of the women were symptomatic within 6 weeks of surgery.[6] Swelling was the most common complaint, followed by a feeling of heaviness, tightness and discomfort. Patients with lymphoedema experience negative body image perception and social inhibition. The condition tends to be chronic and, once developed, treatment can be difficult, costly and time-consuming. Lymphoedema is often exacerbated by the addition of adjuvant radiotherapy following lymphadenectomy.

Surgery for the primary tumour can range from a wide excision of a small lesion resulting in minimal disruption of the normal anatomy to extirpation of the vulva and occasional exenteration or anovulvectomy. Irrespective of the degree of excision, surgery is associated with significant psychosexual problems relating to the resulting 'disfigurement'.[7] Physical morbidity is also common and increases with the extent of surgery. Numerous studies have tried to evaluate the role of neoadjuvant radiotherapy and/or chemotherapy in this disease to reduce the extent of surgery.

Cochrane reviews of surgery and radiotherapy

Since 1999 there have been three Cochrane reviews of clinical trials looking at the role of surgery and radiotherapy in the treatment of vulval cancer and these are summarised below:

- Surgical interventions for early squamous cell carcinoma of the vulva (1999).[8]
  Conclusions: The available evidence regarding surgery for early vulval cancer is generally poor. From the studies of sufficient quality, the reviewers concluded that radical local excision is a safe alternative to radical vulvectomy for women with early vulval carcinoma. Contralateral groin node dissection can be omitted in women with a lateralised tumour, and the triple incision technique is as safe as an en bloc dissection. However, omission of femoral lymph node dissection results in a higher incidence of groin recurrences. Further good-quality studies are required, although conducting randomised controlled trials (RCTs) on vulval cancer treatment may not be realistic owing to the rarity of the disease. However, observational studies of higher quality could provide more reliable evidence.
- Primary groin irradiation versus primary groin surgery for early vulval cancer (2001).[9]
  Conclusions: As shown in the 1992 RCT by Stehman *et al*,[10] primary radiotherapy to the groin results in less morbidity but also in a higher number of groin recurrences compared with surgery. Although the technique of radiotherapy in the RCT was criticised, other uncontrolled data do not give evidence for a similar or better groin control for radiotherapy when compared with surgery. This means that surgery is still to be considered the first-choice treatment for the groin nodes in women with vulval cancer. Individual patients not physically able to withstand surgery can be treated with primary radiotherapy.
- Neoadjuvant chemoradiation for advanced primary vulval cancer (2006).[11]
  Conclusions: Women with inoperable primary tumours or lymph nodes benefit from chemoradiation if surgery is then possible. In women with large tumours that can only be treated with anterior and/or posterior exenteration, complications of neoadjuvant therapy might outweigh complications of exenterative surgery. Neoadjuvant therapy is not justified in women with tumours that can be adequately treated with radical vulvectomy and bilateral groin node dissection alone.

Trials relating to lymphadenectomy

Reducing morbidity of lymphadenectomy

There has been a recent systematic review and meta-analysis of the surgical techniques used to reduce leg lymphoedema following radical groin node dissection.[12] The reviewers did not identify any randomised trials but did identify four studies related to preservation of the saphenous vein that were suitable for a meta-analysis. They concluded that preservation of the long saphenous vein in inguinal lymphadenectomy may reduce the rate of lymphoedema as well as the rate of acute cellulitis and wound breakdown.

Judson *et al.*[13] conducted a randomised trial analysing sartorius muscle transposition following lymphadenectomy, with 28 women randomised to sartorius muscle transposition and 33 to the control arm. The sartorius muscle was mobilised from the anterior superior iliac spine and translocated medially over the femoral artery and vein and fixed to the inguinal ligament and adductor longus muscle. The minimum duration of follow-up was 6 months and they found no statistically significant differences in the incidence of wound cellulitis, wound breakdown, lymphocyst formation, lymphoedema or rehospitalisation. The incidence of lymphocyst formation was higher in the sartorius transposition group.

In 2008, the GOG published a randomised phase III trial of Tisseel VH fibrin sealant to reduce lymphoedema after inguinal lymph node dissection.[14] Tisseel VH fibrin is a surgical fibrin 'glue' used to help stop bleeding and seal tissues. The trial randomised 150 women undergoing an inguinal lymphadenectomy during the management of vulval malignancy to receive sutured closure of the skin versus VH fibrin sealant sprayed into the groin followed by sutured closure. There was no difference in the incidence of lymphoedema, at 67% in the control arm and 60% in the VH fibrin arm ($P = 0.4779$). The incidence of lymphoedema was strongly associated with inguinal infection but not statistically increased in those who received adjuvant radiation. There was no significant difference in duration of drains, drain output or incidence of inguinal infections, wound breakdowns or seromas. However, there was a higher incidence of vulval infections in the VH fibrin sealant arm ($P = 0.0098$).

Sawan *et al.*[15] published a small randomised pilot study in 2009 looking at the feasibility of prophylactic compression garments and validation of leg volume measurement in women undergoing inguino-femoral lymphadenectomy for vulval cancer. Fourteen women were randomised to best supportive care or best supportive care plus the use of graduated compression stockings for 6 months. The conclusion was that the prophylactic use of stockings in this population was feasible. Despite the small number of cases, they noted a significantly greater increase in mean leg volume in the control group than in the study group (953 versus 607 ml; $P = 0.010$). Furthermore, the women in the treatment group showed better performance as judged by leg symptoms ($P = 0.031$ at 3 months) and clinical examination ($P = 0.039$ at 4 weeks and $P = 0.004$ at 6 months). This may be worth pursuing in a larger randomised trial.

Avoiding lymphadenectomy

There have been numerous studies looking at the role of imaging to try to differentiate negative groin nodes from those involved with metastatic disease. These were reviewed by Oonk *et al.*[16] in 2006 and their conclusion was that ultrasound, magnetic resonance imaging (MRI), computed tomography (CT) and positron emission tomography (PET) could not predict lymph node metastases with a negative predictive value that was high enough to safely omit lymphadenectomy. They felt that ultrasound combined with fine-needle aspiration showed promising results but that small metastases would eventually be missed by this procedure.

Sentinel lymph node sampling

From a surgical perspective, the most exciting studies recently have been those investigating the role of sentinel lymph node sampling. The sentinel lymph node is the first lymph node draining a tumour and, if free of metastatic disease, the other lymph nodes draining the tumour should also be negative. Initial studies involved injecting a blue dye around the tumour and identifying the blue sentinel lymph nodes during the dissection. In subsequent pilot studies, a combined technique with a preoperative lymphoscintigram following injection with ^{99m}technetium-labelled nanocolloid followed by an operative injection of blue dye has been used.

Plante *et al.*[17] has published an excellent review of the technique and published studies in gynaecological cancer up to 2003. In the studies for vulval cancer, a full groin node dissection was performed immediately following removal of the sentinel lymph nodes. Using the combined technique of lymphoscintigraphy with blue dye, the sentinel node detection rate was nearly always 100% and, in all the studies bar one, the negative predictive value of a negative sentinel node was 100%.

In March 2000, van der Zee *et al.*[18] commenced a multicentre observational study on sentinel node detection using ^{99m}technetium-labelled nanocolloid and blue dye in women with T1/2 squamous cell cancer of the vulva of less than 4 cm in diameter. When the sentinel node was found to be negative at pathological ultrastaging, inguino-femoral lymphadenectomy was omitted and the patient was observed for 2 years at intervals of every 2 months. Stopping rules were defined for the occurrence of groin recurrences in case these were higher than would be expected after a standard groin node dissection. In the 6 years to June 2006, a sentinel node procedure was performed in 623 groins of 403 women, the largest study on surgical techniques ever performed in vulval cancer. In 259 women with a unifocal lesion and a negative sentinel node, six groin recurrences (2.3%) were diagnosed, and the 3 year survival was 97%. Wound breakdown and cellulitis was significantly less in patients after sentinel node dissection than in patients with a positive sentinel node who underwent lymphadenectomy. Long-term morbidity in the form of erysipelas and lymphoedema was also significantly less frequently observed. The authors' conclusion was that sentinel node dissection, performed by a quality-controlled multidisciplinary team, should be part of the standard treatment in selected patients with early-stage vulval cancer. In the trial, a positive sentinel lymph node was identified in 26.2% of groin node procedures and, of those patients going on to full lymphadenectomy, residual microscopic disease in non-sentinel nodes was found in approximately 20%.

A second observational study, GROINSS-V II, which is currently recruiting, aims to answer the question as to whether these women with a positive sentinel node can be spared the morbidity of a full lymphadenectomy by treating their groins with primary radiotherapy. However, as mentioned earlier, a Cochrane review comparing prophylactic surgery with radiotherapy concluded that surgery is still to be considered the first-choice treatment for the groin nodes in women with vulval cancer.[9] GROINSS-V II is due to close to recruitment in the near future and it will be interesting to see whether it shows that when radiotherapy is given appropriately it can replace full groin node dissection in women with a positive sentinel lymph node.

Trials relating to non-surgical management

Chemoradiation

The 2006 Cochrane review by van Doorn *et al.*[11] looked at whether using concurrent neoadjuvant chemoradiation followed by surgery is effective and safe in vulval cancer patients with advanced primary disease. The reviewers did not identify any randomised trials but did identify five studies that met their inclusion criteria. Although chemotherapy was given uniformly within each of the five selected studies, four different chemoradiation schedules were used. Skin toxicity was observed in nearly all women, and wound breakdown, infection, lymphoedema and lymphocysts were common. The conclusion was that if primary surgery is feasible there is probably little benefit for neoadjuvant chemoradiation because of the toxicity. However, it improves the chances of surgical excision in women with initially inoperable primary tumours or fixed lymph nodes, though adverse effects are considerable.

Since the review, the GOG-0205 study, a phase II trial of radiation therapy and weekly cisplatin chemotherapy for the treatment of locally advanced squamous cell carcinoma of the vulva, closed to recruitment in September 2009. An interim analysis has shown that 50% of patients had pathological complete responses and 64% had clinical complete responses.[19]

Chemotherapy

There have been very few studies looking at the role of chemotherapy in vulval cancer. Drugs used have included cisplatin, bleomycin, methotrexate, 5-fluorouracil, mitomycin C and paclitaxel as single agents or in combination, with response rates up to 60% in chemo-naïve patients. In 2009, the EORTC published a phase II study using single-agent paclitaxel with only a 13.8% response,[20] while, in 2010, a small retrospective review from Coimbra, Portugal, reported a 60% response with single-agent bleomycin.[21]

Targeted therapies

A study presented at the 41st Annual Meeting of the Society of Gynecologic Oncologists (SGO) looked at the role of the epidermal growth factor receptor (EGFR) inhibitor erlotinib.[22] Twelve of 14 women with locally advanced or recurrent vulval cancer responded or had stable disease during neoadjuvant therapy with erlotinib.

Trials on preventing vulval cancer

Treatment of vulval intraepithelial neoplasia

Imiquimod

Imiquimod is an immune response modifying agent that activates immune cells through stimulation of Toll-like receptors on the surface of antigen-presenting cells. This causes synthesis and release of endogenous proinflammatory cytokines such as interferon-α (IFN-α), tumour necrosis factor α (TNF-α) and interleukin (IL)-6 and IL-12, which in turn stimulate both the innate and acquired immune pathways, resulting in upregulation of natural antiviral and anti-tumour activity.

There have been two randomised trials comparing imiquimod 5% cream with placebo. In the study by Mathiesen *et al*,[23] 32 women were randomised, with 21 receiving active treatment for 16 weeks. Seventeen women (81%) in the treatment group showed complete response and two (10%) partial response while none responded in the placebo group when evaluated by a biopsy 2 months after treatment. Long-term follow-up was not reported.

In the second study, by van Seters *et al*,[24] 52 women with high-grade VIN were randomised to receive imiquimod or placebo twice-weekly for 16 weeks. The primary endpoint was a greater than 25% reduction in lesion size at 20 weeks and this was found in 21 of the 26 women (81%) treated with imiquimod and in none of those treated with placebo ($P<0.001$). The lesion progressed to invasion in three of 49 women (6%) followed for 12 months (two in the placebo group and one in the imiquimod group). Nine women, all treated with imiquimod, had a complete response at 20 weeks and remained free from disease at 12 months.

Two studies using imiquimod followed by photodynamic therapy or therapeutic HPV vaccination with TA-CIN (a fusion protein of HPV 16 L2-E6-E7) have both shown promise as non-surgical therapies for VIN.[25,26]

Cidofovir

Cidofovir is an acyclic nucleoside analogue with broad-spectrum antiviral activity. Its activity in HPV-related disease may result from the induction of apoptosis in HPV-infected cells. A topical formulation of 1% cidofovir was used in a pilot study of 12 women with vulval, vaginal or perianal intraepithelial neoplasia, of whom ten completed follow-up.[27] Four women had complete regression of disease and three had a partial response. One woman made a complete symptomatic response but was found to have invasive disease at final biopsy.

RT3VIN is a randomised phase II trial currently running in the UK looking at topical treatment in women with VIN. Women with biopsy-proven VIN3 are randomised to receive either topical imiquimod or topical cidofovir. The purpose of the study is to determine whether there is evidence that either (or both) of these topical treatments is active, safe and feasible to use and would therefore warrant further investigation in a phase III setting.

Therapeutic vaccines

To eliminate existing lesions, a therapeutic HPV vaccine should target HPV antigens that are expressed in the infected and cancer cells. Consequently, many vaccine strategies have focused on stimulating the production and activation of T cells that can recognise infected cells expressing the target antigens E6 and E7. Significant progress has been made in pre-clinical models, which has resulted in several early-phase clinical trials.

In a study using a synthetic long-peptide vaccine containing nine HPV 16 E6 and four HPV 16 E7 synthetic peptides, 15 of 19 women with VIN3 had clinical responses, with a complete response in nine of them that was maintained at 24 months of follow-up.[28]

Ma *et al.*[29] have written an excellent overview of the current status of therapeutic vaccines.

Prophylactic vaccines

Cervarix and Gardasil are two licensed vaccines that have been shown to be highly effective in preventing persistent infections with HPV 16 and HPV 18, which are two high-risk HPVs that cause approximately 70% of cervical cancers. Gardasil also prevents infection with HPV 6 and HPV 11, which cause 90% of genital warts.

A combined analysis of three randomised clinical trials on the efficacy of Gardasil against high-grade vulval and vaginal lesions was published in 2007 by Joura *et al.*[30] In total, 18 174 women were enrolled and randomised to receive either Gardasil or placebo and the mean follow-up time was 3 years. The primary endpoint was the combined incidence of VIN2–3 or vaginal intraepithelial neoplasia (VaIN2–3) associated with HPV 16 or HPV 18. Among women naïve to HPV 16 or HPV 18 through 1 month after vaccination, the vaccine was 100% effective against VIN2 and

VIN3 and VaIN2 and VaIN3 associated with HPV 16 or HPV 18. The vaccine was also found to be 49% effective against all VIN2 and VIN3 or VaIN2 and VaIN3, irrespective of whether or not HPV DNA was detected in the lesion.

Data for Cervarix in relation to VIN are awaited but similar results would be expected.

Conclusion

Vulval cancer is a rare disease and thus randomised phase III trials in the treatment of the disease are almost non-existent. There is currently only one large international trial recruiting, the GROINSS-V II study, which is an observational trial looking at whether it is safe to omit full inguino-femoral lymphadenectomy in women with vulval cancer who have a negative sentinel node and to replace full lymphadenectomy with radiotherapy in those with a positive sentinel node. From a surgeon's perspective, studies looking at the role of sentinel node sampling are currently the most exciting trials relating to management of vulval cancer.

The Cochrane review by van Doorn *et al.*[11] identified the lack of studies relating to neoadjuvant chemoradiation but the suggestion was that its role was probably limited to inoperable tumours owing to the toxicity. It would be useful to see larger studies investigating the role of neoadjuvant chemotherapy alone because of the potential reduced morbidity when combined with surgery. Targeted therapies are in their infancy and require further pilot studies to look at response.

Early studies involving the medical treatment of VIN with imiquimod, cidofovir and especially therapeutic vaccines appear promising in the prevention of vulval cancer. However, the greatest effect on preventing cancer is likely to arise as a result of vaccination programmes of the prophylactic HPV vaccines, assuming adequate uptake of the vaccine.

Finally, the international gynaecological oncology community must work together to recruit the number of women with vulval cancer required for appropriate large trials, be they observational or randomised.

References

1. Sankaranarayanan R, Ferlay J. Worldwide burden of gynaecological cancer: The size of the problem. *Best Pract Res Clin Obstet Gynaecol* 2006;20:207–25.
2. Cancer Research UK. Vulval cancer – UK incidence statistics [info.cancerresearchuk.org/cancerstats/types/%20vulva/incidence].
3. Bodelon C, Madeleine M, Voigt L, Weiss N. Is the incidence of invasive vulvar cancer increasing in the United States? *Cancer Causes Control* 2009;20:1779–82.
4. Baumann KH, Müller O, Naujok HB, Mann E, Barth P, Wagner U. Small-area analysis of incidence and localisation of vulvar cancer. *J Oncol* 2010;2010:512032.
5. Pecorelli S. Revised FIGO staging for carcinoma of the vulva, cervix, and endometrium. *Int J Gynaecol Obstet* 2009;105:103–4.
6. Abang Mohammed DK, de B Lopes A, Regnard C, Monaghan JM. Lymphoedema following surgical treatment of vulva cancer: short term follow up. *Int J Gynecol Cancer* 1999;9:130.
7. Green MS, Naumann RW, Elliot M, Hall JB, Higgins RV, Grigsby JH. Sexual dysfunction following vulvectomy. *Gynecol Oncol* 2000;77:73–7.
8. Ansink A, van der Velden J, Neoplasms-surgery V. Surgical interventions for early squamous cell carcinoma of the vulva. *Cochrane Database Syst Rev* 1999;(4):CD002036.
9. van der Velden K, Ansink A. Primary groin irradiation vs primary groin surgery for early vulvar cancer. *Cochrane Database Syst Rev* 2001;4:CD002224.

10. Stehman FB, Bundy BN, Thomas G, Varia M, Okagaki T, Roberts J, *et al.* Groin dissection versus groin radiation in carcinoma of the vulva: A Gynecologic Oncology Group study. *Int J Radiat Oncol Biol Phys* 1992;24:389–96.
11. van Doorn H, Ansink A, Verhaar-Langereis M, Stalpers L. Neoadjuvant chemoradiation for advanced primary vulvar cancer. *Cochrane Database Syst Rev* 2006;3:CD003752.
12. Abbas S, Seitz M. Systematic review and meta-analysis of the used surgical techniques to reduce leg lymphedema following radical inguinal nodes dissection. *Surg Oncol* [Epub ahead of print].
13. Judson PL, Jonson AL, Paley PJ, Bliss RL, Murray KP, Downs LS, *et al.* A prospective, randomized study analyzing sartorius transposition following inguinal-femoral lymphadenectomy. *Gynecol Oncol* 2004;95:226–30.
14. Carlson JW, Kauderer J, Walker JL, Gold MA, O'Malley D, Tuller E, *et al.* A randomized phase III trial of VH fibrin sealant to reduce lymphedema after inguinal lymph node dissection: a Gynecologic Oncology Group study. *Gynecol Oncol* 2008;110:76–82.
15. Sawan S, Mugnai R, Lopes Ade B, Hughes A, Edmondson RJ. Lower-limb lymphedema and vulval cancer: feasibility of prophylactic compression garments and validation of leg volume measurement. *Int J Gynecol Cancer* 2009;19:1649–54.
16. Oonk MH, Hollema H, de Hullu JA, van der Zee AG. Prediction of lymph node metastases in vulvar cancer: a review. *Int J Gynecol Cancer* 2006;16:963–71.
17. Plante M, Renaud MC, Roy M. Sentinel node evaluation in gynecologic cancer. *Oncology (Williston Park)* 2004;18:75–87; discussion 88–90, 95–6.
18. van der Zee AG, Oonk MH, de Hullu JA, Ansink AC, Vergote I, Verheijen RH, *et al.* Sentinel node dissection is safe in the treatment of early-stage vulvar cancer. *J Clin Oncol* 2008;26:884–9.
19. Moore DH, *et al.* A phase II trial of radiation therapy and weekly cisplatin chemotherapy for the treatment of locally advanced squamous-cell carcinoma of the vulva. 2011 Annual Meeting on Women's Cancer. Society of Gynecologic Oncologists. 6–9 March 2011, Orlando, USA. Abstract 1.
20. Witteveen P, van der Velden J, Vergote I, Guerra C, Scarabeli C, Coens C, *et al.* Phase II study on paclitaxel in patients with recurrent, metastatic or locally advanced vulval cancer not amenable to surgery or radiotherapy: a study of the EORTC-GCG (European Organisation for Research and Treatment of Cancer–Gynaecological Cancer Group). *Ann Oncol* 2009;20:1511.
21. Domingues AP, Mota F, Durão M, Frutuoso C, Amaral N, de Oliveira CF. Neoadjuvant chemotherapy in advanced vulvar cancer. *Int J Gynecol Cancer* 2010;20:294–8.
22. Horowitz NS, Olawaiye A, Growdon W, Borger D, Dizon DS, Brard L, *et al.* Phase II trial of erlotinib (Tarceva) in women with squamous cell carcinoma of the vulva. *Gynecol Oncol* 2010;116(3 Suppl 1):S14.
23. Mathiesen O, Buus SK, Cramers M. Topical imiquimod can reverse vulvar intraepithelial neoplasia: a randomised, double-blinded study. *Gynecol Oncol* 2007;107:219–22.
24. van Seters M, van Beurden M, de Craen AJ. Is the assumed natural history of vulvar intraepithelial neoplasia III based on enough evidence? A systematic review of 3322 published patients. *Gynecol Oncol* 2005;97:645–51.
25. Winters U, Daayana S, Lear J, Tomlinson A, Elkord E, Stern P, *et al.* Clinical and immunologic results of a phase II trial of sequential imiquimod and photodynamic therapy for vulval intraepithelial neoplasia. *Clin Cancer Res* 2008;14:5292–9.
26. Daayana S, Elkord E, Winters U, Pawlita M, Roden R, Stern PL, *et al.* Phase II trial of imiquimod and HPV therapeutic vaccination in patients with vulval intraepithelial neoplasia. *Br J Cancer* 2010;102:1129–36.
27. Tristram A, Fiander A. Clinical responses to Cidofovir applied topically to women with high grade vulval intraepithelial neoplasia. *Gynecol Oncol* 2005;99:652–5.
28. Kenter GG, Welters MJ, Valentijn AR, Lowik MJ, Berends-van der Meer DM, Vloon AP, *et al.* Vaccination against HPV-16 oncoproteins for vulvar intraepithelial neoplasia. *N Engl J Med* 2009;361:1838–47.
29. Ma B, Xu Y, Hung C, Wu T. HPV and therapeutic vaccines: where are we in 2010? *Curr Cancer Ther Rev* 2010;6:81–103.
30. Joura EA, Leodolter S, Hernandez-Avila M, Wheeler CM, Perez G, Koutsky LA, *et al.* Efficacy of a quadrivalent prophylactic human papillomavirus (types 6, 11, 16, and 18) L1 virus-like-particle vaccine against high-grade vulval and vaginal lesions: a combined analysis of three randomised clinical trials. *Lancet* 2007;369:1693–702.

Section 5

Consensus views

Chapter 18

Consensus views arising from the 60th Study Group: Gynaecological Cancers: Biology and Therapeutics

Biology

1. There is a pressing need to reclassify gynaecological cancers. Through recent work we have begun to realise that the most common type of 'ovarian cancer', high-grade serous cancer, is characterised by mutation of the p53 (*TP53*) gene. This has allowed the identification of precursor lesions in the fallopian tube and the realisation that in fact much, if not all, of this type of cancer probably originates in the tube itself. Thus serous cancer of the corpus, tube, ovary and peritoneum are almost certainly variants of the same disease. Similarly, clear-cell and endometrioid cancers also share many molecular characteristics, including driver mutations of *PTEN*, and this is irrespective of whether they appear to originate in the ovary or the uterine corpus.
2. Changing the taxonomy and nomenclature of gynaecological cancers is not just an academic exercise. If we are to make serious inroads into improving the management of these diseases then we need to think about these cancers as distinct entities, types not sub-types of cancer, and initially design our clinical trials to reflect this. Ultimately, based on the results of these trials, we would envisage the development of different management strategies for each type.

Clinical care

3. All women with newly diagnosed high-grade serous ovarian carcinoma should have an accurate family history taken, and be referred for genetic assessment and considered for *BRCA1* and *BRCA2* mutation testing if appropriate. This is of increasing relevance considering the new therapeutic options that are likely to become available as a result of current clinical trials.
4. Strategies to ensure the availability of fast-tracked genetic testing should be part of standard care of women with cancer to ensure access to novel therapeutic strategies based on genetic information.

5. Patient data collection, in both clinical care and clinical trials, should routinely include toxicity and quality of life measurements.
6. A histological diagnosis should be obtained in all women with suspected ovarian cancer before systemic treatment, with therapy based on cytology alone only in rare situations.
7. Improvements in radiotherapy delivery are needed particularly for women with cervical cancer. Radiotherapy should be individualised using conformal techniques, to increase doses to the primary tumour and nodal groups to improve local control and to reduce damage to the surrounding normal tissues.
8. In women being considered for exenterative surgery, an ^{18}F-fluoro-2-deoxy-D-glucose positron emission tomography/computed tomography (FDG-PET/CT) scan should be undertaken routinely as part of the preoperative assessment.

Clinical trials/research

9. Within clinical trials, central pathological review is needed when treatment depends on morphological sub-type or other pathological parameters. The British Association of Gynaecological Pathologists has a representative on the National Cancer Research Institute (NCRI) Gynaecological Oncology Clinical Studies Group who should be the initial point of contact to arrange pathological review.
10. Clinical trial design needs to reflect the growing realisation that the various sub-types of ovarian cancer are distinct biological entities and therefore selection of patients for clinical trials and for individualised therapy should be based on histological sub-type and molecular biomarkers. New trial designs are increasingly being used, such as tumour/molecular marker-specific expansions at phase I and stratified randomised phase II studies rather than large phase III trials.
11. Translational endpoints (predictive biomarker studies) should be incorporated in all future clinical trials in gynaecological cancers, where possible, in order to stratify patients to targeted therapies.
12. Clinical trials of polyadenosine diphosphate-ribose polymerase (PARP) inhibitors for women with homologous recombination-defective tumours should be further developed. Studies of PARP inhibitors in PTEN-deficient endometrioid endometrial cancers are continuing.
13. Functional imaging in multicentre trials should be implemented with strict quality control to ensure standardisation and reproducibility.
14. FDG-PET should be incorporated into clinical trials where relevant, particularly in cervical cancer. The role of FDG-PET in ovarian cancer should be further investigated.
15. Diffusion-weighted magnetic resonance imaging (DW-MRI) in conjunction with conventional MR sequences has shown potential to improve assessment and should be further evaluated in preoperative assessment and in clinical trial settings.
16. Evaluation of novel surgical strategies, such as robotics, should occur through well-conducted clinical trials.

Specific cancer types

Vulval cancer

17. Sentinel lymph node sampling should be incorporated as part of standard care in women with vulval carcinoma with depth of invasion more than 1 mm.

Cervical cancer

18. In cervical cancer, non-surgical strategies to predict disease spread (or not) should be further investigated in order to modify surgery accordingly, with the aim of reducing morbidity.

Ovarian cancer

19. In surgery for ovarian cancer, whether carried out as a primary or a delayed procedure, the aim should be to remove all visible disease. This requires a formalisation of training. In particular competencies for extended surgery, including upper abdominal surgery, should be established. All gynaecological oncologists should have teams of surgeons available to aid them, including colorectal and urological surgeons. What procedures they actually perform themselves will be a matter for local agreement and subject to usual clinical governance procedures. Adequate facilities for surgery must also be provided. Surgeons do not work in isolation – they require appropriately skilled anaesthetic teams and adequate critical care facilities.
20. Given the equivalent survival rates in the published randomised controlled trial between primary and delayed ovarian cancer surgery, a test or series of tests is urgently needed that could be used as a decision aid in clinical practice, not just to predict optimal cytoreduction, which is only one part of the overall question, but also to select those women who would be best served by surgery before chemotherapy as opposed to those who would benefit from receiving half of their chemotherapy first.

Index

Lightning Source UK Ltd.
Milton Keynes UK
UKOW05f0037140114

224545UK00002B/148/P

9 781906 985448